Practical Canine Dermatology
Third Edition

Lowell J. Ackerman, DVM

Editor: Paul W. Pratt, VMD
Production Manager: Elisabeth S. Stein
Cover Design: Elizabeth R. Mason

American Veterinary Publications, Inc.
5782 Thornwood Drive
Goleta, CA 93117

©**1989** by 309425 Ontario, Inc. All rights reserved. No part of this book may be used or reproduced in any manner whatsoever without written permission of the publisher.

Notice

The author has exerted every effort to ensure that drug selections and dosages mentioned in this text are in accord with current recommendations and practice at the time of publication. However, in view of the ongoing advances in medicine, in dermatology in particular, the reader is urged to check the package insert of all medications for indications, dosage, warnings and precautions. In addition, some drugs mentioned have been used by the author in experimental or trial circumstances. Others have been used after official clearance for use in one species but not in others. Readers are cautioned to view this information with discretion until evidence of safety and efficacy is substantiated.

Library of Congress Catalog Card Number 89-80544
ISBN 939674-23-8
Printed in the United States of America

About the Author

Dr. Ackerman is a Diplomate of the American College of Veterinary Dermatology and operates dermatology referral practices in Mesa and Tucson, Arizona, and in Markham, Ontario. He completed an undergraduate degree in biology at the University of Western Ontario and later graduated from the Ontario Veterinary College.

After graduation from OVC, Dr. Ackerman was in general veterinary practice in the Toronto area, doing postgraduate work in immunology, and completing an alternate residency program in dermatology. He successfully completed the certifying examinations of the American College of Veterinary Dermatology, becoming a Diplomate of that college and the first board-certified veterinary dermatologist in Canada.

Dr. Ackerman has written 2 other books, *Practical Equine Dermatology* and *Practical Feline Dermatology*, and numerous articles in the veterinary literature. Readers may contact Dr. Ackerman at the following addresses:

Lowell Ackerman, DVM
Mesa Veterinary Hospital
858 N Country Club Drive
Mesa, Arizona 85201

Denison Veterinary Services
1151 Denison Street, Suite 2
Markham, Ontario L3R 3Y4
Canada

Contents

Introduction

Basic anatomy and physiology of the skin 1
The immune system and its relationship to skin 2

Diagnostic tests	Approach to diagnosis 7	
	Skin scrapings 26	
	Bacterial culture and sensitivity testing 27	
	Fungal culture 29	
	Allergy testing 30	
	Biopsy for histopathologic examination 31	
	Immunopathologic examination 39	
	Cytologic examination 41	
	Serologic testing 42	
	Titers 42	
	Antinuclear antibody testing 42	
	LE cell test 43	
	Complement fixation 44	
	Immunodiffusion 44	
	Latex agglutination 44	
	Circulating immune complex assays 45	
	Fibronectin assay .45	
	Hair analysis 46	

Chapter 1
Parasitic Skin Disorders

Flea infestation 47
Tick infestation 51
Lice infestation 52
Demodectic mange 52
Sarcoptic mange 56
Cheyletiellosis 57
Otodectic mange 57
Trombiculiasis 58
Fly-related dermatoses 58
Helminth-related dermatoses 59
Protozoan-related dermatoses 61

Chapter 2
Bacterial Skin Disorders

Pyodermas	Superficial 66	
	Intermediate 67	
	Deep 69	
Atypical pyodermas	Acne 70	
	Bacterial hypersensitivity 71	
	Callus pyoderma 72	
	Interdigital pyoderma 72	

	Nasal pyoderma	72
	Perianal pyoderma	73
	Bacterial granuloma (botryomycosis)	74
	Actinomycotic mycetoma	74
	Atypical mycobacteriosis	75
	Cutaneous tuberculosis	76
How to select an antibacterial		76

Chapter 3
Fungal Skin Disorders

Dermatophytosis		81
Intermediate mycoses	Eumycotic mycetoma	86
	Aspergillosis	87
	Phaeohyphomycosis	88
	Phycomycosis	89
	Rhinosporidiosis	89
	Sporotrichosis	90
Systemic mycoses	Blastomycosis	91
	Coccidioidomycosis	93
	Cryptococcosis	95
	Histoplasmosis	96
Diagnosis of systemic mycoses		97

Chapter 4
Allergic Skin Disorders

Inhalant allergies	99
Allergy therapy	114
Adverse reactions to food	124
Allergic contact dermatitis	129
Drug eruption	131
Hormonal hypersensitivity	132

Chapter 5
Immune-Mediated Skin Disorders

Lupus erythematosus	135
Pemphigus	139
Pemphigoid	144
Uveodermatologic (Vogt-Koyanagi-Harada-like) syndrome	146
Alopecia areata	146
Scleroderma	147
Sjogren's syndrome	148

Chapter 6
Endocrine Skin Disorders

Hypothyroidism	151
Hyperadrenocorticism (Cushing's disease)	156
Growth hormone-responsive dermatosis	162
Sex hormone disorders	164

Chapter 7
Nutritionally Related Skin Disorders

Protein deficiency 167
Fatty acid deficiency 168
Zinc-responsive dermatosis 169
Generic dog food disease 171
Vitamin A deficiency 172
Vitamin E deficiency 173
Dalmatian bronzing syndrome 174
Nutritional supplements 175
Omega 3 fatty acids 177
Omega 6 fatty acids 177
Dimethylglycine 178
Germanium 179
Bromelain 180

Chapter 8
Congenito-Hereditary Skin Disorders

Breed predispositions 183
Color mutant alopecia 192
Cutaneous asthenia 192
Dermatomyositis/epidermolysis bullosa simplex 193
Dermoid sinus 195
Disorders of pigmentation 195
Hair follicular defects 196
Ichthyosis 198
Lethal acrodermatitis 199
Acral mutilation syndrome 200

Chapter 9
Skin Tumors

Basal-cell tumor 202
Cutaneous cysts 202
Fibroma, fibrosarcoma, nodular dermatofibrosis 203
Hemangioma, hemangiosarcoma 205
Hemangiopericytoma 206
Histiocytic tumors 207
Intracutaneous cornifying epithelioma 210
Keratoses 210
Lipoma 211
Liposarcoma 212
Infiltrating lipoma 212
Lymphosarcoma 212
Mammary tumors 215
Mast-cell tumor 217
Melanoma 219
Myxoma/myxosarcoma 220
Nasal tumors 221
Nevi 223
Oral tumors 224

Papillomas/papillomatosis	226
Perianal-gland tumor	227
Periocular tumors	228
Pilomatrixoma	228
Plasmacytoma	229
Sebaceous-gland tumor	230
Squamous-cell carcinoma	231
Sweat-gland tumor	232
Transmissible venereal tumor	233
Trichoepithelioma	234

Chapter 10
Miscellaneous Skin Disorders

Acanthosis nigricans	237
Acral lick dermatitis	238
Alopecia	239
Anal sac disorders	241
Cutaneous vasculitis	243
Dermatitis herpetiformis	244
Ear problems	245
Eosinophilic granuloma	253
Erythema multiforme	253
Focal mucinosis	254
Footpad diseases	255
Juvenile cellulitis	257
Keratinization disorders	257
Lethal acrodermatitis	256
Lichenoid dermatoses	260
Lichenoid-psoriasiform dermatitis	261
Metabolic dermatosis	261
Nail and nailbed diseases	263
Nasal dermatitis	264
Nodular panniculitis	265
Pododermatitis	268
Periappendageal dermatitis	269
Sterile eosinophilic pustulosis	270
Sterile pyogranuloma	271
Subcorneal pustular dermatosis	271
Toxic epidermal necrolysis	272
Tumoral calcinosis (calcinosis circumscripta)	273

Appendix 1
Systemic Therapy

Antiparasitics	275
Antimicrobials	280
Antifungals	285
Immunostimulants	288
Corticosteroids	292
Antihistamines	294
Omega 3 fatty acids	295
Omega 6 fatty acids	295

Retinoids 297
Chemotherapy 297
Chrysotherapy 302
Dapsone 302
Plasmapheresis 303
Cyclosporine A 304

Appendix 2
Topical Products

Antibacterials 306
Antifungals 306
Antiseptics 308
Corticosteroids 309
Medicated shampoos 313
Hypoallergenic shampoos 316
Moisturizers 317
Aloe vera 318

Appendix 3
Pharmaceutical Companies

Appendix 4
Diagnostic Laboratories

Appendix 5
Board-Certified Veterinary Dermatologists

Appendix 6
Dermatologic Terms, Conversion Tables

Definitions 341
Root words 346
Prefixes 347
Suffixes 348
Conversion tables 348

Color Plates
Index

Preface

Skin diseases in dogs account for a large percentage of visits to the veterinarian. Not infrequently, these cases result in frustration on the part of the veterinary practitioner as well as the pet owner over the chronic nature or refractoriness of the problem. Clients tend to request opinions from anyone who will listen, and veterinarians are tempted to use symptomatic therapy that may pose other health concerns to the animal.

Dermatology is an ever-expanding science, and since it encompasses so many other disciplines (*eg*, immunology, parasitology, microbiology, oncology, endocrinology, nutrition, genetics, etc), it is sometimes difficult for practitioners to assimilate all the new advances as they pertain to private practice. The approach to diagnosis is also very different than in most other specialty areas. The skin can only manifest disease in a few different ways (*ie*, primary and secondary lesions). Thus, myriad different disorders often share many clinical similarities despite quite different etiologies. This absolutely necessitates a logical approach to diagnosis.

The purpose of this book is to serve as a primer of canine dermatology for private practitioners. It is neither a comprehensive text nor an encyclopedia of dermatology. It contains little information on pathophysiology and almost none on pathology. It is an easily read, quick reference for the most common dermatoses, with emphasis on clinical description, diagnostic testing and therapeutic options. Key references are provided and, where possible, the references are taken from literature commonly subscribed to by general veterinary practitioners.

The formulation of this book has been a rewarding experience for me, and the thoughtful comments from practitioners have been most appreciated. I dedicate this book to my late mother, Mary Ackerman, who served as a constant source of inspiration throughout my studies and career. Her caring and vitality are deeply missed. I wish also to acknowledge my canine son, Beau, who took shorter runs and walks to allow me time to write.

Lowell Ackerman, DVM

Introduction

Basic Anatomy and Physiology of the Skin

The skin is the largest organ in the body and serves many functions, including protection from the environment, thermoregulation (heat conservation and loss) and water balance. The importance of the skin in providing these functions is demonstrated by the life-threatening situations that arise when it is damaged (*eg*, severe burns).

The skin is well adapted to performing its specialized functions. The surface is covered by a tough layer of keratinized (shingle-like) cells (the stratum corneum), that provides a waterproof barrier to the environment. Deep to this are columns of cells (keratinocytes) that replace the overlying layers as they are shed from the skin surface. The basal cell layer is the base from which all of these cells originate and then migrate toward the surface. These keratinocytes rise until they reach a transitional zone, where they die and become part of the surface stratum corneum. This collection of keratinizing cells is known as the epidermis. The epidermis has no blood supply and receives all of its nutritive needs from the underlying tissue.

Deep to the epidermis is the dermis, composed of connective tissue fibers, blood vessels, nerves and a ground substance, which is gel-like and enables the dermis to be firm and supportive yet still flexible. The boundary between the epidermis and the dermis, called the dermal-epidermal junction or the basement membrane zone, performs important stabilizing, barrier and filtering functions.

The hypodermis, panniculus or subcutis is a collection of fat deep to the dermis. It provides a cushioning effect to the wear and tear of everyday life.

Hair follicles and the glands that supply them are collectively termed pilosebaceous units. Production of a hair is a joint venture between the dermis and epidermis. The base of the hair follicle (hair matrix) rests in the deep dermis or subcutis. Cells of epidermal origin, which are specialized for hair production, extend down into the dermis during fetal life to form a follicle. Following birth, no new hair follicles are produced; therefore, hair follicles that have been destroyed never produce more hair. Since epidermal cells do not have their own blood supply, a specialized structure arising from the dermis (the dermal papilla) becomes intimately involved with the epidermal hair matrix to supply it with blood and nutrition.

There are 2 main types of hair: the long bristly guard hairs and the downy vellus hairs. Whiskers (vibrissae) are specialized sensory hairs with an elaborate blood and nerve supply. Three types of glands are related to skin function. All are located in the dermis. The most conspicuous are sebaceous glands, which secrete sebum into the hair follicles via ducts. Sebum is composed of cholesterol and waxes. It imparts water resistance to the skin surface and adds luster to the haircoat. In people, overproduction of sebum in sebaceous follicles is an important component of acne. Apocrine glands secrete a form of sweat via ducts into the hair follicle and are the major sweat glands in animals. In people, these glands are present only in the armpits, anogenital regions, abdomen, face and scalp, but in animals they are present everywhere.

The eccrine sweat glands are similar in structure to the apocrine glands, and in people are important in temperature regulation. Though they are distributed over the entire body surface in people, with different regional densities, they are rare in animals, being prevalent only on the footpads and nose of dogs. Thus, dogs obviously do not sweat in the same manner as people and must dissipate heat by other mechanisms.

The Immune System and its Relationship to Skin

With the continued advances in dermatology, it becomes apparent how important the immune system is to the well-being of not only certain organ systems but the whole body. When the immune system is perfectly balanced, it wards off microorganisms (bacteria, parasites, fungi) and produces antibodies against many other invaders, especially viruses. For these 2 different roles, 2 different arms of the immune system function independently and in unison.

Immune responses arise as a result of exposure to foreign stimuli. An immunogen is any agent capable of inducing an immune response, while an antigen is any agent capable of binding specifically to components of the immune system, such as lymphocytes and antibodies. Thus, all immunogens are antigens, but not all antigens are immunogens. To be immunogenic, a compound must be exogenous ("foreign"), of high molecular weight, and chemically complex. Animals normally do not respond defensively to endogenous tissues ("self") and must recognize a substance as foreign before mounting an immune response against it. In general, compounds with a molecular weight of <1,000 daltons are not immunogenic, while those with molecular weights between 1,000 and 6,000 daltons may be immunogenic, and most compounds >6,000 daltons are usually immunogenic. Despite large molecular weights, molecules must be complex enough to be immunogenic.

The *T-cell system* consists of lymphocytes that patrol the body and keep invading foreign material at bay. The name "T-cell system" comes from the fact that most of these cells were programmed in the thymus gland to recognize the difference between the body (self) and everything else (nonself). Thus, every cell in the body bears a unique marker that informs the T-cell system that it is "self," and everything else T-cells encounter is considered foreign, so is destroyed. This process poses some problems to transplant patients, since T-cells attempt to destroy the transplanted organ. On the other hand, patients with defective T-cell systems (*eg*, people with AIDS) fail to ward off foreign material effectively and are more prone to a variety of infections, parasitic conditions and certain cancers.

T-cells perform a vast array of functions, including helping B-cells make antibody (T-helper cells), suppressing the production of antibody by B-cells (T-suppressor cells), directly attacking target cells, mediating delayed-type (Type-IV) hypersensitivity reactions, and modulating the immune response through production of lymphokines. Animals with partially defective T-cell systems may have problems ranging from recurrent infections to demodectic mange.

The *B-cell system* involves a group of lymphocytes that produce immunoglobulins (IgG, IgM, IgA, IgE) to a variety of substances, especially viruses. Viruses act as parasites within the body's cells and therefore are usually not vulnerable to the T-cell system. The body therefore produces antibodies that circulate in the bloodstream and prevent virus spread. Unfortunately, when the B-cell system becomes overactive, it produces unnecessary antibodies that may harm the system. In allergic patients, antibodies of a special type (IgE) are produced to a variety of pollens, molds, house dust, foods, etc, to cause some disturbing signs. In autoimmune diseases, autoantibodies are produced that selectively attack parts of the animal's own body.

The skin is the site for numerous inflammatory reactions that may involve a variety of inflammatory cells. As discussed above, there are 2 main types of lymphocytes. The B-cells have surface immunoglobulins, Fc receptors and C3b receptors. They differentiate into plasma cells, which produce the various immunoglobulins (IgG, IgM, IgA, IgE).

Immunoglobulin G (IgG), with a half-life of about 23 days, is the predominant immunoglobulin of internal components, such as blood, cerebrospinal fluid and peritoneal fluid. The major function of IgG is to remove microorganisms and neutralize toxins.

IgM, with a serum half-life of 5 days, accounts for 5-15% of the total immunoglobulin and is the initial immunoglobulin formed in the primary response. Because of its large size, IgM is an excellent complement-fixing or complement-activating antibody and is the most efficient initiator of complement-mediated lysis of microorganisms and other cells.

IgA, with a serum half-life of 5.5 days, constitutes 5-10% of the plasma immunoglobulin concentration and is the most important immunoglobulin in respiratory, genital and intestinal tract secretions. Secretory IgA can neutralize toxins, adhere to bacteria and viruses, and interact with the surfaces of parasites. Apparently its major function is to prevent attachment of bacteria and viruses to mucosal surfaces.

IgE, with a serum half-life of 2 days, has the unique ability to bind to specific receptors on the surface of mast cells and basophils, and is important in the immunopathogenesis of allergic disease and in the effector mechanism against parasites.

The T-cells are responsible for so-called cell-mediated immunity, as well as elaborating B-cell helper and suppressor substances.

Introduction

Monocytes, macrophages and histiocytes belong to the mononuclear-phagocyte or reticuloendothelial system. They are necessary for processing antigen, secreting a variety of proteins and factors (enzymes, monokines, complement components), and acting as phagocytes. The monokines (lymphocyte-activating and suppressor factors, neutrophil chemotactic factor, interferon) are responsible for modulating many inflammatory reactions.

Mast cells are responsible for recruitment of other inflammatory cells, mainly through releasing their contents of inflammatory mediators, such as histamine, proteolytic enzymes, slow-reacting substance of anaphylaxis and eosinophil chemotactic factor. These substances increase vascular permeability to permit access of other inflammatory cells, elaborate chemotactic substances to draw inflammatory cells to the area, and finally modulate release of additional mediators. Slow-reacting substance of anaphylaxis is now known to consist of leukotrienes (LT). LTB4, LTC4 and LTD4 cause prolonged constriction of smooth muscle and are considered the cause of much antihistamine-resistant asthma in people.

Neutrophils are present to some extent in most inflammatory reactions. They are attracted by a number of stimuli, including bacterial proteins, lymphokines, monokines, immune complexes, neutrophil chemotactic factor from mast cells, and other mediators, but are most prominent in microbial dermatoses. Their granules contain lysozyme, myeloperoxidase, a variety of proteases, hydrolases, eosinophil chemotactic factor, prostaglandins and thromboxanes.

Eosinophils are primarily responsible for attenuating the immune response, but other functions include phagocytosis and defense against parasites. Eosinophils are attracted to an area by histamine, eosinophil chemotactic factor (from mast cells and lymphocytes), immune complexes and other factors, and produce a variety of substances that downgrade the immune response (arylsulfatase inactivates slow-reacting substance of anaphylaxis, collagenase breaks down collagen, histaminase degrades histamine, prostaglandins inhibit mast-cell degranulation, etc).

Langerhans cells are considered cells of the mononuclear phagocyte system located in the epidermis. Their primary function is to present antigens to lymphocytes for further processing.

Table 1. Protein factors related to immune function in people.

Family	Members	Other Names
Interferons (IFN)	IFN-alpha	Leukocyte interferon
	IFN-beta	Fibroblast interferon
	IFN-gamma	Immune interferon
Tumor necrosis factors (TNF)	TNF	TNF-alpha, cachectin, lymphotoxin TNF-beta
Interleukins (IL)	IL-1 alpha	Endogenous pyrogen
	IL-1 beta	Lymphocyte-activating factor, leukocyte endogenous mediator, hemopoietin 1
	IL-2	T-cell growth factor
	IL-3	Multipotential CSF, mast-cell growth factor
	IL-4	B-cell stimulatory factor 1 (BSF-1)
	IL-5	T-cell-replacing factor (TRF), eosinophil differentiation factor, B-cell growth factor-II (BCGF-II)
	IL-6	B-cell stimulatory factor 2 (BSF-2), interferon-beta-2, hepatocyte-stimulating factor (HSF)
Colony-stimulating factors (CSF)	Granulocyte Macrophage-CSF	CSF-2
	Granulocyte-CSF	Pluripoietin
	Macrophage-CSF	CSF-1
		Erythropoietin
Other growth and regulatory factors	Epidermal growth factor (EGF)	
	Fibroblast growth factor	
	Insulin-like growth factor 1	Somatomedin C
	Insulin-like growth factor 2	Somatomedin A
		Nerve growth factor
		Platelet-derived growth factor
		Transforming growth factor-alpha
		Transforming growth factor-beta

Mediator substances, such as leukotrienes, prostaglandins, complement, lymphokines, free radicals, adaptagens and other factors, are also important in the inflammatory process but are beyond the scope of this book.

This of course is a great simplification of immune system function. Many protein factors are also involved in inflammation and immunity. Most are produced by either lymphocytes or macrophages. Table 1 lists the families of protein factors found in people, members of those families, and other names by which they are known. Not all of these substances have been demonstrated in dogs.

Classically, hypersensitivity reactions have been divided into 4 types.

Type-I hypersensitivity reactions (immediate, anaphylactic) are mediated almost exclusively by IgE (occasionally by IgG), such that when a specific antigen (allergen) comes in contact with a specific immunoglobulin bound to a mast cell or basophil, mediators are released and inflammation results. This hypersensitivity reaction often also involves genetic predilection. The classic example in inhalant allergies (atopy).

Type-II hypersensitivity reactions (cytotoxic) involve immunoglobulins (usually IgG or IgM) binding to complete tissue antigens, resulting in cell death. An example is pemphigus.

Type-III hypersensitivity reactions (immune complex) involves deposition of circulating antigen-antibody complexes (in antigen excess). The classic example is lupus erythematosus.

Type-IV hypersensitivity reactions (cell-mediated or more appropriately, lymphokine-mediated) involve interaction of an incomplete antigen (hapten) with a tissue protein to form a complete antigen that sensitizes T-lymphocytes that respond to further challenge by elaborating lymphokines that ultimately result in inflammation. A classic example is contact sensitivity.

Thus, in dermatology we must be concerned with a number of disorders of the immune system that might involve the B-cell or T-cell system, a variety of other inflammatory cells or elaborated substances.

Diagnostic Tests

Approach to Diagnosis

Dermatology is a medical science that requires no less diagnostic acumen than internal medicine, ophthalmology or any other specialty. It is amazing then that many practitioners are so confused by dermatology. As a specialist in a referral practice, I hear inquiries from veterinarians, such as "This dog is itchy and scaly. What do you think it could be?" If these same practitioners consulted with an ophthalmologist, they would not say "This dog has an eye problem. What do you think it is?" Therefore, like any other medical science, we must orient ourselves in dermatology, take the time to learn how to properly describe lesions, and use this information to select suitable differential diagnoses.

Algorithms in veterinary dermatology have limited usefulness, since so many conditions are manifested in a similar fashion. Regional dermatoses (nasal dermatitis, pododermatitis) and descriptive terms (alopecia, exfoliative dermatoses) lend themselves most to algorithmic approaches, but a good physical examination and minimum data base go much further than any algorithm could. For instance, pruritus is so common and so subjective as to have the same diagnostic specificity as a fever. The rectal temperature is often elevated in many different conditions, but alone a fever is never diagnostic.

One must take the time to examine the dog completely and search for significant primary and secondary lesions. (Appendix 6 contains a glossary of common dermatologic terms.) Primary lesions include macules, patches, papules, nodules, plaques, tumors, pustules, wheals, vesicles, bullae, petechiae and purpura. Tumor is usually included as a primary lesion but nodule is usually sufficient and a better descriptor, since it does not imply a diagnosis. Secondary lesions include excoriations, scales, crusts, scars, ulcers, hyperpigmentation, lichenification, induration and sclerosis. Erythema constitutes a nebulous intermediate.

Primary Skin Lesions

Macule: A circumscribed, flat discoloration of the skin up to 1 cm in diameter.

Patch: Macules >1 cm.

Papule: A circumscribed, elevated, superficial, solid lesion up to 1 cm in diameter.

Plaque: A circumscribed, elevated, superficial solid lesion >1 cm. A papule that has enlarged in 2 dimensions.

Wheal: An edematous, transitory papule or plaque.

Nodule: A solid lesion with depth. A papule that has enlarged in 3 dimensions.

Vesicle: A circumscribed elevation of the skin, up to 1 cm in diameter, containing serous fluid.

Bulla: A vesicle >1 cm in diameter.

Pustule: A circumscribed elevation of skin containing purulent fluid.

Petechia: A circumscribed deposit of blood or blood pigment up to 1 cm in diameter.

Purpura: A circumscribed deposit of blood or blood pigment >1 cm in diameter.

Secondary Skin Lesions

Scale: Shedding dead epidermal cells that may be dry or greasy.

Crust: Variously colored collections of skin exudates.

Excoriation: Abrasions of the skin, usually superficial and traumatic in origin.

Fissure: A linear break in the skin, sharply defined with abrupt walls.

Erosion: An excavation in the skin limited to the epidermis and not breaking the integrity of the dermal-epidermal junction.

Ulcer: An irregularly sized and shaped cavitation in the skin extending into the dermis.

Scar: A formation of connective tissue replacing tissue lost through injury or disease.

Lichenification: A diffuse area of thickening and scaling, with resultant increase in the skin lines and markings.

Induration: Palpable thickening of the skin.

Sclerosis: Hardening.

Hyperpigmentation: Increased coloration (darkening) of skin.

Margination is the shape of a lesion as it is viewed in cross-section and represents the transition from normal to lesional skin. The lesions are said to be sharply marginated if it is dome shaped, or flat topped, or the transition takes place over 1 mm or so. A lesion is poorly or diffusely marginated if its transition occurs over several millimeters.

Introduction

Configuration is the outline of a lesion as it is viewed from above. Lesions may have a circular, oval, linear, angular, gyrate (polycyclic), anular (arciform) or serpiginous configuration. Anular configurations occur when central lesional clearing creates a ring-like border.

If you do not know how to relate clinical signs with differential diagnoses, review the remainder of this book and appreciate what features are associated with which conditions. Understanding the diagnostic value of a good physical examination, I often recommend using a chart so you do not overlook any relevant conditions because "you just didn't think of them at the time" (Table 2).

For every skin disorder you see in practice and can't immediately identify, try this diagnostic exercise: Do a thorough physical examination and then ask yourself, chart in hand, which conditions it could be. For example, a dog has a papular eruption, hair loss in a follicular pattern and moderate pruritus. Ask yourself, "Could it be parasitic?" Yes: demodectic mange. "Could it be bacterial?" Yes: bacterial folliculitis. Run through the entire list and create a list of differential diagnoses. These differentials can be prioritized based on additional information, such as age, breed, sex, and medical and therapeutic history. Using your list of differentials and their order of likelihood, you

Table 2. Chart to aid diagnostic considerations during dermatologic examination.

Condition	Diagnostic Tests	Differential Diagnoses
Parasitic		
Bacterial		
Fungal		
Allergic		
Immune-mediated		
Endocrine		
Nutritional		
Neoplastic		
Congenito-hereditary		
Miscellaneous		

can then suggest appropriate diagnostic testing. The test results should help suggest a diagnosis. The chart is nothing new; it is just a reminder to help you consider all possibilities and get the proper tests done before initiating therapy.

To create differential diagnoses, one can take several approaches. One can formulate lists based on clinical presentation regarding types of lesions, location of lesions or clinical signs. Additionally, differentials can be considered on the basis of histopathologic characteristics, responses to therapy, etc.

Differential Diagnoses Based on Clinical Presentation

One approach I like is to accurately describe morphologic characteristics of different disorders and categorize them into variations of 8 different themes as presented in Table 3. Obviously, dermatologic disorders may manifest in more than one of the described features.

Maculopapular eruptions include the most innocuous of clinical lesions, which are basically spots and bumps. Maculopapular eruptions are typically somewhat scaly and may also be pruritic. Epithelial disruption (excoriations) may be seen secondary to scratching or rubbing. Chronically, this might result in lichenification. Most often maculopapular eruptions have diffuse margination (*ie*, the transition between normal skin and lesional skin occurs over a space of ≥2 mm) and thus have many similarities to the eczematous dermatoses of people. This group can be subdivided into *macular* or *papular*, depending on which primary lesion predominates according to Table 4.

The second morphologic category is *papulonodular dermatoses*, which may then be further subdivided into those that are basically *nodular*, are *plaques*, or are *vegetative* in nature. This entire category is a progression in severity from the papular subdivision of the maculopapular eruptions. The nodular category is pretty straightforward, but the plaque and vegetative categories may need further definition. Plaques are flat-topped palpable lesions >1 cm in diameter and may be considered papules that have enlarged in 2 dimensions. Nodules are papules that have enlarged in 3 dimensions. Nodules may be solid, edematous or cystic. Vegetative describes lesions with projections or proliferations above the skin surface. Causes of papulonodular dermatoses are outlined in Tables 5 and 6.

Parasitic Causes of Papular Dermatoses

Fleas	Flea bite dermatitis/hypersensitivity
Mites	Demodectic mange, sarcoptic mange, cheyletiellosis, trombiculiasis
Ticks	Ixodidae, Argasidae infestation
Lice	*Mallophaga, Anoplura* infestation
Helminths	Hookworm dermatitis, *Dirofilaria* dermatitis, *Pelodera strongyloides* dermatitis

Table 3. Morphologic classification of cutaneous lesions.

Category	Subgroups
Maculopapular	Macular
	Papular
Papulonodular	Nodular
	Plaques
	Vegetative
Vesiculopustular	Vesicular
	Pustular
Alopecia	Focal/multifocal
	Patchy
	Regional
	Generalized
Erosive-ulcerative	Parasitic
	Microbial
	Immune-mediated
	Neoplastic
	Miscellaneous
Exfoliative	Patchy
	Regional
	Generalized
Indurated	Turgid
	Solid
Pigmented	Red
	White
	Dark
	Skin-colored

Table 4. Maculopapular eruptions.

Macular	Papular
Allergic inhalant dermatitis	Parasitic dermatoses
Food allergy	Bacterial folliculitis
Allergic contact dermatitis	Drug eruption
Irritant contact dermatitis	Food allergy
Drug eruption	Dermatophytosis
Erythema multiforme	Comedones
Lupus erythematosus	Hormonal hypersensitivity
Alopecia areata	Erythema multiforme
Acanthosis nigricans	Vitamin A-responsive dermatosis
Endo/ectoparasitism	Dermatitis herpetiformis

Table 5. Papulonodular eruptions.

Nodular	Plaque	Vegetative
Parasitic	Bacterial hypersensitivity	Pemphigus vegetans
Intermediate pyoderma	Callus pyoderma	Mast-cell tumor
Deep pyoderma	Dermatophytosis	Cutaneous papilloma
Atypical pyoderma	Lupus profundus	Sebaceous gland hyperplasia
Dermatophytosis	Viral papillomatosis	Squamous-cell carcinoma
Intermediate mycoses	Calcinosis cutis	Transmissible venereal tumor
Deep mycoses	Calcinosis circumscripta	Fibroma
	Histiocytoma	Nevi
Lupus profundus	Histiocytosis	
Neoplastic	Keratoses	
Miscellaneous	Nevi	
	Lymphoma	
	Urticaria	
	Lichenoid dermatoses	
	Mucinosis	
	Erythema multiforme	
	Acanthosis nigricans	
	Dermatitis herpetiformis	

Introduction

Table 6. Specific causes of nodular dermatitis.

Parasites
Demodicosis
Cuterebriasis
Dirofilariasis
Dracunculiasis
Leishmaniasis

Bacteria
Furunculosis
Acne
Interdigital pyoderma
Nasal pyoderma
Bacterial pyoderma (Botryomycosis)
Abscess
Actinomycotic mycetoma
Atypical mycobacteriosis
Cutaneous tuberculosis

Fungi
Dermatophytosis (Kerion reaction)
Majochi's granuloma
Hyalohyphomycosis
Eumycotic mycetoma
Phaeohyphomycosis
Phycomycosis
Sporotrichosis
Blastomycosis
Coccidioidomycosis
Cryptococcosis
Histoplasmosis

Neoplasia
Basal-cell tumor
Fibroma/fibrosarcoma
Hemangiopericytoma
Hemangioma/hemangiosarcoma
Perianal-gland tumor
Histiocytic tumor
Lymphoma
Mast-cell tumor
Melanoma
Cysts
Nodular dermatofibrosis
Sebaceous-gland tumors
Sweat-gland tumors
Transmissible venereal tumor
Trichoepithelioma
Pilomatrixoma
Intracutaneous cornifying epithelioma
Lipoma
Collagenous nevi

Miscellaneous
Lupus profundus
Dermoid sinus
Nodular panniculitis
Juvenile cellulitis
Mucinosis
Eosinophilic granuloma
Periappendageal dermatitis (sebaceous adenitis)
Sterile pyogranuloma
Calcinosis circumscripta

Table 7. Vesiculopustular skin diseases.

Vesicular	Pustular
Pemphigus	Demodicosis
Pemphigoid	Bacterial folliculitis
Dermatomyositis	Dermatophytosis
Epidermolysis bullosa simplex	Subcorneal pustular dermatosis
Dermatitis herpetiformis	Sterile eosinophilic
Erythema multiforme	Lupus erythematosus pustulosis

Table 8. Alopecic disorders.

Focal/Multifocal	Patchy	Regional	Generalized
Demodicosis	Demodicosis	Discoid lupus erythematosus	Demodicosis
Dermatophytosis	Lice infestation	Hypothyroidism	Dermatophytosis
Bacterial folliculitis	Cheyletiellosis	Hyperadrenocorticism	Systemic lupus erythematosus
Scleroderma	Dermatophytosis	Growth hormone-responsive	Drug eruption
Cutaneous asthenia	Drug eruption	Hyperestrogenism	
Alopecia areata	Lupus erythematosus	Hypoestrogenism	
	Telogen defluxion	Pattern baldness	
	Protein deficiency	Testicular neoplasia	
	Bronzing syndrome	Dermatomyositis	
	Color mutant alopecia	Follicular dysplasia	
	Spiculosis	Toxicity	

Vesiculopustular eruptions are so grouped because in animals vesicles very quickly evolve into pustules, thus confusing diagnostic efforts. Vesicles are small fluid-filled structures (blisters), while pustules are white or yellow-white from their very inception. Bullae are the result of enlarging vesicles. When vesicles or pustules burst, they create either erosions (if only the epidermis is involved) or ulcers (if the integrity of the dermal epidermal junction has been disturbed). The *vesicular* and *pustular* subgroups are outlined in Table 7. One must appreciate that most vesicular disorders are mistakenly identified initially as pustular.

Introduction

Alopecia or hair loss is a common clinical finding and may result from several causes. Any process that results in folliculitis, or disturbs the growth cycle of the hair follicle, results in hair loss. Alopecia has been subdivided into *focal/multifocal, patchy, regional* and *generalized.* Focal/multifocal and patchy reflect a certain nonspecificity of hair loss. Regional alopecias have certain geographic limitations that may include such areas as the dorsum, head, tail, neck, legs, etc. Generalized alopecias include more extensive progressions of the former groupings. Alopecic disorders are listed in Table 8.

The *erosive-ulcerative* category reflects the secondary changes that may occur with many underlying processes; thus they are subcategorized by their potential underlying cause. Subgroupings include *parasitic, microbial, immune-mediated, neoplastic* and *miscellaneous* dermatoses. Erosive-ulcerative dermatoses are listed in Table 9.

Exfoliative dermatoses include excessively scaly disorders. This accumulation of scale may be *patchy, regional* or *generalized.* Ex-

Table 9. Erosive-ulcerative dermatoses.

Parasitic	Fleas
	Demodicosis
	Sarcoptic mange
Microbial	Skin-fold pyoderma
	Pyotraumatic dermatitis
	Perianal pyoderma
	Bacterial granuloma
Miscellaneous	Acral lick dermatitis
	Acral mutation syndrome
	Metabolic dermatoses
	Lethal acrodermatitis
	Tyrosinemia
	Dermatomyositis
Immune-Mediated	Pemphigus
	Pemphigoid
	Cutaneous vasculitis
	Toxic epidermal necrolysis

Table 10. Exfoliative dermatoses.

Patchy	Regional	Generalized
Lice infestation	Pemphigus foliaceus	Demodicosis
Demodicosis	Pemphigus erythematosus	Dermatophytosis
Cheyletiellosis	Hypothyroidism	Drug eruption
Dermatophytosis	Zinc-responsive dermatosis	Systemic lupus erythematosus
Pagetoid reticulosis	Tyrosinemia	Pemphigus foliaceus
Drug eruption	Nasodigital hyperkeratosis	Hypothyroidism
Sjogren's syndrome	Discoid lupus erythematosus	Keratinization defects
Color mutant alopecia		Vitamin E deficiency
Hyperestrogenism		Ichthyosis
Fatty acid deficiency		T-cell lymphoma
Vitamin A-responsive dermatosis		Metabolic disorders
Periappendageal dermatosis		Keratinization defects
Generic dog food disease		
Subcorneal pustular dermatosis		
Chronic maculopapular dermatoses		
Parapsoriasis		

Table 11. Indurated dermatoses.

Turgid	Solid
Urticaria	Scar
Angioedema	Cellulitis
Myxedema	Amyloidosis
Mucinosis	Bacterial granuloma
Juvenile cellulitis	Intermediate mycoses
	Deep mycoses
	Scleroderma
	Calcinosis cutis
	Calcinosis circumscripta (tumoral calcinosis)
	Neoplasia
	Periappendageal dermatitis
	Chronic maculopapular dermatoses (lichenification)

foliative dermatoses may also be described as eczema, seborrhea or erythroderma, but the implication is that scaling encompasses a significant part of the dermatosis. Exfoliative dermatoses are included in Table 10 under their appropriate subgrouping.

Indurated dermatoses are conditions in which the skin is thickened by accumulation of fluid, cells or matter (Table 11). It is at best arbitrary to try to delineate further the clinical subgroupings of induration; in rough terms, if the lesion feels compressible or fluid-filled and perhaps pits to the touch, it is classified as *turgid*. If the lesion feels firm, as though there is increased cellularity or material present, it is classified as *solid*.

The last category describes lesions that are *pigmented*. This category is further subgrouped into lesions that are red, white, dark or skin-colored(Table 12).

Red lesions are subgrouped as *focal/multifocal, patchy* or *extensive*. White lesions are subgrouped as *focal, patchy* or *extensive*. Dark lesions are subgrouped as the result of *hyperpigmentation* or describing the color of *dark pigmented masses*.

A final category includes *skin-colored* lesions.

Pigmented dermatoses are listed in Table 12.

Differential Diagnoses Based on Distribution

Many dermatoses have certain regional trends on the body surface, breed predispositions or sex predilections and therefore our clinical examination may also turn up helpful clues towards formulating differential diagnoses.

Conditions Often with a Facial Distribution

Parasites: demodicosis, trombiculiasis, fly bites, cuterebriasis, *Dirofilaria* dermatitis

Bacteria: skin-fold pyoderma, pyotraumatic dermatitis, acne, nasal pyoderma, atypical mycobacteriosis

Fungi: hyalohyphomycosis, cryptococcosis

Immune: Allergic inhalant dermatitis, food hypersensitivity, contact dermatitis, lupus erythematosus, pemphigus foliaceus/erythematosus, Vogt-Koyanagi-Harada-like syndrome

Introduction

Table 12. Pigmented lesions and dermatoses.

Red

Focal	Patchy	Extensive
Fold pyoderma	Demodicosis	Demodicosis
Pyotraumatic dermatosis	Drug eruption	Systemic lupus
Drug eruption	Systemic lupus	Toxicosis
Histiocytoma	Drug eruption	Photodermatitis
Petechiae	Erythema multiforme	
Purpura	Petechiae	
Vasculitis	Photodermatitis	
	Vasculitis	

White

Focal/Multifocal	Patchy	Extensive
Systemic lupus	Vogt-Koyanagi-Harada	Vogt-Koyanagi-Harada
Vogt-Koyanagi-Harada	Vitiligo	Albinism
Scleroderma	Tyrosinase deficiency	
Vitiligo		
Tyrosinase deficiency		

Dark

Hyperpigmentation	Pigmented Masses
Postinflammatory	Melanoma
Hypothyroidism	Basal-cell tumor
Hyperadrenocorticism	Vascular nevi
Growth hormone-responsive	Hemangioma
Acanthosis nigricans	Hemangiosarcoma
Lentigines	Organoid nevus
	Melanocytic nevus

Skin-Colored

Scleroderma	Callus
Papilloma	Epidermal nevus
Sebaceous-gland hyperplasia	Sebaceous nevus

Neoplasia: squamous-cell carcinoma, hemangiosarcoma, malignant histiocytosis, fibrous histiocytoma, actinic keratosis, melanoma, papilloma, transmissible venereal tumor

Other: zinc-responsive dermatosis, dermatomyositis, epidermolysis bullosa simplex, spiculosis, viral papillomatosis, juvenile cellulitis, metabolic dermatosis

Conditions Manifested as Nasal Dermatitis

Parasites: demodicosis, cuterebriasis, cutaneous dirofilariasis

Bacteria: nasal pyoderma, dermatophilosis, actinomycotic mycetoma

Fungi: dermatophytosis, hyalohyphomycosis, rhinosporidiosis, blastomycosis, coccidioidomycosis, cryptococcosis, histoplasmosis

Immune: allergic inhalant dermatitis, food allergy, contact sensitivity, lupus erythematosus, pemphigus foliaceus/erythematosus, bullous pemphigoid, Vogt-Koyanagi-Harada-like syndrome, drug eruption

Neoplasia: malignant histiocytosis, transmissible venereal tumor, cutaneous T-cell lymphoma, squamous-cell carcinoma

Other: vitamin A-responsive dermatosis, zinc-responsive dermatosis, generic dog food disease, dermatomyositis, epidermolysis bullosa simplex, tyrosinemia, trauma, photodermatitis, nasodigital hyperkeratosis

Conditions Involving the Eyelids

Parasites: demodicosis, sarcoptic mange

Bacteria: juvenile pyoderma, bacterial blepharitis

Fungi: dermatophytosis, intermediate mycoses, blastomycosis

Immune: pemphigus, pemphigoid, lupus erythematosus, dermatomyositis, Vogt-Koyanagi-Harada-like syndrome, allergic inhalant dermatitis, food hypersensitivity, parasite hypersensitivity, drug eruption

Endocrine: hypothyroidism, hyperadrenocorticism

Nutritional: vitamin A-responsive dermatosis, zinc-responsive dermatosis, generic dog food disease

Neoplasia: cutaneous lymphoma, T-cell-like lymphoma, acrocordon, squamous-cell carcinoma, adenocarcinoma

Miscellaneous: irritation, seborrheic dermatitis, thallium toxicosis

Conditions Involving the Head

Parasites: flea infestation, cuterebriasis

Bacteria: pyotraumatic dermatitis, atypical mycobacteriosis

Fungi: dermatophytosis, intermediate mycoses

Immune: Pemphigus foliaceus/erythematosus, lupus erythematosus

Neoplasia: basal-cell tumor, histiocytoma, actinic keratosis, collagenous nevi, nodular dermatofibrosis, papilloma, sebaceous-gland hyperplasia, apocrine cyst

Other: zinc-responsive dermatosis, dermatomyositis, epidermolysis bullosa simplex, juvenile cellulitis, periappendageal dermatitis, subcorneal pustular dermatosis

Conditions Involving the Ears

Parasites: tick infestation, lice infestation, demodicosis, sarcoptic mange, otodectiasis, fly bites

Immune: allergic inhalant dermatitis, pemphigus foliaceus/ erythematosus, lupus erythematosus, cutaneous vasculitis, cold agglutinin disease

Other: dermatomyositis, histiocytoma, psoriasiform-lichenoid dermatitis, idiopathic lichenoid dermatitis, hyperestrogenism, pinnal alopecia, periodic alopecia

Conditions Involving the Neck Region

Parasites: flea infestation, tick infestation, cuterebriasis

Neoplasia: basal-cell tumor, hemangioma, malignant fibrous histiocytoma, apocrine cyst, intracutaneous cornifying epithelioma, lipoma

Other: dermoid sinus, dermatitis herpetiformis

Introduction

Conditions Involving the Dorsum

Parasites: fleas, lice, cheyletiellosis

Microbes: bacterial folliculitis, dermatophytosis

Endocrine: hypothyroidism, hyperadrenocorticism, growth hormone-responsive dermatosis

Neoplasia: apocrine adenoma, trichoepithelioma, pilomatrixoma, intracutaneous cornifying epithelioma, dermoid sinus, hepatoid-gland tumor

Other: vitamin A-responsive dermatosis, Dalmatian bronzing syndrome, nodular panniculitis, periappendageal dermatitis, metabolic dermatoses, dermatitis herpetiformis

Conditions Involving the Ventrum

Parasites: sarcoptic mange, *Pelodera* dermatitis, trombiculiasis, dracunculiasis

Microbes: bacterial folliculitis, atypical mycobacteriosis, actinomycotic and eumycotic mycetoma

Immune: allergic inhalant dermatitis, contact dermatitis erythema multiforme

Neoplasia: lipoma, liposarcoma

Other: calcinosis cutis, generic dog food disease, eosinophilic granuloma, lichenoid dermatoses

Conditions Involving the Perineum

Microbes: skin-fold pyoderma, pyotraumatic dermatitis, perianal pyoderma

Neoplasia: perianal tumors, apocrine adenocarcinoma of anal sac origin, mast-cell tumor, fibroma, melanoma

Other: sex hormone-responsive disorders, hyperestrogenism

Conditions Involving the Genitalia

Neoplasia: melanoma, vascular nevi, squamous-cell carcinoma, transmissible venereal tumor, genital neoplasms, Sertoli-cell tumor, seminoma, interstitial-cell tumor, maligant histiocytosis

Other: estrogen-responsive disorders, hyperestrogenism, metabolic dermatoses

Conditions Involving the Legs

Parasites: demodicosis, sarcoptic mange, cutaneous dirofilariasis, dracunculiasis

Bacteria: callus pyoderma, actinomycotic mycetoma

Fungi: sporotrichosis, blastomycosis

Neoplasia: fibroma, fibrosarcoma, lipoma, hemangiopericytoma, hemangioma, histiocytoma, malignant fibrous histiocytoma, mast-cell tumor, collagenous nevi, nodular dermatofibrosis, squamous-cell carcinoma, transmissible venereal tumor, pilomatrixoma

Other: zinc-responsive dermatosis, calcinosis circumscripta, generic dog food disease, spiculosis, acral lick dermatitis, acral mutilation syndrome, erythema multiforme, dermatitis herpetiformis

Conditions Involving the Feet

Parasites: demodicosis, ticks, trombiculiasis, *Pelodera* dermatitis, hookworm dermatitis

Microbes: interdigital pyoderma, eumycotic mycetoma, blastomycosis, candidiasis, furunculosis, bacterial granuloma, dermatophytosis

Immune: allergic inhalant dermatitis, food allergy, contact dermatitis, pemphigus vulgaris, cutaneous vasculitis, drug eruption

Neoplasia: squamous-cell carcinoma, papilloma, melanoma, pilar cysts

Other: sterile pyogranuloma, foreign body reaction, lethal acrodermatitis, immunodeficiency, acral mutilation syndrome

Conditions Involving the Footpads

Parasites: hookworm dermatitis, *Pelodera* dermatitis

Microbes: dermatophytosis, intermediate, systemic mycoses

Introduction

Immune: pemphigus foliaceus, pemphigus erythematosus, lupus erythematosus, contact dermatitis

Neoplasia: pagetoid reticulosis, eccrine adenoma, eccrine adenocarcinoma, squamous-cell carcinoma

Other: zinc-responsive dermatoses, generic dog food disease, tyrosinemia, nasodigital hyperkeratosis, acral mutilation syndrome, lethal acrodermatitis, metabolic dermatoses, foreign body penetration, epidermolysis bullosa simplex

Conditions Involving the Nails and Nail Beds

Microbes: bacterial paronychia, dermatophytosis, candidal paronychia, sporotrichosis, blastomycosis, coccidioidomycosis

Immune: pemphigus vulgaris, lupus erythematosus, bullous pemphigoid, cutaneous vasculitis, erythema multiforme, drug eruption

Other: demodicosis, nutritional imbalances, cardiopulmonary disease, lethal acrodermatitis

Conditions Involving the Mucocutaneous Junctions

Immune: pemphigus vulgaris, bullous pemphigoid, cicatricial pemphigoid, systemic lupus erythematosus, Vogt-Koyanagi-Harada-like syndrome, vitiligo, Sjogren's syndrome, erythema multiforme, drug eruption

Other: candidiasis, melanoma, fibrous histiocytoma (see also oral, periocular and nasal tumors)

Conditions More Common in Males Than Females

Neoplasia: testicular tumors, hemangiosarcoma, perianal-gland adenoma, perianal-gland adenocarcinoma, malignant histiocytosis, liposarcoma, B-cell lymphoma, melanoma, vascular nevi, cutaneous papilloma, apocrine adenoma, intracutaneous cornifying epithelioma

Other: acne, growth hormone-responsive dermatosis, eosinophilic granuloma, spiculosis

Introduction

Conditions More Common in Females Than Males

Neoplasia: fibrosarcoma, hemangiopericytoma, apocrine adenocarcinoma of anal sac origin, fibroma, lipoma

Other: estrogen-responsive dermatosis, hyperestrogenism, vulvar fold pyoderma, discoid lupus erythematosus, focal mucinosis

Conditions More Common in Younger Dogs

Parasites: demodicosis, cheyletiellosis, otoacariasis

Microbes: viral papillomatosis, acne, impetigo, dermatophytosis

Immune: allergic inhalant dermatitis, food allergy, Vogt-Koyanagi-Harada-like syndrome

Neoplasia: histiocytoma, sebaceous nevi, epidermal nevi, fibrous histiocytoma, intracutaneous cornifying epithelioma

Inherited: color mutant alopecia, cutaneous asthenia, dermatomyositis, epidermolysis bullosa simplex, ichthyosis

Other: zinc-reponsive dermatosis, growth hormone-responsive dermatosis, dermoid sinus, albinism, vitiligo, tyrosinase deficiency, follicular dysplasia, spiculosis, eosinophilic granuloma, acral mutilation syndrome, lethal acrodermatitis, juvenile cellulitis, juvenile panniculitis, lichenoid dermatoses, periappendageal dermatitis, sterile pyogranuloma, tyrosinemia

Conditions with a Breed Predilection

Conditions with a breed predilection are covered in the chapter on congenito-hereditary skin diseases.

Additional Reading

1. Ackerman, L: A new approach to dermatologic diagnosis in the dog. *Vet Focus* 1(1):6-11, 1989.

2. August, JR: Taking a dermatologic history. *Comp Cont Ed Pract Vet* 8:510-518, 1986.

3. Scott, DW: Examination of the integumentary system. *Vet Clin No Am* 11:499-510, 1981.

4. Lynch, PJ: *Dermatology for the House Officer.* 2nd ed. Williams & Wilkins, Baltimore, 1987. p 353.

Introduction

Skin Scrapings

Skin scrapings are, or should be, the most common diagnostic test performed in veterinary dermatology. A dull scalpel blade or similar instrument is moistened with mineral oil and used to scrape away some of the epidermis, in which may reside a number of different parasites. The epidermis has no blood supply of its own, so if the scraping goes deep enough so that blood just begins to appear, one can be assured that a reasonable amount of epidermis has been collected for examination. After the scraping is obtained, the blade is then wiped onto a clean microscope slide and a microscope used to scan the slide for parasites.

Parasites that might be recovered on skin scrapings include mites (*Demodex, Sarcoptes, Cheyletiella, Otodectes*, chiggers) and worms (*Pelodera*, hookworms, heartworms). Skin scraping is a quick and sometimes very rewarding procedure. A negative scraping does not mean that parasites are not present, only that they were not present in the area scraped. Some parasites, such as *Sarcoptes*, the scabies mite, are notoriously difficult to recover even with multiple scrapings. When they are found, the diagnosis can be readily confirmed. Multiple skin scrapings should always be an important part of a thorough examination of the skin.

If a specific parasite is suspected, the process can be even more selective. For demodicosis, deep scrapings must be made, as *Demodex* inhabits hair follicles. Only superficial scrapings are needed if sarcoptic mange or cheyletiellosis is suspected, as these parasites inhabit the superficial layers of skin.

An alternative to routine skin scraping was evaluated at Michigan State University using a portable vacuum cleaner. A filter was inserted in the cleaner hose and after 10 minutes of vacuuming the animal with a crevice attachment, the filter was examined under a microscope. The 206 animals examined yielded fleas, flea feces, forage mites, *Cheyletiella, Sarcoptes, Chorioptes, Psoroptes, Otodectes, Demodex* and *Damalinia* spp, suggesting that the sensitivity of this technique is greater than that for routine skin scraping.

When parasitism is suspected, it is also worthwhile to perform a fecal evaluation. Some internal parasites may cause dermatoses, and some external parasites may be ingested by the chewing animal.

Additional Reading

1. Klayman, E and Schillhorn van Veen, TW: Vacuum cleaner method for diagnosis of ectoparasitism. *MVP* 62:767-771, 1981.

2. Yang, J and Scholten, T: A fixative for intestinal parasites permitting the use of concentration and permanent staining procedures. *Am J Clin Pathol* 67:300-304, 1977.

Bacterial Culture and Sensitivity Testing

Bacteria can be beneficial to the animal (*eg*, aid in digestion), harmless (saprophytic) or produce disease (pathogenic). When a bacterial disease is suspected, one may obtain a sample of those bacteria (by swab, pricking a pustule or biopsy) and culture them for further evaluation. Blood agar is used as an initial culture medium for bacteria. After 18-24 hours of incubation, numerous colonies of bacteria may indicate an infection. The bacteria are then identified, and samples from 4-5 well-isolated colonies of the same type are inoculated into 4-5 ml of trypticase soy broth and incubated at 35 C for 2-5 hours until the medium becomes slightly turbid. The sample's turbidity is adjusted to that of a standard (McFarland 0.5) by diluting with normal saline.

A sterile cotton swab is then used to streak some of the sample onto a Muller-Hinton agar plate. Small paper discs saturated with different antibacterials are then placed on the agar plate. The antibacterial in each disc diffuses out into the agar (the heaviest concentration of antibacterial being closest to the disc), inhibiting the growth of susceptible bacteria surrounding each disc. Colonies of bacteria growing close to an antibacterial disc over the next 16-18 hours are presumed resistant to that drug. A region of no growth (zone of inhibition) surrounding a disc indicates sensitivity to that antibacterial. These zones are measured and interpreted, and bacteria are classified as sensitive, intermediate or resistant, according to a standard table (Table 13). The antibacterials selected for the discs are a matter of convention, such that lincomycin is assessed with a clindamycin disc, cephalexin with a cephalothin disc, etc.

This entire procedure constitutes bacterial culture and sensitivity testing. This test should only be considered in light of other diagnostic information, and may be misleading if considered alone. For example, an animal with a skin disorder is very likely to have secondary bacterial complications. These bacteria may be cultured, but even treatment with an appropriate antibacterial will not correct the underlying problem. Therefore, treatment failures using therapy indicated by culture and sensitivity testing should prompt the investigator to consider underlying disorders.

A second pitfall is that the antibacterial discs and zones of inhibition have been standardized according to blood levels of antibacterials in people, exerting an effect on a standard number of bacteria. Therefore, if the antibacterials are applied to the surface of the skin or into the ear canal, the amount of drug in contact with the bacteria is independent of the blood levels. Also, the antibacterial must reach the site of bacterial infection, encounter a standardized number of bacteria and be fully potent when it does engage bacteria.

Abscesses and granulomas tend to "wall off" infectious agents, making them poorly accessible to antimicrobials. Some drugs are inactivated by contact with blood, pus or damaged tissue and may not exert any antibacterial effect. Other drugs cannot penetrate to the skin surface in an adequate concentration to be effective. Thus, treatment of bacterial infections of the skin must

Table 13. Zones of inhibition for various antibacterials.

	Disc Content (μg)	Zone of Inhibition (mm)		
		Resistant	Intermediate	Sensitive
Amoxicillin-clavulanate	30	<20	—	>20
Ampicillin	10	<21	21-28	>28
Carbenicillin	50	<18	18-22	>22
Cephalothin	30	<15	15-17	>17
Chloramphenicol	30	<15	15-17	>17
Clindamycin	2	<17	17-20	>20
Cloxacillin	1	<10	10-13	>13
Enrofloxacin	46	<16	16-20	>20
Erythromycin	15	<14	14-17	>17
Gentamicin	10	<13	—	>13
Kanamycin	30	<14	14-17	>17
Nitrofurantoin	300	<15	15-16	>16
Rifampin	5	<25	—	>25
Streptomycin	10	<12	12-14	>14
Sulfonamides	300	<13	13-16	>16
Tetracyclines	30	<15	15-18	>18
Trimethoprim-sulfa	1.25	<11	11-15	>15

involve a more holistic approach than just relying on the information provided by culture and sensitivity testing.

Additional Reading

1. Faler, K: Standardizing antimicrobial disk sensitivity testing. *MVP* 65:197-201, 1984.

2. Prescott, JF and Baggot, JD: Antimicrobial susceptibility testing and antimicrobial drug dosage. *JAVMA* 187:363-368, 1985.

3. Jones, RN and Edson, DC: Antibiotic susceptibility testing accuracy. *Arch Pathol Lab Med* 109:595-601, 1985.

4. Dow, SW *et al:* Bacteriologic specimens: Selections, collection, and transport for optimum results. *Comp Cont Ed Pract Vet* 11:686-702, 1989.

Fungal Culture

In most veterinary practices, fungal cultures are used predominantly to identify various fungi that cause dermatophytosis (ringworm). Dermatophyte culture media often use a specially formulated agar (Sabouraud's) to which has been added antibacterials (usually gentamicin or chloramphenicol), antifungals (cycloheximide) that inhibit growth of most nonpathogenic fungi, and sometimes a pH color indicator that reflects changes in the acid/alkaline balance of the medium. Ringworm-causing fungi (dermatophytes) grow as white fluffy colonies in 3-14 days. Since they use the protein in the medium preferentially, they produce alkaline waste products that change the pH color indicator from yellow to red.

The fungi can then be isolated from the medium and identified by microscopic examination. Some of the fungal growth can be immersed in water placed on the slide or can be highlighted with a number of stains, including lactophenol cotton blue, new methylene blue, or a stain containing KOH, DMSO and chlorazol dye. This last stain can be purchased commercially (Dermatologic Lab and Supply) or prepared by dissolving 100 mg chlorazol black E dye in 10 ml DMSO, then adding 90 ml water containing 5 g KOH. With this stain, hyphae stain green against a gray background. The KOH is not a necessary component but the stain created by its addition is then also very useful for fungal wet mounts of material scraped directly off the animal's skin.

Fungal cultures for intermediate and deep fungi are normally performed at diagnostic laboratories rather than in private practices, not only because of the difficulty in identifying these fungi but also because of the considerable public health concerns in working with them. Dermatophyte test medium is usually not suitable for growing intermediate and deep fungi because the cycloheximide and antibacterials may interfere with the growth of these fastidious organisms.

Additional Reading

1. Carroll, HF: Evaluation of dermatophyte test medium for diagnosis of dermatophytosis. *JAVMA* 165:192-195, 1974.

2. Burke, WA and Jones, BE: A simple stain for rapid office diagnosis of fungus infections of the skin. *Arch Dermatol* 120:1519-1520, 1984.

Allergy Testing

Allergy testing is performed in a manner modified from the human procedure (Chapter 4). Substances that can cause inhalant allergies include tree, grass and weed pollens, molds, house dust, house dust mites, feathers and dander. Before the test is commenced the animal must be properly prepared. This means not only preparing the site to be tested, but also ensuring that the animal is no longer receiving drugs that might interfere with the test. Such substances include corticosteroids, hormones, antihistamines, anesthetics and tranquilizers. There must be a sufficient interval between the last dose of any of these products and the testing date. Use of injectable corticosteroids, such as methylprednisolone acetate (Depo-Medrol, Depocoid 40, MP 40, Methysone 40), must be discontinued at least 4-8 weeks before testing, while oral corticosteroids should not be given for at least 2 weeks before testing. Ideally, the withdrawal time should consist of 1 week for every month that oral corticosteroids were used.

The classic antihistamines and tranquilizers should not be given for at least 48 hours (preferably 10 days) before testing, while some of the newer antihistamines (Seldane, Hismanal) may require an even longer withdrawal period. In general, it is advisable to use a 10-day withdrawal period for all antihistamines except astemizole (Hismanal), which requires at least a 1-month withdrawal period and preferably 6 months. Note that these withdrawal times reflect minimum intervals. It is not unusual to require many months of withdrawal from all drugs in an animal that has received corticosteroids for a long period before testing is productive.

Skin testing is accomplished by shaving a rectangular patch on the side of the animal's chest and injecting small amounts of potential allergens into the skin (intradermal) in a predetermined sequence. The amount of allergen varies from 0.02 to 0.1 ml but should be consistent for each bleb. The concentration of pollen and mold allergens used is 1000-1500 PNU/ml or 1:1000 weight/volume. Glycerine must not be a component of a test solution, as it can cause irritation. Most animals can be tested without tranquilization/sedation or anesthesia if they can be coaxed to lie on their sides quietly without fussing. If not, they can be given a mild sedative that does not interfere with testing (*eg*, xylazine: Rompun).

When the injections have been completed, the results are evaluated 15-30 minutes later. The interpretation is made by comparing the height, diameter and redness of the reactions with 2 controls: a positive (*eg*, histamine, 48/80) that produces a large reaction and a negative (*eg*, saline, sterile water) that produces no reaction. The reactions to individual allergens injected can then be compared subjectively or actually measured. Formulation of immunotherapy is then based on the reaction pattern and the animal's individual history.

A less specific alternative to skin testing is *in-vitro* diagnostic tests for allergen-specific IgE. Radioallergoabsorbent testing (RAST) or enzyme-linked immunosorbent assay (ELISA) may be used.

Allergy testing is covered more completely in Chapter 4.

Additional Reading

1. Ackerman, L: Diagnosing inhalant allergies: Intradermal or *in vitro* testing? *Vet Med* 83:779-789, 1989.

Biopsy for Histopathologic Examination

Biopsy for histopathologic examination (microscopic tissue evaluation) is especially important in dermatology, since the tissue to be sampled (skin) is so readily accessible. Biopsies are valuable diagnostic tools but should not be expected to tell the entire story. They reveal the changes only in a small region of skin surface at a particular point in time.

Skin samples may be removed by excision with a scalpel blade or more commonly with a special punch to remove a small core of tissue. The most commonly used punch is the Baker disposable biopsy punch. A 4-mm or 6-mm punch is preferred.

Unlike a skin scraping, which removes only stratum corneum and epidermis, a biopsy must include all skin layers, including the epidermis, dermis and subcutis. For most skin biopsies the procedure can be painlessly performed by injecting some local anesthetic beneath the skin, removing the sample, and closing the small defect with 1-2 sutures. Only occasionally is it necessary to induce general anesthesia to gather samples. The material collected is blotted clean of excess blood and added to a container of buffered formalin.

Obtaining multiple biopsies of different lesions greatly increases the chances of finding diagnostic changes. When possible, primary lesions should be selected for biopsy. Biopsy of chronic, excoriated, infected, scarred or ulcerated lesions rarely leads to a diagnosis. Crusts, however, may offer important clues to diagnosis and should never be stripped from the skin before biopsy. Samples from inflammatory dermatoses should be obtained with important lesions in the center of site, rather than at the junction with normal skin. Additional peripheral biopsies are helpful in neoplastic processes to provide further prognostic information.

The carefully selected biopsy samples should be sent to a competent and patient pathologist who is prepared to view multiple sections in search of diagnostic changes. Accordingly, veterinarians must provide the pathologist with well-chosen material, a complete history and a list of suspected diagnoses. The biggest mistake made by practitioners is to take a large sample for biopsy, plop it in formalin and send it off for the pathologist to cut into more workable pieces. When a large sample arrives, it is often completely decolorized by the formalin; what may have once been obvious no longer appears so. The technician, who has never seen the patient, then cuts more workable pieces to be embedded and stained for the pathologist, and the remaining material is discarded. Take the time to properly assess the tissue to be biopsied, and preferably obtain multiple small samples rather than a single large chunk.

While practitioners need not be proficient at reading biopsies, it is often helpful if you understand the limitations of the procedure. Categorizing inflammatory dermatoses into different patterns of inflammation can help turn otherwise nonspecific findings into important diagnostic clues. Following is a generalized grouping of dermatologic disorders based on their representative patterns of inflammation on biopsy.

Perivascular Dermatitis

Superficial perivascular dermatitis without significant epidermal changes:

The most common of the inflammatory patterns. Further information can be gleaned by the cell types involved.

Monomorphous: atopy, food hypersensitivity, drug eruption, dermatophytosis, Rocky Mountain spotted fever, postinflammatory dermatoses

Polymorphous: all of the above plus urticaria, parastism (ecto- and endo-), and early cellulitis

Superficial and deep perivascular dermatitis without epidermal changes:

Consider all of the above as well as systemic diseases, infections and immune-mediated disorders

Interface dermatitis includes perivascular dermatitis and a process obscuring the dermal-epidermal junction.

Hydropic: lupus erythematosus, drug eruption, toxic epidermal necrolysis (TEN), graft-vs-host, dermatomyositis, erythema multiforme, epidermolysis bullosa simplex

Lichenoid: lupus erythematosus, drug eruption, pemphigus, pemphigoid, idiopathic lichenoid dermatosis, metabolic dermatopathy, cutaneous T-cell-like lymphoma, erythema multiforme, Vogt-Koyanagi-Harada-like syndrome, psoriasiform-lichenoid dermatosis of Springer Spaniels

Spongiotic dermatitis, which includes perivascular dermatitis and epidermal intercellular edema (spongiosis)

Monomorphous: atopy, food hypersensitivity, contact hypersensitivity, drug eruption, dermatophytosis

Polymorphous: all of the above plus ectoparasitism, endoparasitism, seborrheic dermatoses, pemphigus, erythema multiforme, cutaneous T-cell-like lymphoma

Hyperplastic dermatitis, which includes perivascular dermatitis with hyperkeratosis, epidermal hyperplasia and little or no intercellular edema

Orthokeratotic hyperkeratosis implies an accumulation of surface scale in which the cells of the stratum corneum are devoid of nuclei. It may be further characterized as basket-weave, compact or laminated.

Parakeratotic hyperkeratosis (parakeratosis) implies an accumulation of surface scale in which the cells of the stratum corneum still contain nuclei.

Follicular hyperkeratosis implies an accumulation of scale within hair follicles.

Though orthokeratotic, parakeratotic and follicular hyperkeratosis are chronic nonspecific findings implying altered keratinization, their description may be of some benefit. Orthokeratotic hyperkeratosis is most commonly seen in keratinization disorders, endocrinopathies, dermatophytosis, chronic allergic reactions, lichenoid dermatoses, Vitamin A-responsive dermatosis, and ichthyosis. Generalized parakeratotic hyperkeratosis is seen most commonly in zinc-responsive dermatoses, Vitamin A-responsive dermatoses, ectoparasitism, metabolic dermatopathies, dermatophytosis, seborrheic dermatoses, and thallium toxicosis. Epidermal hyperplasia can be further classified as regular, irregular, papillomatous, or pseudocarcinomatous.

Conditions that may be manifested as hyperplastic dermatitides include atopy, food hypersensitivity, parasitism (ecto- or endo-), contact allergy, drug eruption, seborrheic dermatoses, dermatophytosis, acral lick dermatitis and postinflammatory dermatoses.

Vasculitis

An inflammatory reaction involving blood vessels and including conditions in which inflammatory cells are present within blood vessel walls, assuming some degree of vessel damage.

Neutrophilic vasculitis:

Leukocytoclastic: often from immune complex deposition

Nonleukocytoclastic: lupus erythematosus, drug eruption, polyarteritis nodosa, bacterial hypersensitivity, septicemia, thrombophlebitis, Rocky Mountain spotted fever, lymphocytic drug eruption, ectoparasitism, immune-mediated disorders

Introduction

Nodular and Diffuse Dermatitis

Nodular dermatitis implies formation of dermal nodules by discrete clusters of cells. *Diffuse dermatitis* implies a more generalized trend such that discrete nodules are no longer discernible.

Granulomatous inflammation implies a circumscribed region of inflammation in which the histiocyte is a predominant cell type. Granulomatous infiltrates that contain large numbers of neutrophils are called *pyogranulomatous*. *Granulomas* can be further classified as:

Palisading granulomas are characterized by alignment of histiocytes around a central focus of collagen degeneration. This is most commonly seen with collagenolytic granuloma (eosinophilic granuloma), xanthoma, calcinosis circumscripta (tumoral calcinosis) and dystrophic calcinosis cutis.

Histiocytic granulomas describe a tissue reaction pattern characterized by an infiltrate composed predominantly of histiocytes and perhaps smaller numbers of lymphocytes, plasma cells and multinucleated giant cells. This pattern is most commonly seen with histoplasmosis, rheumatoid nodule, sterile pyogranuloma and leishmaniasis.

Epithelioid granuloma describes a reaction pattern characterized by epithelioid cells within clusters and groups variably associated with histiocytes, lymphocytes and multinucleated giant cells. Reactions may be subdivided further as *tuberculoid* when epithelioid cells are surrounded by giant cells, followed by a layer of lymphocytes, then an outer layer of fibroblasts, or *sarcoidal* with just collections of epithelioid cells. Epithelioid granulomas may result from cutaneous mycobacterial infections including cutaneous tuberculosis.

Mixed inflammatory granulomas describe a pattern that may have elements of an acute, chronic and granulomatous process. Infiltrations of neutrophils, eosinophils, lymphocytes, histiocytes and multinucleated giant cells may be seen against a background of fibrocapillary proliferation. Mixed inflammatory granulomas may result from blastomycosis, cryptococcosis, coccidioidomycosis, sporotrichosis, prototheccosis and atypical mycobacteriosis.

Foreign body granulomas represent a large number of tissue reactions in which the giant cell is the most conspicuous member of the granulomatous infiltrate. The most common causes are dislodged keratin, such as might be seen in furunculosis, dermatophytosis, demodicosis, Majocchi's granuloma and foreign body penetration (*eg*, plant products, insect parts).

Another approach to defining nodular to diffuse dermatitides is to categorize the condition according to the predominating cell types as follows:

Predominantly neutrophilic dermatitis: aerobic bacterial infection, mycobacterial infection, actinomycotic mycetoma, fungal infection (superficial, intermediate, deep), *Prototheca* infection, foreign body reaction, sterile pyogranuloma

Predominantly histiocytic dermatitis: chronic stages of the above, xanthoma, dystrophic calcification, rheumatoid nodule, calcinosis circumscripta (tumoral calcinosis)

Predominantly eosinophilic dermatitis: so-called eosinophilic granulomas appear to be immune-mediated phenomena and may be seen with eosinophilic granuloma associated with collagenolysis, intermediate and deep mycoses, furunculosis.

Intraepidermal Vesicular and/or Pustular Dermatitis

Clefting occurs within the epidermis and the location sometimes suggests possible causation.

Intraepidermal: spongiotic dermatitis, metabolic dermatopathy, pemphigus vegetans, viral infections, cutaneous T-cell-like lymphoma, linear IgA dermatosis, sterile eosinophilic pustulosis.

Subcorneal: superficial (juvenile) pustular dermatitis (impetigo), subcorneal pustular dermatosis, lupus erythematosus, pemphigus foliaceus/erythematosus, sterile eosinophilic pustulosis, linear IgA dermatosis.

Intragranular: pemphigus foliaceus/erythematosus

Suprabasilar: pemphigus vulgaris.

Intrabasal: lupus erythematosus, epidermolysis bullosa simplex, drug eruption, toxic epidermal necrolysis.

Subepidermal Vesicular and/or Pustular Dermatitis

Clefting occurs beneath the epidermis.

Secondary to hydropic degeneration (see above).

Secondary to dermal-epidermal separation (eg, pemphigoid, dermatomyositis)

Secondary to severe dermal edema

Secondary to severe spongiotic dermatitis (see above)

As a disease process (eg, dermatitis herpetiformis)

Perifolliculitis, Folliculitis and Furunculosis

This pattern reflects inflammatory reactions centered about the hair follicle. The most common cause is bacterial infections secondary to a number of causes, such as allergies, endocrinopathies, keratinization defects, though dermatophytes, parasites (*Demodex, Pelodera,* etc) and immune-mediated disorders (alopecia areata, sterile eosinophilic pustulosis) must be considered. The hair follicles can also be involved as extensions of the epidermis (pemphigus, cutaneous T-cell-like lymphoma, vitamin A-responsive dermatosis, etc).

Panniculitis

This pattern reflects inflammatory reactions centered about the subcutaneous fat.

Lobular panniculitis: microbial infections, immune-mediated processes, foreign body reactions, nodular panniculitis.

Septal panniculitis: erythema nodosum, systemic lupus erythematosus, vasculitis, scleroderma.

Fibrosing Dermatitis

A secondary scarring phenomenon that might be a sequel to a number of different processes, including microbial infections, immune-mediated diseases (lupus erythematosus, vasculitis), foreign body reactions, lymphedema, dermatomyositis, scleroderma, alopecia areata and periappendageal dermatitis (sebaceous adenitis.

Endocrinopathy

A nonspecific noninflammatory pattern characterized by orthokeratotic and follicular hyperkeratosis, telogen hair follicles predominating and adnexal atrophy. Endocrine conditions to be considered include hypothyroidism, hyperadrenocorticism, growth hormone-responsive dermatosis, and sex hormone-related dermatosis. Nonendocrine differential diagnoses include telogen effluvium, alopecia areata, black hair follicular dysplasia, color mutant alopecia and hypotrichosis.

Biopsy Interpretation

Skin biopsies may be interpreted at a few centers including:

Dr. Lowell Ackerman
858 N Country Club Dr
Mesa, AZ 85201
(602) 833-7330

Dr. Patrick Breen
4725 Cornell Rd
Cincinnati, OH 45241
(513) 489-4644

Dr. E.G. (Ted) Clark
Western College of Veterinary Medicine
Department of Veterinary Pathology
University of Saskatchewan
Saskatoon, Saskatchewan S7N 0W0
(306) 966-7286

Dr. James Conroy
DVM Pathology Laboratory
PO Box 5407
Mississippi State, MS 39762

Dr. Thelma Lee Gross
Dermatopathology Services
Veterinary Pathology Consultants
3911 West Capitol Ave
West Sacramento, CA 95691
(916) 372-4200

Histovet, Veterinary Histopathology Consultants
Attention: Drs. J. Yager and B. Wilcock
309 Edinburgh Rd South
Guelph, Ontario N1G 2K3

Introduction

Michigan State University
Attention: Dr. R. Dunstan
PO Box 30076
Lansing, MI 48909-7576
(517) 353-0621

Dr. Emily Walder
A & E Clinical Veterinary Laboratory
11518 Pico Blvd
Los Angeles, CA 90064
(213) 477-9725

These are only a few facilities; inclusion in this book should not be construed as an endorsement. Veterinary dermatohistopathology is in its infancy and many highly competent individuals are emerging in this field. Please contact me if you are aware of others that do a good job with skin biopsies.

Additional Reading

1. Austin, VH: Skin biopsies: When, where, and why. *Comp Cont Ed Pract Vet* 2:531-536, 1980.

2. Rojko, JL et al: Histologic interpretation of cutaneous biopsies from dogs with dermatologic disorders. *Vet Pathol* 15:579-589, 1978.

3. Withrow, SJ and Lowes, N: Biopsy techniques for use in small animal oncology. *JAAHA* 17:889-902, 1981.

Immunopathologic Examination

Immunopathologic techniques include direct immunofluorescence testing (DIT) and immunoperoxidase testing. They are used to identify autoantibodies and/or complement in tissue sections. The pattern of antibody deposition is of diagnostic significance. Immunofluorescence at the intercellular spaces (ICS) is most consistent with pemphigus although it may occur as a false positive with other conditions. Conditions which result in staining at the dermal-epidermal junction (DEJ), also designated as the basement membrane zone (BMZ) include bullous pemphigoid, cicatricial pemphigoid, systemic and discoid lupus erythematosus, linear IgA disease and (if it exists in the dog) dermatitis herpetiformis. A third pattern in which immunoglobulins with or without complement is deposited about blood vessels may be seen with the myriad conditions that cause cutaneous vasculitis.

Samples taken for direct immunofluorescence testing are placed in Michel's solution, a transport medium that preserves tissue proteins such that samples can be mailed, without refrigeration, to laboratories that perform these specialized tests. This medium can be purchased commercially (Zeus Scientific, Foot of Thompson St, Raritan, NJ 08869), prepared (mix 2.5 ml of 1-M potassium citrate pH 7 with 5 ml of 0.1-M magnesium sulfate, 5 ml of 0.1-M N-ethyl maleimide, 87.5 ml of distilled water and 55 g of ammonium sulfate and adjust pH to 7.0 with 1-M KOH), or acquired from laboratories that perform this specialized test. Since formalin fixation destroys tissue antibodies, immunofluorescence tests cannot be performed on samples submitted for histopathologic examination.

Biopsies submitted from the nose or footpads are often positive on direct immunofluorescence testing using IgM even in the absence of actual autoimmune disease.

Indirect immunofluorescence testing is designed to detect disease-specific antibodies circulating in the blood; however, it has proven unreliable in its veterinary applications.

Immunopathologic examination is available at several different facilities, including:

> Department of Veterinary Microbiology & Immunology
> Attention: Dr. Roger Johnson
> University of Guelph
> Guelph, Ontario N1G 2W1
>
> Immunopathology Laboratory
> 306 Veterinary Research Tower
> NYS College of Veterinary Medicine
> Cornell University
> Ithaca, NY 14853
>
> Immunopathology Laboratory
> College of Veterinary Medicine
> University of Florida
> Gainesville, FL 32601
>
> Veterinary Pathology Consultants
> 3911 West Capitol Ave
> West Sacramento, CA 95691
> (916) 372-4200

Immunoperoxidase testing is a newer alternative to direct immunofluorescence testing. It can be performed at some special facilities. Preliminary studies indicate this technique is suitable for use with animal tissues but it is not yet readily available to veterinary practitioners. Immunoperoxidase testing is used exclusively as an immunopathologic assay at the following facility.

>Western College of Veterinary Medicine
>Department of Veterinary Pathology
>University of Saskatchewan
>Saskatoon, Saskatchewan S7N 0W0
>(306) 966-7286

Additional Reading

1. Wolfe, MJ et al: Immunofluorescent staining of cutaneous and renal biopsy specimens: A comparison of preservation by quick-freezing with or without storage in transport medium of Michel. *JAAHA* 18:444-448, 1982.

2. Penneys, NS: Immunoperoxidase methods and advances in skin biology. *J Am Acad Dermatol* 11:284-290, 1984.

3. Seiler, RJ: Staphylococcal protein A labeled with horseradish peroxidase for the immunohistologic diagnosis of canine autoimmune diseases. *Am J Vet Res* 44: 195-200, 1984.

4. Medleau, L and Miller Jr, WH: Immunodiagnostic tests for small animal practice. *Comp Cont Ed Pract Vet* 5:705-714, 1983.

5. Medleau, L et al: Complement fluorescence in sera of dogs with pemphigus foliaceus. *Am J Vet Res* 48:486-487, 1987.

Cytologic Examination

Cytology is the study of free cells from tissues. Samples may be obtained in various ways. Fine-needle aspiration involves inserting a needle into a tissue, applying gentle suction with a syringe, and withdrawing the needle while maintaining back pressure on the syringe plunger. The needle is then detached and the barrel of the syringe is filled with air. The needle is then reattached to the syringe, and the material in the hub of the needle is expressed onto a clean microscope slide. In dermatology, this is most commonly used to evaluate masses in or beneath the skin.

An impression smear is made by touching a microscope slide to the tissue being evaluated. The smear may then be stained to highlight certain cell types and products. A preferred stain for cytologic examination is Diff-Quik (Dade Diagnostics). Additional unstained slides can be preserved with a cytologic preservative spray or alternatively, with hair spray. These may then be sent to a laboratory for evaluation.

Additional Reading

1. Roszel, JF: Cytologic procedures. *JAAHA* 17:903-910, 1981.

2. O'Rourke, LG: Cytologic technics: Sampling, slide preparation and staining. *MVP* 64:185-189, 1981.

3. Barr, RJ: Cutaneous cytology. *J Am Acad Dermatol* 10:163-180, 1984.

4. Mills, JN: Diagnoses from lymph node fine-needle aspiration cytology. *Aust Vet Practit* 14:14-17, 1984.

5. Cowell, RL and Tyler, RD: *Diagnostic Cytology of the Dog and Cat.* American Veterinary Publications, Goleta, CA, 1989.

Serologic Testing

Titers

Titers are serum levels of antibodies against specific entities of viral, bacterial, fungal or immunologic origin. Titers are prepared by diluting the blood serum and exposing these dilutions to known amounts of the agent being tested for. If a reaction is noted at even high dilutions of serum, there must be very high levels of that specific antibody in the bloodstream. Thus, a titer of 1:1000 indicates a much higher concentration of antibodies than a titer of 1:10.

Additional Reading

1. Jackson, JA: Immunodiagnosis of systemic mycoses in animals: A review. *JAVMA* 188:702-705, 1986.

2. Tyler, JW and Cullor, JS: Titers, tests, and truisms: Rational interpretation of diagnostic serologic testing. *JAVMA* 194:1550-1558, 1989.

Antinuclear Antibody Testing

The antinuclear antibody (ANA) test, performed on blood serum, detects antibodies directed against cell nuclei. The test is intended to diagnose lupus erythematosus but has been reported positive (false positive?) in a number of other conditions, including pemphigus erythematosus, thrombocytopenia, endocarditis, heartworm disease, generalized demodicosis, cholangiohepatitis, various cancers, autoimmune hemolytic anemia, rheumatoid arthritis, myeloma, autoimmune thyroiditis, atopy, aural hematoma and glomerulonephritis, as well as in some normal dogs. It is, however, the best screening test for systemic lupus erythematosus, since it is positive in up to 90% of dogs with this condition. The value is normally expressed as a titer that represents a concentration of antibody in the blood. ANA titers of ≥1:20 are usually considered significant in dogs, though each laboratory must establish its own normal limits.

In human medicine, the concept of antinuclear antibodies has advanced to the point where autoantibodies to specific nuclear components can be assayed. Thus, antibodies to Sm antigen are considered markers for SLE (though they only occur in about 30% of cases) since they are not found in other autoimmune disorders, including discoid lupus erythematosus (DLE). Autoantibodies to histones are seen in about 95% of drug-induced lupus cases, while autoantibodies to ribonucleoprotein (RNP) are seen most commonly in mixed connective tissue diseases, as well as some cases of SLE.

Autoantibodies to single-stranded DNA are most common in Sjogren's syndrome. Anticentromere antibodies are seen in 80-90% of scleroderma patients with the CREST variation. Antibodies to the newly discovered PM-1 and Jo-1 antigens appear to be the ANAs of polymyositis and dermatomyositis. Veterinary applications of these different ANAs are still in their infancy but will undoubtedly be available to practitioners in the future.

Additional Reading

1. Schultz, RD: ANA diseases. *Calif Vet* 7(2):23-26, 1984.

2. Sontheimer, RD *et al*: Antinuclear and anticytoplasmic antibodies. *J Am Acad Dermatol* 9:335-343, 1983.

3. Medleau, L and Miller Jr, WH: Immunodiagnostic tests for small animal practice. *Comp Cont Ed Pract Vet* 5:705-714, 1983.

4. Shull, RM *et al*: Investigation of the nature and specificity of antinuclear antibody in dogs. *Am J Vet Res* 44:2004-2008, 1987.

5. Bennett, D and Kirkham, D: The laboratory identification of serum antinuclear antibody in the dog. *J Comp Pathol* 97:523-539, 1987.

LE Cell Test

The lupus erythematosus (LE) cell test is performed on clotted or heparinized blood. The tube containing the blood sample is shaken gently to slightly damage the white blood cells such that nuclei are available to be acted upon by autoantibodies. Other white blood cells that ingest these damaged nuclei are known as LE cells.

It takes an experienced eye to differentiate LE cells from other WBC. They may be seen in about 60% of animals with systemic lupus erythematosus. The test has also been positive in cases of autoimmune hemolytic anemia, rheumatoid arthritis, lymphosarcoma, lymphoblastic leukemia, pulmonary granulomatosis and warfarin poisoning. This test is too subjective and not sensitive enough to be recommended as an important diagnostic test for lupus erythematosus.

Complement Fixation

The complement-fixation test is based on competition for complement between various antigen-antibody complexes and red blood cell-specific antibodies. The complement-fixation test consists of 2 parts. First, the antigen and the serum being tested are mixed and incubated in the presence of normal guinea pig serum (a source of complement). The serum to be tested is heated to destroy its own complement activity and to ensure that this serum complement does not interfere with the fixation test. The second part of the test involves assessing the amount of free complement remaining in the above mixture.

Appropriate controls must be established for every complement-fixation assay because some antigens bind complement by themselves, in the absence of antibodies. A large percentage (perhaps 25%) of canine serum samples is anticomplementary. This means that complement can be fixed in the apparent absence of antigen, as demonstrated by other tests (usually immunodiffusion). Most anticomplementary problems are associated with alterations by other antigen-antibody complexes, drug interference (amphotericin B, tetracycline), hemolysis or bacterial contamination. Detergents can also alter the test; therefore, cleaned and reused syringes should not be used for blood collection for complement-fixation tests. Because of these potential "false-positive" anticomplementary results, complement fixation should only be performed with adequate controls.

Immunodiffusion

Immunodiffusion tests operate on the principle that when antigen contacts antibody, a band of precipitate forms. This principle can be used when wells are cut in agar and 1 well is filled with soluble antigen and the other with patient's serum. Ideally, a third well contains specific antibody-containing serum to act as a positive control. Antigen and antibody each diffuse out of the wells in a radial fashion. A visible line of precipitation implies the presence of antigen-specific antibody in the patient's serum.

Latex Agglutination

Reactions of antibody with antigen on an insoluble particle (*eg*, latex) result in cross-linking of the various antigen particles by the antibodies and consequent clumping (agglutination).

Agglutination titers can be determined by serial dilution of the patient's serum. The titer is only semiquantitative and represents the ability of a certain dilution of the antibodies in the serum to cause agglutination. Significant titers must be determined for each agglutination assay, since the titer depends on a variety of factors, such as size, charge and density of epitopes on an antigen.

Additional Reading

1. Schalm, OW: Lupus erythematosus (LE) cells in the dog. *Canine Pract* 5(1):20-25, 1978.

Circulating Immune Complex Assay

Circulating immune complexes (CICs) are a heterogeneous group of immmunoreactants formed by the union of antigen and antibody. They can mediate tissue damage in certain pathologic states, and in other instances may form in response to tissue injury and subsequently modify the immune response.

Assay for CICs in people may have important implication in a variety of diseases, including SLE, cutaneous vasculitis and dermatitis herpetiformis. As with ANAs, veterinary application of CIC assay is still in its infancy. Preliminary research suggests that dogs with lupus erythematosus, generalized demodicosis, dermatomyositis, rheumatoid arthritis or pyoderma have significantly higher CIC levels than normal dogs.

Additional Reading

1. Yancey, KB and Lawley, TJ: Circulating immune complexes: Their immunochemistry, biology and detection. *J Am Acad Dermatol* 10:711-731, 1984.

2. Jegasothy, BV: Immune complexes in cutaneous disease. *Arch Dermatol* 119:795-798, 1983.

3. Deboer, DJ *et al*: Circulating immune complex concentrations in selected cases of skin disease in dogs. *Am J Vet Res* 49:143-146, 1988.

4. Wu, C-C *et al*: Purification and characterization of the 1q subcomponent of canine complement and its use in the 125I-C1q binding assay for detection of immune complexes. *Am J Vet Res* 49:865-869, 1988.

Fibronectin Assay

Fibronectin is a dimeric protein with binding sites for fibrin, fibrinogen, heparin, cell surfaces, *Staphylococcus aureus*, collagen, gelatin and yeast. It is involved in opsonization, adhesion, phagocytosis, hemostasis, oncogenic transformation and modulation of the reticuloendothelial system. As such, it appears to be involved in a nonspecific host defense mechanism for removal of foreign particles from blood.

Low plasma levels may be associated with sepsis, neoplasia, trauma, burns, malnutrition, and disseminated intravascular coagulation (DIC). Fibronectin levels are not diagnostic of any disorder but may have prognostic value if they remain abnormal or return to normal following successful therapy.

Additional Reading

1 Feldman, BF *et al*: Plasma fibronectin concentration associated with various types of canine neoplasia. *Am J Vet Res* 49:1017-1019, 1988.

2 Hauptman, JG *et al*: A turbidimetric method for fibronectin assay in the dog. *Am J Vet Res* 49:1935-1936, 1988.

Hair Analysis

I hesitate to even mention this topic but am including my opinions for the sake of completeness. It is well recognized by dermatologists and many nutritionists that mineral and trace element analysis of hair samples is not a clinically useful tool to assess nutritional status. There is no standardization of so-called "normal" hair mineral levels in people, and certainly not in animals. Also there is very little information that attempts to correlate hair concentration of elements with other tissue mineral concentrations.

Perhaps the most doubtful aspect of hair analysis is that in every instance I have used the procedure, alleged imbalances have been detected and megadose nutritional therapy recommended by the companies performing the tests. Hair analysis may have some validity (I'm not convinced as yet) but the results must be interpreted in conjunction with other better-defined forms of assessment.

Additional Reading

1. Sherertz, EC: Misuse of hair analysis as a diagnostic tool. *Arch Dermatol* 121:1504-1505, 1985.

2. Barrett, S: Commercial hair analysis: Science or scam? *JAMA* 254:1041-1045, 1985.

Chapter 1
Parasitic Skin Disorders

External parasites are one of the main reasons why clients consult veterinarians. It is thus important that information provided be comprehensive, current and correct.

Recommended Reading

1. Fadok, VA: Miscellaneous parasites of the skin (Part I). *Comp Cont Ed Pract Vet* 2: 707-712, 1980.

2. Fadok, VA: Miscellaneous parasites of the skin (Part II). *Comp Cont Ed Pract Vet* 2: 782-787, 1980.

3. Reedy, LM: Common parasitic problems in small animal dermatology. *JAVMA* 188: 362-364, 1986.

4. Moriello, KA: Common ectoparasites of the dog. Part 1: Fleas and ticks. *Canine Pract* 14(2):6-18, 1987.

5. Moriello, KA: Common ectoparasites of the dog. Part 2: *Sarcoptes scabiei* var *canis* and *Demodex canis*. *Canine Pract* 14(3):25-41, 1987.

Flea Infestation

Fleas are wingless insects, 1.0-2.5 mm long, with laterally compressed bodies and mouthparts structured for puncturing the skin to suck blood. Because of a superelastic protein (resilin) located in the thorax above the hind legs, the flea can jump 150X its own length (about 2.5 ft).

The major species infesting both dogs and cats are *Ctenocephalides felis* and *Ctenocephalides canis*. The average lifespan of a flea is 6-24 months. In that time, a female flea may lay up to 500 eggs in the environment. Though the life cycle may be completed in as little as 3 weeks, this time is quite variable, depending upon environmental conditions. Optimal features include temperatures of 18-27 C (65-80 F) and relative humidities above 70%. The eggs laid by the adult female flea hatch in 4-7 days, the first-stage larvae feeding on organic material and fecal pellets. The second-stage larvae emerge after a week, then molt to the third larval stage within another week. The pupal stage then follows in response to a decrease in endogenous juvenile major growth hormone. If artifically high levels of juvenile growth hormone are maintained in the environment by application of an insect growth regulator (*eg,* methoprene), larvae never pupate and eventually die. The adult flea emerges from the pupal stage in several days to 2 weeks. An emerging adult flea may survive as long as a year before its first blood meal, but after this time it must feed on a regular basis. The flea also serves as the intermediate host for the tapeworm, *Dipylidium caninum.*

Only adult fleas are parasitic and spend about 10% of their time actually feeding on the animal. Fleas rarely leave an animal unless they die or are mechanically removed. It has been estimated that for every flea on an animal, at least 100 live in the immediate environment.

Not all animals appear sensitive to flea bites, and cats especially may be asymptomatic carriers. Most infested dogs and cats develop a maculopapular crusting eruption in the area of flea bites (usually around the base of the tail, Fig 1). Some animals develop flea-bite hypersensitivity to the allergenic material in flea saliva. Flea saliva contains a low-molecular-weight hapten (4000-10,000 daltons) that binds to dermal collagen to form a complete antigen. Flea saliva also contains histamine-like compounds and enzymes that cause nonimmunologic reactions. In these cases, the bite of only 1 flea every 4-5 days is sufficient to perpetuate flea-bite dermatitis indefinitely.

Proper management of flea infestation requires treating the animal and the premises. Treatment of the animal is best accomplished with insecticidal dips, sprays, topicals and powders available from veterinary suppliers. The most effective products include pyrethrins, pyrethroids, carbamates, malathion, organophosphates or rotenone, individually or in combination (Appendix 1).

Flea shampoos usually contain pyrethrins or pyrethroids. Though they effectively kill fleas on contact, there is no residual activity once the shampoo is rinsed off.

Spray products may be water or alcohol based. The alcohol allows the insecticide to be transported more rapidly through the insect cuticle and have more immediate knockdown effect but tends to be more flammable, odoriferous, irritating, and potentially more drying to the skin.

Dips provide the most complete flea kill and residual action but are restricted in the frequency that they may be administered. Most dips contain organophosphates, synergized pyrethrins or combinations of synergized pyrethrins and pyrethroids. The pyrethrin/pyrethroid dips may be applied more often than organophosphate preparations. Animals should not be rinsed following application of the dip to obtain maximum efficacy.

Powders are less frequently used flea control products probably because they are aesthetically displeasing. They also have the potential for insecticide "buildup" with overenthusiastic application.

Foggers are concentrated insecticide products in pressurized containers. Their ingredients might include one or more of the following: synergized pyrethrin, pyrethroid, organophosphates, carbamates or methoprene. Foggers offer convenience but their dispersion does not provide uniform coverage of the environment.

Corticosteroids may be necessary to control the prominent pruritus until flea control is achieved. Allergy shots with flea extract have been, for the most part, of little benefit to infested animals. The main reason for this is undoubtedly that flea saliva is the allergenic component but flea vaccines are comprised of whole-body extracts.

Flea collars contain toxic chemicals and do not come close to meeting their claims as flea deterrents. The best place for a flea collar is in a vacuum cleaner bag where, with limited air flow, they have some flea-killing ability. Such use of flea collars is not recommended by manufacturers and should be considered extra-label use of the products.

"Electronic" flea collars purportedly alter flea behavior and kill fleas with high-frequency compressional wave energies. However, the efficacy of this "high-tech" approach has not been validated by controlled studies.

Despite repeated testing and the enthusiastic reports of some pet owners, neither supplementation with brewer's yeast nor thiamin appears to have any real effect on fleas. Environmental application of borax appears to have some antiparasitic effects.

Management of flea-infested premises is a major challenge to all concerned. Integral to any control program is the realization that available insecticides generally only kill adult fleas, not eggs or larvae, and so procedures must be regularly repeated to kill newly emergent adult fleas.

A new product, methoprene (Precor: Zoecon), is an insect growth regulator that inhibits development of flea larvae to adult stages and has a long residual effect of up to 3 months. The product on its own will not kill adult fleas, since it is not an insecticide, and therefore is usually sold in combination with an insecticide to give quick-kill (Siphotrol Plus: Vet-Kem). Bear in mind that methoprene does not kill adult fleas, and pyrethrins are short-lived in the environment. Thus, new adult fleas entering the home after an application can still cause problems. Safe insecticides, such as pyrethrins, may therefore still need to be used for ongoing control.

Recently, a topical form of methoprene has become available (Ovitrol: Vet-Kem) that prevents eggs laid on pets from hatching, even after falling off the pet into the environment.

Potent environmental sprays, powders and foggers are available from veterinary distributors. Since the ingredients can have toxic consequences, the manufacturer's directions should be followed. Products that are microencapsulated have the advantage of offering timed release of insecticides slowly into the environment, thereby minimizing the risk of toxicity and increasing the residual effect. When using these products, it is important not to vacuum between treatments or the insecticides in encapsulated form will be removed from the environment.

When carpets are vacuumed, the dust bag should be immediately thrown out or, as an alternative, moth balls or a flea collar can be added to the bag to kill the trapped fleas before they can escape. Professional exterminators occasionally are required to treat extensively infested premises.

Hyposensitization with flea extract has never been regarded as terribly effective. This is probably a consequence of the use of whole body flea extracts rather than the allergenic (actually haptenic) component, the flea saliva, as discussed earlier. Effective flea vaccines will likely follow refinement of the hapten into an immunomodulatory form.

The flea problem appears to be becoming more troublesome with each passing year, and effective flea control products are barely keeping pace.

Additional Reading

1. Melman, SA and Hutton, P: Flea control on dogs and cats indoors and in the environment. *Comp Cont Ed Pract Vet* 7:869-887, 1985.

2. Schick, MP and Schick, RO: Understanding and implementing safe and effective flea control. *JAAHA* 22:421-434, 1986.

3. Bledsoe, B *et al*: Current therapy and new developments in indoor flea control. *JAAHA* 18:415-422, 1982.

4. Mason, KV *et al*: Fenthion for flea control on dogs under field conditions: Dose response efficacy studies and effect on cholinesterase activity. *JAAHA* 20:591-595, 1984.

5. Baker, NF and Farver, TB: Failure of brewers' yeast as a repellent to fleas on dogs. *JAVMA* 183:212-214, 1983.

6. Halliwell, REW: Ineffectiveness of thiamine (Vitamin B1) as a flea-repellent in dogs. *JAAHA* 18:423-426, 1982.

Tick Infestation

Ticks are members of the spider family (arachnids) and are blood-sucking parasites capable of transmitting a variety of protozoal (*eg,* babesiosis, anaplasmosis, cytauxzoonosis, hemobartonellosis), rickettsial (*eg,* Rocky Mountain spotted fever, ehrlichiosis), viral (*eg,* St. Louis encephalitis) and bacterial (*eg,* tularemia, borreliosis, coxiellosis) diseases, in addition to producing toxins, dermatologic disorders, paralysis and anemia. Ticks also transmit the newly recognized "Lyme disease."

There are 2 major families of ticks. Soft (argasid) ticks (*eg, Otobius megnini, Ornithodorus talaje*) have no shield, and the larvae and nymphs are parasitic. *Otobius megnini* parasitizes the external ear canal of small animals, while *Ornithodurus talaje* is the cause of Mexican-American relapsing fever. Hard (ixodid) ticks (*eg, Rhipicephalus sanguineus, Dermacentor, Ixodes, Amblyomma, Boophilus* and *Haemaphysalis*) are the most common ticks affecting dogs. Their larvae, nymphs and adults are all parasitic. Most species require 3 hosts to complete the 4-stage, relatively slow life cycle. *Rhipicephalus* is the only tick that reproduces in and infests buildings and is also infamous as the only species that develops resistance to insecticides.

Ticks can live up to 200 days and females can lay thousands of eggs in walls, cracks and crevices after a blood meal.

Diagnosis of tick-related dermatoses is by clinical signs of a maculopapular eruption and finding the ticks. Skin scrapings may reveal larvae and nymphs.

Treatment is not difficult, as the ticks are susceptible to many common flea products. It is important, however, that treatment be thorough. To be effective, dips, sprays or powders must make direct contact with the tick to kill it. Since *Rhipicephalus sanguineus* can survive indoors and the female often lays eggs on vertical surfaces, infestation with this species of tick may necessitate environmental treatment at 2-week intervals or even require professional exterminators.

Additional Reading

1. Hoskins, JD and Cupp, EW: Ticks of veterinary importance. Part I.The Ixodidae family: Identification, behavior and associated diseases. *Comp Cont Ed Pract Vet* 10:564-580, 1988.

2. Hoskins, JD and Cupp, EW: Ticks of veterinary importance. Part II. The Argasidae family: Identification, behavior and associated diseases. *Comp Cont Ed Pract Vet* 10:699-708, 1988.

Lice Infestation

Lice are wingless insects that are host specific and live only on certain species. They are transmitted by direct contact or via contaminated objects. The entire life cycle, egg (nit) to nymph to adult, requires about 3 weeks. There are 2 different types of lice: biting lice (*eg, Trichodectes canis, Heterodoxus spiniger*) feed on epidermal debris and hair; sucking lice (*eg, Linognathus setosus*) pierce the skin and feed on body fluids. Infested animals have a dull, dry coat, with hair loss, scales and crusts. Adult lice and nits can be seen on the haircoat. Animals infested with sucking lice may also be anemic because of blood loss.

Treatment is not difficult, since most lice are sensitive to flea products, but treatment must include all animals in the household. Though people may be bitten by canine lice, they do not require any specific treatment if the lice are completely eradicated from the dogs.

Demodectic Mange

Demodex canis is a mite that is a normal resident of canine skin. It lives within the hair follicles and only appears on the skin surface when travelling between follicles. Demodicid mites of one species or another are present in small numbers on the skin of all normal mammals, including people, and are therefore considered noncontagious. In small numbers, they do not cause any disease but simply feed on debris within the hair follicles. The complete life cycle lasts 20-35 days.

Though demodicosis (demodectic mange) is generally considered a disease of young animals, transmission does not occur across the placenta. Infestation is normally acquired from the bitch by nursing pups during the first 2-3 days of life. After this time, infestation is unlikely. So, pups delivered by cesarean section and raised away from the dam do not have *Demodex* mites. Many breeds appear predisposed to demodicosis; the following appear to be overrepresented: Doberman Pinscher, Shar Pei, Boxer, Great Dane, German Shepherd, Collie, Bull Terrier, English Bulldog, Boston Terrier, Dalmatian, Old English Sheepdog, Afghan, Dachshund, Beagle and Staffordshire Terrier.

If *Demodex* mites are present on all normal animals, why do some animals develop mange and most do not? Animals with demodectic mange may have an inherited or acquired immune defect that fails to keep the mite numbers in check. The result is a demodectic mite population explosion. Though stress may be a triggering mechanism for clinical episodes, in large numbers the mites produce substances that further suppress the immune system. This secondary immunosuppression can be reversed once the mite population is eliminated, but any underlying primary immune defect cannot be corrected.

The degree of immunologic impairment determines the extent of skin disease, be it localized or generalized. The skin disease itself is caused by the mites crowding out the hairs within the hair follicles, eventually destroying the hair follicle. Release of the contents of the follicle (hair, debris, bacteria, mites) into the dermis causes infection, and the redness, hair loss and infection are what we refer to as demodectic mange (Fig 2). In fact, the old name for demodicosis was "red mange."

About 90% of cases of demodicosis are localized and resolve without treatment in a few months. The remaining 10% of localized cases fail to resolve and develop into the generalized form, characterized by large areas of hair loss, redness, scaling and infection. The areas affected most often are the legs and face. Clinically, the disorder makes the transition from a maculopapular eruption to a papulonodular dermatosis with increased follicular involvement.

Diagnosis: Diagnosis of demodicosis is not difficult. A scalpel blade or similar instrument is used to remove the top layers of epidermis and dermis by scraping, and the characteristic mites, larvae and eggs are viewed under the microscope. This can be facilitated by squeezing the skin before scraping to express the mites from the hair follicles. If scrapings are not done, the mites are easily seen on biopsy specimens within the hair follicles. Biopsy is occasionally necessary to reveal the mites in some breeds, especially the Shar Pei.

Since 90% of localized demodicosis cases resolve without treatment, it is often advisable to take a wait-and-see attitude and treat conservatively with antiseborrheic shampoos, which remove the scale that forms on the skin surface. Animals in which mange does not resolve by 18 months of age (perhaps 3 years in the larger breeds) with conservative therapy should be considered to have major immunologic defects that will likely be passed on to future generations.

These animals may be effectively treated in many instances, but under no conditions should these animals be used for breeding. As veterinarians we are faced with an ethical dilemma in this regard. If we successfully treat an animal, it looks entirely normal but still has a defective immune system. If the owner then breeds the now normal-looking dog, the hereditary immune defect is propagated. It is therefore recommended that owners agree to have their pet neutered once it is safe to do so. This should help eliminate the inherited immunoincompetence that allows generalized demodicosis to occur.

Management: Specific treatment for generalized demodicosis is usually accomplished with amitraz (Mitaban: Upjohn), the only product currently licensed specifically for this use. Treatment is successful in 60-80% of cases. It is a fairly safe compound but must be applied exactly as recommended by the manufacturer. Many veterinary dermatologists have found that frequently the dosage must be doubled or the treatment interval halved to eradicate the mites in problem cases; this is considered extra-label drug use and must be done at the practitioner's risk, since it is not the manufacturer's recommended use.

A protocol for use of amitraz follows:

Parasitic Skin Disorders

1. Clip the hair to facilitate penetration of the drug.

2. Use an antiseborrheic shampoo to remove crust and scales. Ideally, this should be done the night before the amitraz dip.

3. Empty the contents of the Mitaban vial into 7.5 L (2 gal) of water. This amount may need to be doubled for very large dogs or in chronic cases.

4. Slowly sponge on the entire amount of solution prepared, concentrating on problem areas.

5. Allow the animal to air dry; do not rinse or blow dry.

6. Do not allow the animal to get wet between treatments or the dip must be repeated.

7. Repeat the dips every 2 weeks (perhaps weekly) until the condition has been adequately controlled. The dog should not be stressed after dipping.

8. Do skin scrapings before each dip. When scrapings are negative on 2 successive occasions, no further treatment is indicated.

9. For demodectic pododermatitis, apply a mixture of 0.5 ml of Mitaban in 30 ml of propylene glycol or mineral oil every 3-4 days.

10. Outdated or opened bottles of Mitaban should not be used in treatment, since the breakdown products are more toxic than the Mitaban itself.

Unresponsive cases may be treated with the old standard of ronnel (Ectoral) as a 4% solution with propylene glycol (60 ml of Ectoral in 330 ml propylene glycol) or alternatively with trichlorfon (Neguvon) diluted to a 3% solution with water. The mix is applied to a third of the body daily and not rinsed off. Solutions must be made up fresh each time. Once again, be aware that neither trichlorfon nor ronnel has been approved for use in dogs.

Some safer alternatives include 1% rotenone in alcohol, vitamin E therapy (200 IU 4-5 times daily) and ivermectin (0.2 mg/kg every 2 weeks). Insufficient documentation has been presented to comment on the efficacy of these alternatives.

Additional Reading

1. Folz, SD: Demodicosis (*Demodex canis*). *Comp Cont Ed Pract Vet* 5:116-121, 1983.

2. Folz, SD *et al*: Long-term use of amitraz in treating chronic generalized demodicosis. *MVP* 66:241-243, 1985.

3. Kwochka, KW et al: The efficacy of amitraz for generalized demodicosis in dogs: A study of two concentrations and frequencies of application. *Comp Cont Ed Pract Vet* 7:8-17, 1985.

4. Scott, DW and Walton, DK: Experiences with the use of amitraz and ivermectin for the treatment of generalized demodicosis in dogs. *JAAHA* 21:535-541, 1985.

5. Bussieras, J and Chermette, R: Amitraz and canine demodicosis. *JAAHA* 22:779-782, 1986.

Sarcoptic Mange

Sarcoptic mange is caused by the scabies mite, *Sarcoptes scabiei* var *canis*, a burrowing mite that causes intense pruritus. These mites cause a maculopapular eruption and prefer lightly haired areas of the body. They are most commonly recovered from the ear margins, elbows, hocks, sternum and abdomen (Fig 3). The condition is quite contagious and about one-third of people in contact with infested dogs acquire the mites, though the mites have difficulty reproducing on people.

Diagnosis is based on the history, intense pruritus, multiple skin scrapings and possibly biopsy. The mites are exceedingly difficult to recover, and it is not unusual for multiple skin scrapings to be negative. Similarly, biopsies are only informative if a section of mite actually appears on the microscope slide. Therefore, the credo of many veterinary dermatologists has become, "If you suspect scabies, treat for it!"

Treatment can be safely accomplished with 2.5% lime sulfur, phosmet or amitraz (Mitaban) dips. Such products as ivermectin have been used to treat scabies (at 0.2-0.4 mg/kg SC or PO) but ivermectin is not licensed for this use; therefore, the risk must be borne by practitioners using the product. The product in general is quite safe, except with the Collie, in which many side effects, including death, have been reported. Licensure will probably eventually be granted for treatment of a number of parasitic conditions with this agent, but until then it should be used with caution.

Additional Reading

1. Folz, SD: Canine scabies (*Sarcoptes scabiei* infestation). *Comp Cont Ed Pract Vet* 6:176-180, 1984.

2. Arlian, LG et al: Survival and infestivity of *Sarcoptes scabiei* var *canis* and var *hominis*. *J Am Acad Dermatol* 11:210-215, 1984.

3. Folz, SD et al: Clinical evaluation of amitraz for treatment of canine scabies. *MVP* 65:597-600, 1984.

Cheyletiellosis

Cheyletiella mites (*Cheyletiella yasguri, C blakei, C parasitivorax*) are nonburrowing surface-dwelling parasites. They are highly contagious and infest people, though they cannot reproduce on people. Pets acquired from kennels, pet stores or any other place where large numbers of dogs are housed in close proximity to one another are most likely to acquire this important parasite. The clinical presentation is quite variable. Some dogs may just have a dry, dandruffy, flaky coat, while other dogs scratch themselves almost incessantly.

Diagnosis is not difficult if the mites and their eggs can be demonstrated on skin scrapings, but this is not always an easy task (Fig 4). The mites are white and barely visible to the naked eye, and have been given the nickname, "walking dandruff." Still, they are not always easy to recover. A variety of techniques, from dragging combs and toothbrushes through the coat to applying adhesive tape to multiple sites, have been employed to reveal the parasites.

Once acquired, *Cheyletiella* mites are sometimes quite difficult to eliminate. After removing the scales with an antiseborrheic shampoo, all animals in the household must be treated. Dipping once weekly for about 6 treatments with either lime sulfur or phoxim, as well as treating the environment (occasionally exterminators must be called in), usually solves the problem. Though they are not licensed for this use, amitraz and ivermectin effectively kill *Cheyletiella* mites when used 2 weeks apart. The products are currently not licensed for this purpose and should be used with appropriate caution.

Additional Reading

1. Carroll, HF and Theis, JH: *Cheyletiella* mite dermatitis: A review. *JAAHA* 9:573-576, 1973.

2. Rivers, JK *et al*: Walking dandruff and *Cheyletiella* dermatitis. *J Am Acad Dermatol* 15:1130-1133, 1986.

3. Paradis, M and Villeneuve, A: Efficacy of ivermectin against *Cheyletiella yasguri* infestation in dogs. *Can Vet J* 29:633-635, 1988.

Otodectic Mange (Ear Mite Infestation)

Otodectes cynotis, the common ear mite, is a major cause of otitis externa. These mites are highly contagious and feed on superficial epidermal debris and waxes in the ear canal. There is a great deal of variability in clinical signs, since some animals have intensely itchy ears and others remain almost asymptomatic. In most cases, there is a dark black waxy accumulation (like coffee grounds) in the ear canal and considerable flapping of the ears. Possible consequences include extension of the infection through the ear drum, and aural hematoma from head shaking.

Diagnosis is on the basis of clinical signs and examination of the ear canal with an otoscope. Treatment includes flushing the ear canal to remove accumulated debris and then instilling antiparasitic medications designed specifically for ear mites. Since these mites can survive on the skin surface outside of the ear canal, it is also important to treat the entire body of all animals in the household with an appropriate flea powder or spray to contain the infestation.

Trombiculiasis (Chigger Infestation)

The larvae of chiggers (*eg, Eutrombicula alfreddugesi, Trombicula batatas,* and perhaps *Walchia americana*) usually parasitize rodents, birds, snakes and lizards in well-wooded areas. The adults are free living and do not feed on animals. Dogs and cats roaming through infested environments may acquire the parasitic larval forms. This problem is more prevalent in the late summer and fall. The bites of chigger mites are quite irritating and pruritic; most bites occur on the head and feet.

Diagnosis is by the history (exposure to forests in late summer or fall), clinical examination (larvae may occasionally be seen as orange dots) and skin scrapings (to reveal larvae). The larvae are susceptible to most common insecticides and eradication is usually not difficult, though irritation from the bites may persist for several days.

Fly-Related Dermatoses

Flies undergo a complete metamorphosis in their life cycles, from egg to larva, to pupa to adult. Some flies may cause dermatologic conditions from their irritating bites, some from laying eggs within wounds (myiasis) and others by completing their life cycles under the skin.

Fly bites, especially those of stable flies (*Stomoxys calcitrans*) or black flies (*Simulium* spp), can be very irritating. Dogs may be bitten anywhere, but the flies prefer the head, ears and lightly haired skin. The lesions appear as little red bumps, with or without associated bleeding.

Treatment involves cleansing the affected area and, if necessary, applying some topical preparation (*eg*, corticosteroid creams, baking soda and water, cooling lotions). If the bites are very bothersome, oral antihistamines or corticosteroids can be given. Applying insect repellents or a thin layer of petroleum jelly to susceptible areas should lessen the problem.

Some flies lay eggs in organic matter, and any skin wound may provide access so flies can deposit their eggs. The eggs hatch in a day or so and the larvae (maggots) then begin to feed on the damaged tissue. Most larvae only feed on dead tissue and do not invade living skin. Toxins released from the larvae, however, may further damage surrounding tissue to the extent that it is then suitable for continued feeding. Treatment involves extensive clipping of the affected area and flushing with an appropriate antiseptic. All larvae must be removed, the damaged skin debrided and the area treated as an open wound. A broad-spectrum antibiotic is indicated, as well as continued fly control.

The botfly, *Cuterebra*, lays its eggs in soil. The larvae then penetrate the skin of passing rabbits and rodents, where they mature to the pupa stage beneath the skin. The larvae create a breathing pore and eventually enlarge the hole, emerge and pupate on the ground. Dogs may be affected accidentally if exposed to the larvae. Treatment involves surgically removing the subcutaneous larva and treating the remaining pocket as an open wound. Larvae must not be crushed during extraction, since the material can be extremely irritating.

Helminth-Related Dermatoses

Nematodes, such as *Pelodera (Rhabditis) strongyloides*, the hookworm (*Ancylostoma caninum*), the heartworm (*Dirofilaria immitis*) and *Dracunculus insignis*, may cause skin disorders. Ascarids, coccidia, tapeworms and whipworms also reportedly cause pruritus in dogs.

Pelodera Dermatitis

Pelodera (Rhabditis) strongyloides is a free-living nematode often found in organic matter, such as damp hay or straw. The larvae may actively penetrate a dog's skin during direct contact, such as when these materials are used as bedding (Fig 5). Diagnosis is based on the history and clinical signs, and is confirmed by finding the characteristic larvae on skin scrapings. Therapy includes removing the infested bedding and treating affected animals with parasiticidal dips, such as lime sulfur, phoxim or amitraz. Amitraz (Mitaban) is not licensed for this purpose and therefore should only be used with this explicit understanding.

Hookworm Dermatitis

The hookworm (*Ancylostoma caninum, Uncinaria* spp) may penetrate the dog's skin as part of its normal migration, especially between the toes. Diagnosis is based on the history and clinical signs, and is supported by finding hookworm larvae on skin scrapings or hookworm eggs on fecal examination. Therapy involves use of anthelmintics effective against hookworms, such as pyrantel pamoate (5 mg/kg) or fenbendazole (55 mg/kg for 3 days). Environmental control may also be warranted.

Heartworm Dermatitis

The heartworm (*Dirofilaria immitis*) only occasionally causes skin disorders. The exact mechanism by which this occurs has not been elucidated. Most affected dogs show pruritic, erythematosus nonfollicular papules and nodules on the face, neck and trunk. Diagnosis is based on the history and clinical signs, and is supported by finding heartworm microfilariae on skin scrapings or biopsy, by blood tests and by response to therapy. Treatment with caparsolate, levamisole or ivermectin should result in remission of the skin disorder.

Dracunculiasis

Infection with *Dracunculus insignis* is uncommon in dogs, but these slender nematodes may be mistaken for adult heartworms on microscopy. The parasite typically causes a large fluid-filled subcutaneous swelling. Surgical removal is the treatment of choice.

Additional Reading

1. Horton, ML: Rhabditic dermatitis in dogs. *MVP* 61:158-159, 1980.

2. Scott, DW and Vaughn, TC: Papulonodular dermatitis in a dog with occult filariasis. *Compan Anim Pract* 1(1):31-35, 1987.

3. Panciera, DL and Stockham, SL: *Dracunculus insignis* infection in a dog. *JAVMA* 192:76-78, 1988.

4. Moriello, KA: Dermatologic manifestations of internal and external parasitism. *Compan Anim Pract* 2(3):12-17, 1988.

Protozoan-Related Dermatoses

Leishmaniasis

Leishmaniasis is a rare protozoal disease but will be covered here in some length because information is scant in most other sources. Leishmaniasis is caused by 5 species of nonmotile flagellated protozoa, *Leishmania canis* (*L donovani, L infantum*), *L chagasi, L tropica, L braziliensis* and *L mexicana* found most commonly in animals imported from enzootic areas exotic to North America (most commonly around the Mediterranean). Recently however, it has also become evident that there may exist a reservoir of infection in the southwestern United States (Oklahoma, Texas).

Sandflies (*Phlebotomus, Lutzomyia, Sergentomyia, Psychodopygus*) are the insect vectors most responsible for the spread of these organisms. Transmission can also occur through blood transfusions, and transmission via direct contact from infected skin lesions on a dog to a person was recently described. Rats, mice, gerbils, dogs and cats are the most common reservoirs. Two rodents found in Texas, the hispid cotton rat (*Sigmodon hispidus*) and the house mouse (*Mus musculus*), serve as reservoirs of *Leishmania* organisms in enzootic areas.

Clinically, leishmaniasis can occur as a strictly cutaneous, mucocutaneous or visceral form, or all of the above. In people, it is considered that *Leishmania donovani* (*L canis, L infantum*) causes visceral (systemic) leishmaniasis, *L braziliensis* causes mucocutaneous leishmaniasis and *L tropica* or *L mexicana* cause cutaneous leishmaniasis. Currently it is being debated whether different organisms or rather variations in host immune competence are actually responsible for the clinical variations evident.

The clinical presentation is highly variable and ranges from a systemic infection of reticuloendothelial cells to localized cutaneous lesions without systemic involvement. The organism parasitizes and multiplies within macrophages. Host immunity plays an important role in clinical expression, and resolution of cutaneous leishmaniasis usually results in permanent immunity.

The cutaneous form includes a papulonodular to erosive-ulcerative presentation with variable pruritus and induration. These lesions occur about the head and ventrum, the most common sites for insect bites. Generalized lymphadenomegaly may also be apparent.

Systemic (visceral) leishmaniasis spreads from cutaneous reticuloendothelial cells to systemic reticuloendothelial cells, and eventually all organs may be involved. Common clinical findings include weight loss, fever, lameness, hepatosplenomegaly, lymphadenomegaly, anemia, thrombocytopenia and ocular manifestations. Corticosteroid administration may greatly exacerbate clinical signs.

Diagnosis of leishmaniasis is made on the basis of clinical findings, cytologic examination, serologic examination, culture and biopsies for histopathologic examination. Cytologic preparations from cutaneous nodules, lymph nodes, splenic aspirates or bone marrow often reveal the *Leishmania* organisms with their rod-like kinetoplast, within macrophages. The organisms are best highlighted by Giemsa stain.

Biopsies should be taken from the edge of the active lesion, as far away from crusting, ulceration and secondary infection as possible. Biopsies should then be bisected, and half used for culture and the other for touch impressions and histopathologic examination. The portion for culture is wrapped in sterile gauze moistened with sterile saline and transferred to appropriate media. Touch impressions of tissue on microscope slides are placed in methyl alcohol for 3 minutes for fixation and then into Wright's-Giemsa stain for 45 minutes. Biopsies for histopathologic examination often reveal nodular to diffuse dermatitis, with organisms present within macrophages. An indirect fluorescent antibody test using *L donovani* promastigotes and rabbit anticanine IgG conjugates has been described but is not commonly available to practitioners. Cultures can be grown on NNN medium to which has been added antibiotics, but this is also not commonly available to practitioners.

Treatment of leishmaniasis should be considered once the owners understand the potential public health risks of having an infected pet in their household. Therapy with pentavalent antimony compounds and ketoconazole are most commonly employed. The antimony compound (Pentostam) may be given IV at 10-50 mg/kg daily for 10 days, then again in 10 days. A liposome-encapsulated meglumine antimonate (Glucantime: Rhodia) has also successfully been evaluated experimentally in the dog. Ketoconazole may be administered at 5-20 mg/kg daily. In people, intralesional injections of emetine hydrochloride, at 0.4 ml/cm diameter of lesion, have also been successfully used. Dapsone and rifampin have also successfully been used.

Additional Reading

1. Swenson, CL *et al*: Visceral leishmaniasis in an English Foxhound from an Ohio research colony. *JAVMA* 193:1089-1092, 1988.

2. Nelson, DA *et al*: Clinical aspects of cutaneous leishmaniasis acquired in Texas. *J Am Acad Dermatol* 12:985-992, 1985.

3. Mancianti, F and Meciani, N: Specific serodiagnosis of canine leishmaniasis by indirect immunofluorescence, indirect hemagglutination, and counterimmunoelectropheresis. *Am J Vet Res* 49:1409-1411, 1988.

4. Ferrer, L *et al*: Skin lesions in canine leishmaniasis. *J Small Anim Pract* 29:381-388, 1988.

Chapter 2
Bacterial Skin Disorders

The skin is not like the sterile surface of the moon, but rather is an ideal culture medium that plays host to a number of normal resident bacteria (*eg, Staphylococcus epidermidis, Corynebacterium* spp, *Clostridium* spp, *Micrococcus* spp), fungi (*eg, Malassezia,* formerly *Pityrosporum* spp) and parasites (*eg, Demodex*). On normal skin, the bacterial count is usually less than 1000 aerobic bacteria per cm^2 of skin surface. These bacteria are normally confined to the skin surface and the immediate openings of the hair follicles, and the hair roots and glandular structures are considered almost sterile.

Bacterial skin diseases are commonly encountered in veterinary practice and are most frequently referred to as "pyodermas," implying pus (pyo-) production. *Staphylococcus intermedius* is involved in over 95% of canine pyodermas from which only 1 organism is isolated. Secondary invaders, such as *Proteus, Pseudomonas* and coliforms, occasionally may be recovered but do not pose a primary concern to treatment.

Most pyodermas have an underlying cause that must be diagnosed before animals can be successfully treated. These include allergies, hormonal imbalances, parasitic infestations and immune defects. Since *Staphylococcus intermedius* is not contagious, a critical question is whether the pyoderma is due to the potency of the bacteria or due to reduced host defenses. Usually some inciting factor allows the bacteria to colonize the skin and keeps the skin overly habitable despite chronic antibiotic administration. Staphylococci are complex organisms that may elaborate a number of important enzymes (*eg,* coagulase, fibrinolysins, hyaluronidase, phosphatase, protease, lipase) and toxins (*eg,* dermonecrotoxin, enterotoxin, hemolysins, leukocidin, lethal toxin), which serve to complicate the situation.

An additional feature of bacterial skin disease, often treated as a separate entity, is that some of the conditions can cause considerable pruritus. This is often referred to as "bacterial" or "staphylococcal hypersensitivity" though this is obviously not hypersensitivity in the traditional use of the word. These conditions are probably best referred to as "pruritic pyodermas" or "pruritic staphylococcal disease," since therapy with antibiotics removes not only the infection but the pruritus as well. However, when practitioners hear the term "hypersensitivity," they often reach for the corticosteroids.

Pyodermas may be arbitrarily subclassified as superficial, intermediate or deep, according to the depth of penetration of bacteria.

Superficial Pyodermas

Superficial or surface pyodermas include skin-fold pyodermas, juvenile pustular dermatitis (impetigo) and pyotraumatic dermatitis (hot spots).

Skin-fold pyodermas involve folds of skin that are continually traumatized by friction and that do not have adequate ventilation. Many different varieties exist, including whole body folds (*eg*, Shar Pei), facial folds (*eg*, Pugs), lip folds (*eg*, Spaniels), vulvar folds (*eg*, older bitches) and tail folds (*eg*, Boston Terriers).

Juvenile pustular dermatitis (impetigo) is commonly referred to as puppy pyoderma and is a relatively benign process. It is most commonly found on the ventrum of young dogs as crops of pustules. The condition in no way adversely affects the health status of affected individuals. Cytologic examination reveals neutrophils and occasionally evidence of phagocytosed cocci. Staphylococci are commonly cultured from intact pustules. Biopsies demonstrate a subcorneal pustular disorder limited to the very superficial levels of the epidermis. Treatment includes therapy with antibacterial products (*eg*, benzoyl peroxide, chlorhexidine, etc) and, rarely, a 7- to 10-day course of antibiotics. Impetigo is a poor name for this disorder because that condition in people is very contagious; this is not at all the case in dogs. There is no problem of contagion or zoonotic potential for juvenile pustular dermatitis in the dog.

Pyotraumatic dermatitis ("hot spot") is an acute superficial infection that evolves over a period of hours due to self-inflicted trauma. The underlying causes include allergies, ear infections, irritated anal sacs, the buildup of humidity within a dense haircoat, borreliosis, or any of a multitude of reasons. Despite their extremely superficial location, they can look terribly inflamed with redness, exudation and associated pain (Fig 6). It is often surprising to owners how quickly the process can evolve, when earlier that day the dog had been apparently normal.

Therapy: Superficial pyodermas can be cured if the underlying problem is corrected. For skin-fold pyodermas, this means resection of the folds so that involved skin is exposed to the air and adequately ventilated. Hot spots can be prevented if the ear problems, allergies, anal sac disorders, etc, have been corrected. For the most part, however, superficial pyodermas are treated symptomatically and controlled rather than cured. Most people select a breed for its appearance, including the skin folds, and are reluctant to surgically alter the animal's appearance to correct a superficial skin disease.

Antibiotics are usually not necessary. Most superficial pyodermas respond adequately to gentle clipping, cleansing and appropriate topical products. Ointments and other occlusive products are poor choices for these conditions, since they tend to seal in the infection. Mild astringents, such as aluminum acetate (Buro Sol: Trans Canada Dermapeutics, Domeboro's: Miles), propylene glycol, chlorhexidine (Hibitane, Savlon) and povidone-iodine (Betadine, Bridine) all have antibacterial as well as drying properties and are much better suited for treating superficial pyodermas. It may be advisable to also treat animals with pyotraumatic dermatitis with a short course (*eg*, 5 days) of corticosteroids to relieve inflammation and minimize self-trauma while the skin is healing.

Intermediate Pyodermas

Intermediate pyodermas consist of infections within the hair follicles (folliculitis) or surrounding the hair follicles (perifolliculitis). These are also common forms of pyoderma and are most easily observed on the sparsely haired skin surfaces, especially on the abdomen. The lesions first appear as small red spots (macules) that progress to little bumps (papules) and then pimples (pustules), then terminate as a circular rim of peeling scale (epidermal collarettes) with a red border surrounding an area of increased pigmentation (Figs 7, 8). To the inexperienced, this circular lesion may be confused with ringworm, but bacteria are usually implicated.

Diagnosis: Diagnosis can normally be made on the basis of clinical signs, cytology, biopsies for histopathologic examination and bacterial culture. The clinical presentation normally involves pustules, epidermal collarettes, erythema and hyperpigmentation. Biopsies of pustules usually demonstrate perifolliculitis and folliculitis. Cytologic examination is also useful. A pustule can be pricked with a needle, and the pus expressed onto a microscope slide and highlighted by a variety of stains. Usually there are abundant neutrophils (pus cells), many of which contain engulfed microorganisms. In many uncomplicated cases this is sufficient, and empiric therapy can be instituted while evaluating for underlying causes.

Alternatively, material can be aseptically collected from an intact pustule and submitted for culture to determine the susceptibility of that organism to a variety of antibacterials. Since there are normally bacteria on the surface of the skin, it does little good to simply swab the skin surface and hope to recover significant microorganisms. Similarly, even if multiple organisms are isolated, it is most suitable to pay particular heed to the information concerning *Staphylococcus intermedius*, since treatment should be based on the sensitivities of this organism preferentially over others. If an intact pustule is not available for sampling, alternatives include culture of a macerated skin biopsy sample, or swabbing affected sites with polysorbate 80 (Tween 80: Becton Dickinson) and hoping that a representative sample has been harvested.

Therapy: Intermediate pyodermas usually require antibiotics for at least 10 days and often 3-4 weeks. Bathing with an antiseptic wash, such as benzoyl peroxide, chlorhexidine or cetrimide, also helps decreases bacterial population on the skin surface, though the skin can never be considered sterile. Once again, if the underlying cause is identified and addressed, the folliculitis should respond entirely to systemic and topical therapy. Such bacteriostatic antibiotics as lincomycin, chloramphenicol and erythromycin are frequently prescribed for treatment of bacterial folliculitis.

Deep Pyodermas

Deep pyodermas most commonly result from extension of an intermediate pyoderma but may also be introduced by skin trauma.

Furunculosis results when infected hair follicles rupture and release their contents into the surrounding dermis. Fistulous tracts may appear at the skin surface and exude trapped pus and serum (Fig 9).

Cellulitis refers to a deep bacterial infection that spreads between tissue planes and fails to "head up" into an abscess.

Abscesses are deep pyodermas that do "head up" and normally result from the traumatic inoculation of microorganisms into the dermis or panniculus. They may appear as firm to fluctuant subcutaneous nodules that may exude pus and may be painful to the touch.

German Shepherds appear to be particularly susceptible to furunculosis and cellulitis. Further effort is necessary to determine if an inherited problem of immunoincompetence is involved.

Deep pyodermas are serious conditions that may require many weeks or months of antibacterial therapy. More potent antibacterials, such as oxacillin, trimethoprim-sulfa, amoxicillin-clavulanate and the cephalosporins, are often employed to penetrate into the deeper tissues involved. Antibacterial resistance is common. In the case of abscesses, surgical drainage and judicious use of hot compresses should precede antibacterial therapy.

Culture and sensitivity tests should always be performed with chronic or deep bacterial infections. Ampicillin, amoxicillin and tetracycline make poor choices for all pyodermas in dogs, regardless of the results of sensitivity testing. Successful treatment depends on identifying and eliminating the underlying cause. If this cannot be accomplished, long-term antibacterial therapy is unavoidable. This is not only expensive but may also lead to resistance to multiple antibacterials and the increased possibility of drug reactions.

Many chronic, recurring pyodermas for which another cause (*eg,* hypothyroidism, allergies, parasites) cannot be determined are associated with impaired immune function. Affected dogs cannot keep their surface bacterial population under control. This once again represents a condition not due to the potency of the organism but rather to reduced host defenses. If this is the case, there may be a history of immunoincompetence-related disease, such as demodicosis as a pup, recurrent ear infections or bladder infections. These animals are immunologic cripples and unlikely to regain their resistance without treatment, which may or may not be effective.

In the section on the immune system, we discussed B- and T-cell function. These animals are often lacking normal T-cell function. A number of products have been used to augment T-cell function, but unfortunately none has been consistently successful (Appendix 1). Most are derivatives of the cell wall of staphylococci (*eg,* Staphoid A-B, Staphage lysate, Lysigen), *Propionibacterium* (*eg,* ImmunoRegulin: Immunovet) or mycobacteria (*eg,* Regressin or Stimune: Vetrepharm), or offer immunostimulation in addition to their primary purpose (*eg,* levamisole is an anthelmintic that augments immune function).

The field of immunology is ever expanding, and no doubt one day there will be products on the market specially formulated to bolster a faltering T-cell system. The products currently available appear to be successful in about 65-70% of cases. Since they all work by different mechanisms, if an animal does not respond to one product, it may respond to another. At present, the only other alternative is long-term antibacterial use, which carries its own disappointments.

Atypical Pyodermas

Acne

Acne is an intermediate to deep bacterial invasion of the hair follicles in certain anatomic distributions. The condition is not wholly the result of bacteria, since even chronic antibiotic therapy fails to resolve the situation. Certain breeds, such as the Great Dane, Doberman Pinscher, Bulldog and Bull Terrier, are particularly at risk, but any animal may be affected.

Acne in dogs is not analogous to the condition in people, but there are certain similarities. Frequently cleansing the areas with such antiseptics as alcohol, benzoyl peroxide, chlorhexidine or povidone-iodine usually keeps the situation under control but is unlikely to effect a cure. Acne is more a cosmetic concern than a health issue. In particularly bad cases, I have had some success with a new vitamin A derivative (Accutane: Roche), but I caution that it is not licensed for this use, has side effects of its own, and is quite expensive.

Bacterial Hypersensitivity

Bacterial hypersensitivity, sometimes referred to as pruritic pyoderma, pruritic superficial folliculitis, or staphylococcal hypersensitivity, is bacterial folliculitis with a marked pruritic component. It is possible that Type-I and/or Type-III hypersensitivity is involved, though documentation has been incomplete.

Clinical signs include erythematous pustules, seborrheic plaques and hemorrhagic bullae, in addition to the lesions of folliculitis. About 50% of cases have some documentable concurrent disease (*eg,* hypothyroidism, allergy, immune dysfunction, keratinization defects, etc) that predisposes them to the pyoderma. Both the lesions and pruritus clear with antibiotics, and this is a most important diagnostic feature.

Biopsies show at least some degree of vasculitis in addition to the folliculitis/furunculosis. A staphylococcal cell wall extract (Staphoid A-B, Coopers, Agropharm) can be used to help substantiate a diagnosis. The suspension is diluted 50/50 with sterile saline and 0.1 ml injected intradermally. A positive reaction consists of erythema and swelling in 24-72 hours. All normal dogs should have at least some immediate reaction to the injected extract in 15-30 minutes. Reactions appearing in 24-72 hours should be considered significant. Animals that fail to react to the injection in 15-30 minutes may be immunologically compromised.

Treatment initially should be attempted with a long course of antibiotics, and any underlying problems eliminated. Long-term maintenance may require daily antibiotics or immune stimulants. For long-term antibacterial use, bactericidal drugs given once daily, such as oxacillin, cephalosporins, trimethoprim-sulfas and amoxicillin-clavulanate, are usually satisfactory, though the possibility of adverse reactions should be anticipated.

Callus Pyoderma

Callus pyoderma refers to bacterial invasion of traumatized calluses. Calluses are commonly found on the elbows and hocks of large breeds (*eg,* Great Dane, St. Bernard) and on the sternum of other breeds (*eg,* Dachshund, Doberman Pinscher). They result from repeated impact of a hard surface, especially in heavy dogs. The continual trauma drives dislodged hair and debris (including bacteria) into the callus, resulting in infection. Therapy is often only symptomatic and includes weight reduction, keeping the animal on a padded surface or having it fitted with protective pads (*eg,* hockey elbow pads or a padded vest for sternal calluses). Surgical alternatives may be considered but they are often more hazardous and less effective than they are worth.

Interdigital Pyoderma

Interdigital pyoderma, a form of pododermatitis, is a bacterial infection between the toes. The condition may begin in the front feet, then eventually involve all of them. The disorder is most common in Great Danes, Bulldogs, German Shepherds, Boxers and Dachshunds, but may occur in any breed.

Pododermatitis, like nasal dermatitis, can occur from a vast array of causes, and only those due to bacterial causes can be expected to respond to antibiotic therapy. A full diagnostic workup should be performed because so many different conditions involving the feet appear identical. Diagnostic testing might include cytologic examination of direct smears and skin scrapings, bacterial and fungal cultures, fecal evaluation for parasites, biopsies, immune panels, evaluation for thyroid function and allergy testing. Treatment often requires therapy for 6-8 weeks with an antibacterial selected on the basis of culture and sensitivity tests, and soaking the feet daily with an appropriate antiseptic. In advanced cases, surgical drainage may be required to expose sites of infection.

Nasal Pyoderma

Nasal pyoderma is a deep pyoderma involving the dorsal aspect of the nose. It is most common in long-nosed breeds (*eg,* Collie, German Shepherd) and may or may not be the result of "rooting" in the dirt. Since this is one of the causes of nasal dermatitis ("Collie nose"), a good workup must be done to arrive at a diagnosis. Therefore, such other tests as skin scrapings, cytologic examination, and bacterial and fungal cultures should be performed. Therapy includes antibiotic treatment, often for 3-8 weeks, gentle cleansing with an antiseptic wash (*eg,* chlorhexidine, benzoyl peroxide, povidone-iodine) and protection against further trauma. Recovery is often complete with appropriate therapy, but scarring may result if the area is not protected.

Perianal Pyoderma

Perianal pyoderma (perianal fistulae, anal furunculosis) is most common in the German Shepherd and Irish Setter breeds. It appears as draining tracts around the anus (Fig 10). Researchers for years have been trying to determine the cause of the condition and have proposed many possibilities, such as overproduction by local secretory glands, poor ventilation associated with low tail carriage, anal sac disease or hip dysplasia. Neither thyroid nor immunologic status appears to be severely compromised in affected dogs according to a recent study. However, nothing conclusive has been determined. A 2:1 male to female ratio has been observed.

Diagnosis is supported by clinical findings, biopsy, and perhaps culture and sensitivity tests. Biopsy findings include epithelium-lined tracts, perifolliculitis, diffuse to nodular dermatitis, and an inflammatory reaction in the perianal gland regions. The most common organisms recovered on culture include *E coli, Staphylococcus aureus,* beta-hemolytic streptococci and *Proteus mirabilis.*

Therapy has been disappointing but successes have been reported with surgical removal of the tracts. Unfortunately, complications are common. Cryosurgery with multiple freezes may be required, or removing part of the tail musculature and sometimes amputating the tail. Though studies have not confirmed it, neutering and extirpation of the anal sacs may also benefit the patient. Even long-term antibacterial therapy is seldom of any real benefit. I have recently had some success using isotretinoin, a vitamin A derivative (Accutane: Roche) at 1.0 mg/kg daily, which is marketed for treatment of chronic severe acne in people. However, treatment is expensive, can be toxic, and is required for many months, though some successes have been realized. No doubt once the condition is better understood, improved forms of therapy will become available.

Bacterial Granuloma

Bacterial granuloma (botryomycosis) is a bacterial infection in which the microorganisms have been effectively walled off but not eliminated (Fig 11). The bacteria, having been walled off, are protected from an immune response. Deprived of a blood supply, the granuloma cannot be readily penetrated by antibacterials. Diagnosis relies on biopsies for histopathologic examination and culture and sensitivity tests. Treatment can be curative if the granuloma can be entirely removed by surgery. Otherwise, the condition poses many therapeutic dilemmas.

I have recently had some success in treating these cases with rifampin, which is used in treatment of human tuberculosis. The drug cannot be used on its own because of rapid development of resistance and must be used in conjunction with another bactericidal such as potentiated penicillins or cephalosporins. The response is only complete in animals in which the underlying problem is identified (*eg*, allergy, hypothyroidism). Treatment is quite costly and some side effects (increased liver enzyme activity, bilirubinuria) occur.

These bacterial granulomas represent a state of impaired immune function in that although the bacteria can be confined by the body, they cannot be eliminated. *Staphylococcus intermedius* is the most common microbe isolated. Though on sensitivity testing many antibacterials may appear effective, they cannot reach the bacteria within the granuloma to exert their effect.

Actinomycotic Mycetoma

Actinomycotic mycetomas are bacterial granulomas caused by *Nocardia*, *Actinomyces* and *Streptomyces griseus* and are rare in dogs. Infections are most commonly caused by contamination of existing wounds. Lesions may include abscesses, cellulitis, ulcers, draining tracts, lumps and scarring. Diagnosis is confirmed by cytologic examination, aerobic and anaerobic bacterial culture, and biopsies for histopathologic examination employing special stains to highlight the organisms. Therapy is usually attempted with penicillins for *Actinomyces* and trimethoprim-sulfas (dosed by trimethoprim fraction at 2.2 mg/kg BID) for *Nocardia* and *Streptomyces*. These organisms are not considered contagious to people or other animals.

Atypical Mycobacterial Infections

Atypical mycobacterial infections are caused by species of mycobacteria (*eg, Mycobacterium fortuitum, M chelonei, M phlei, M xenopi, M smegmatis*) that are not causes of tuberculosis or leprosy. These mycobacteria, unlike their more sinister cousins, are mainly common soil and water inhabitants that may contaminate existing wounds.

In 1959, these atypical mycobacteria were classified by Runyon into 4 categories based on morphology, pigmentation and rate of growth in culture (Table 1).

The resulting granulomas appear as nodules that may ulcerate and cause fistulous tracts. There appears to be a site predilection for the ventral abdominal region and limbs.

Diagnosis requires cytologic examination, sending specimens to special facilities capable of culturing mycobacteria (on Lowenstein-Jensen agar), and obtaining biopsies for histopathologic examination employing special stains (*eg*, rapid Ziehl-Neelsen or Auramine-O fluorescent staining) to highlight the organisms.

Table 1. Mycobacterial groups, as classified by Runyon.

Group Growth	Features	Species
Slow growers	Produce pigment only after exposure to light (photochromogens)	*M marinum* *M kansasii* *M simiae*
Slow growers	Produce pigment only in the dark (scotochromogens)	*M scrofulaceum* *M szulgai*
Slow growers	Produce no pigment (nonchromogens)	*M avium-intracellulare* *M xenopi* *M ulcerans*
Rapid growers	Produce no pigment (nonchromogens)	*M fortuitum* *M chelonei* *M phlei* *M smegmatis* *M vaccae*

Only resection is predictably curative. Spontaneous remission is uncommon. Kanamycin, gentamicin, amikacin, doxycycline and the fluoroquinolones may also be helpful in a limited number of cases. I have also attempted therapy with dapsone and rifampin, antibacterials useful in treatment of human mycobacterial infections, with little success and many adverse side effects.

Cutaneous Tuberculosis

Cutaneous tuberculosis has been documented in dogs and is diagnosed in the same manner as are atypical mycobacterial infections. Most infections are due to *Mycobacterium bovis*, though *M avium* and *M tuberculosis* also have been implicated.

Diagnosis is based on histopathologic examination using special stains to highlight the organisms, submitting samples to special laboratories for culture of the organism, and biochemical tests of frozen tissues, done by special laboratories.

Treatment is not often attempted, however, because of the considerable public health risk.

Additional Reading

1. Kunkle, GA: Canine pyoderma. *Comp Cont Ed Pract Vet* 1:7-13, 1979.

2. Baker, BB: Bacterial dermatoses in dogs. *MVP* 68:472-476, 1986.

3. Berg, JN *et al*: Identification of the major coagulase-positive *Staphylococcus* sp. of dogs as *Staphylococcus intermedius*. *Am J Vet Res* 45:1307-1309, 1984.

4. Hoskins, JD *et al*: What's new in bacteriology? *Staphylococcus intermedius*. *Vet Med* 79:1261-1263, 1984.

5. Kunkle, GA *et al*: Rapidly growing mycobacteria as a cause of cutaneous granulomas: Report of five cases. *JAAHA* 19:513-521, 1983.

6. Ackerman, L: Cutaneous bacterial granuloma (botryomycosis) in 5 dogs: Treatment with rifampin. *MVP* 68:404-409, 1987.

7. Liu, Si-kwang *et al*: Canine tuberculosis. *JAVMA* 177:164-167, 1980.

8. Bloomberg, MS: The clinical management of perianal fistulas in the dog. *Comp Cont Ed Pract Vet* 2:615-623, 1980.

9. Killingsworth, CR *et al*: Bacterial population and histologic changes in dogs with perianal fistula. *Am J Vet Res* 49:1736-1741, 1988.

10. Killingsworth, CR *et al*: Thyroid and immunologic status with perianal fistula. *Am J Vet Res* 49:1742-1746, 1988.

How to Select an Antibacterial

Antibacterials exert a harmful effect on microorganisms (Appendix 1). They may be of natural, semisynthetic or synthetic origin. Antibacterials may be bactericidal (destroy bacteria), bacteriostatic (inhibit growth of bacteria) or either, depending upon their concentration. Some antibacterials, such as ampicillin, amoxicillin and tetracycline, have poor therapeutic value in treatment of skin infections, while others, such as gentamicin and kanamycin, are too toxic to be used for the long periods required for skin infections.

In uncomplicated bacterial infections, it can be assumed that the usual culprit is *Staphylococcus intermedius*, and such drugs as lincomycin or chloramphenicol are usually effective. This is known as an empiric choice of an antibacterial, since the drug was selected on the basis of clinical experience and not by laboratory confirmation. If these antibacterials are not effective initially, bacterial culture and sensitivity tests should be performed to determine the causative organism and the antibacterials likely to be effective in treatment (see also the section on Bacterial Culture and Sensitivity Testing in the Introduction). Samples for culture should not be obtained while animals are receiving antibacterials; a minimum withdrawal time of about 5

Table 2. Antibacterials used in skin infections.

Family	Generic Name	Examples
Cephalosporin	Cephadroxil	Cefa-Tabs
	Cephalexin	Keflex
	Cephalothin	Keflin
	Cephradine	Velosef
Chloramphenicol	Chloramphenicol	Rogar-Mycine
Fluoroquinolone	Ciprofloxacin	Cipro
	Enrofloxacin	Baytril
	Norfloxacin	Noroxin
Lincosamides	Clindamycin	Antirobe
	Lincomycin	Lincocin
Macrolides	Erythromycin	E-Mycin
Penicillin	Amoxicillin-clavulanate	Clavulin
		Clavamox
	Carbenicillin	Geopen
	Cloxacillin	Orbenin
		Tegopen
	Dicloxacillin	Dynapen
	Oxacillin	Prostaphlin
Trimethoprim-sulfa	Trimethoprim-sulfadiazine	Tribrissen
	Trimethoprim-sulfamethoxazole	Apo-Sulfatrim
		Septra

Table 3. Suggested antibacterial dosages.

Drug	Action	Dosage
Amoxicillin-clavulanate	Bactericidal	12-14 mg/kg BID
Cephadroxil	Bactericidal	22 mg/kg BID
Cephalexin	Bactericidal	30 mg/kg BID
Chloramphenicol	Bacteriostatic	50 mg/kg TID
Ciprofloxacin	Bactericidal	11-22 mg/kg BID
Clindamycin	Bacteriostatic	5.5 mg/kg BID
Cloxacillin	Bactericidal	15 mg/kg TID
Enrofloxacin	Bactericidal	2.5 mg/kg BID
Erythromycin	Bacteriostatic	15 mg/kg TID
Flucloxacillin	Bactericidal	15 mg/kg TID
Lincomycin	Bacteriostatic	20 mg/kg BID
Oxacillin	Bactericidal	15 mg/kg TID
Trimethoprim-sulfa	Bactericidal	30 mg/kg BID

days is necessary. In chronic cases, more potent antibacterials, such as trimethoprim-sulfa, beta-lactamase-resistant penicillins and cephalosporins, may be required.

Two very important points must be understood. First, it is very unusual for an animal to develop bacterial infections unless there is some underlying cause (*eg*, allergy, immunoincompetence, hypothyroidism). If this underlying problem is not addressed, it is unlikely that the secondary infection will be completely resolved.

Second, antibacterials often must be given for many weeks or months and at the proper dosage to clear the infection. Cutting corners to save money or time usually results in an incomplete response and development of antibacterial resistance. Considering these 2 points is of far greater importance than simply treating the condition on the basis of culture and sensitivity test results. Such drugs as tetracyclines, ampicillin and amoxicillin are not successful in enough cases to warrant their use in cutaneous infections in dogs. Tables 2 and 3 list some antibacterials used in skin infections. Antibacterials and immunostimulants are more completely covered in Appendix 1.

Additional Reading

1. Ihrke, PJ: Therapeutic strategies involving antimicrobial treatment of the skin in small animals. *JAVMA* 185:1165-1168, 1984.

2. Riviere, JE: Calculation of dosage regimens of antimicrobial drugs in animals with renal and hepatic dysfunction. *JAVMA* 185:1094-1097, 1984.

Chapter 3
Fungal Skin Disorders

Dermatophytosis
(Ringworm)

Ringworm, or more correctly, dermatophytosis, is not a worm, but rather a fungal skin disorder that may infect people as well as animals. The individual type of fungus is classified according to its preferred habitat: zoophilic fungi have animals as their natural host; anthropophilic fungi (*eg,* athlete's foot fungus) are normally adapted to people, and geophilic fungi have the soil as their natural habitat.

Three species of fungi (*Microsporum canis, Microsporum gypseum, Trichophyton mentagrophytes*) are responsible for over 95% of all ringworm cases in pets.

Microsporum canis is the most common cause of ringworm in pets, and cats are the natural reservoir. Cats may be carriers of infection without manifesting the disease and therefore may transmit it to other animals and people. The fungus may also be contracted from spores in the environment or on contaminated objects (*eg,* brushes, combs, toys, furniture, etc).

Microsporum gypseum is normally a soil inhabitant and may be found transiently on the hair and skin of outdoor animals. Infection is usually acquired from direct contact with contaminated soil. Once infected, an animal can transmit the fungus to other animals and people.

Trichophyton mentagrophytes uses rodents as the natural reservoir. Infections thus may occur from contact with infected rodents or exposure to contaminated areas.

Less common causes of dermatophytosis include *Microsporum persicolor, M nanum, Trichophyton verrucosum, T terrestre, T rubrum, T equinum, T schoenleinii* and *Epidermophyton floccosum*.

Dermatophytes can only live on the superficial dead layers of the skin and cannot penetrate living tissue or survive in areas of severe inflammation. In addition, the fungi only penetrate actively growing hairs; therefore, the infection spreads centrifugally as it progresses. Pruritus may or may not be a problem. Inflammatory reactions may result if hair follicle rupture releases hair and fungal elements into the underlying dermis.

Exposure to ringworm fungi is not rare but few animals ever develop dermatophytosis. The body's immune system is remarkably efficient at warding off infections, but a number of circumstances may encourage colonization by fungi, such as a young animal with a naive immune system, trauma, poor nutritional status, contaminated environmental conditions or a depressed immune system.

Dermatophytosis can mimic many other diseases, such as parasitism, bacterial infections, allergies, immunologic diseases, nutritional diseases, hormonal disorders, some skin cancers and disorders of keratinization (seborrhea). In fact, among veterinary dermatologists, disorders we think look most like ringworm usually are not. Thus, clinical presentation may vary from asymptomatic, to patchy hair loss, to a papulocrustous eruption, to an exfoliative dermatosis, to a suppurative nodular disorder (kerion reaction) (Fig 12).

Dermatophytosis may be diagnosed by Wood's lamp evaluation, microscopic examination of hairs, fungal culture or skin biopsy but cannot be confirmed by visual examination alone.

Wood's Lamp Evaluation

A Wood's lamp employs ultraviolet light filtered through nickel oxide to cause some fungi to glow green in a darkened room. Though the test is rapid, it is very unreliable in that, of the 3 common ringworm fungi of dogs and cats, only *Microsporum canis* fluoresces, and then only about 30-40% of the time.

Direct Microscopic Evaluation

The microscopic examination of hairs to identify characteristic spores and hyphae is a relatively specialized test in animals and not commonly performed in general veterinary practice. In people, dermatophytes parasitize the inside of the hair shaft, and potassium hydroxide (KOH) is used to first digest the hairs. In animals, the fungi are usually outside the hairshaft and thus KOH is usually not necessary, mineral oil alone being sufficient for preparation. Specimens may be sent to a laboratory. When viewed by an experienced technician, specimens are diagnostic about 60-70% of the time. The inexperienced may find it difficult to distinguish spores from pigment, and hyphae from keratin.

Use of a solution of KOH, DMSO and chlorazol fungal stain (Dermatologic Lab and Supply) is often helpful in practice, since hyphae stain green against a gray background. A recipe for this formulation is given in the Introduction (see Fungal Culture).

Fungal Culture

Fungal cultures on dermatophyte test medium (DTM) are relatively easy to use but the fungi occasionally take up to 2 weeks to grow. For some ringworm species contracted from farm animals, a source of B vitamins must be added to the medium to permit growth. Dermatophytes produce alkaline metabolites that react with the phenol red in the medium to change the color of the medium from yellow to red with the growth of ringworm fungi. When properly conducted, this test is over 90% reliable in providing definite proof of infection and identifying the species of fungus. It is important that hairs are carefully chosen, correctly applied to the medium and the cap not tightened, since dermatophytes are aerobic and need a supply of oxygen.

Broken or "sick-looking" hairs are the best choice and are frequently found around the periphery of lesions. If the dog is completely asymptomatic (more common in cats than in dogs), I have had some luck by dragging a clean toothbrush through the coat and then touching the bristles lightly to the surface of the medium. One must not put too much material on the medium or contaminants are likely to grow. Specimens should not be imbedded in the medium but gently placed on the surface. Whatever grows and regardless of whether the medium has changed color, any fungal growth should be examined microscopically and identified. This is easily done by taking transparent tape and touching it to some of the growth and then applying this to a clean microscope slide to which has been added either a drop of water or some lactophenol cotton blue. Most fungal culture kits provide a guide to microscopic identification of fungi.

Biopsy

Ringworm occasionally is diagnosed when a biopsy of the skin reveals fungal elements within the hair follicles. The typical histologic pattern is one of perifolliculitis, folliculitis and furunculosis, the fungal elements being present within hair follicles, around hairs and in the stratum corneum. In general, the number of fungal elements present is inversely proportional to the extent of inflammatory response. There is often associated focal parakeratotic hyperkeratosis, intercellular epidermal edema and nonspecific perivascular dermatitis. Visualization of organisms is facilitated with either PAS or acid orcein Giemsa (AOG) staining. A rare presentation is the Majochi's granuloma, in which there is a nodular to diffuse pyogranulomatous response in the deep dermis or panniculus. Mycetomas or pseudomycetomas may also result from dermatophyte infection.

Antifungal Therapy

The significance of dermatophytosis may vary from a mild inconvenience to a major skin disease. Treatment depends on a number of criteria and varies with the particular clinical evaluation of each individual animal. Whereas mild infections are self-limiting and may spontaneously regress, others are chronic, debilitating and poorly responsive to therapy. The aim of treatment is to clear the infection, prevent spread of infection to other animals and people and decontaminate the environment to prevent future infections.

For localized infections, treatment may only involve trimming the area and applying suitable antifungal creams or ointments. Good products for "spot" treatment include miconazole (Conofite) and clotrimazole (Canesten). Nystatin is not effective against ringworm fungi. Other products with at least some antifungal properties include chlorhexidine, povidone-iodine and thiabendazole (included in Tresaderm). Tolnaftate (*eg,* Tinavet) is ineffective on haired skin and is thus a poor choice for any topical antifungal therapy on animals.

For more generalized infections, considerable clipping of hair may be warranted. Some animals may require a total body clip, accompanied by weekly or biweekly dips with antifungal agents, such as lime sulfur, captan, thiabendazole or benzoyl peroxide. Treatment with oral antifungal medication also is often necessary for 6 weeks or longer (Appendix 1). Griseofulvin may be given as a microsize (50-150 mg/kg) or ultramicrosize (25-75 mg/kg) preparation once daily with a fat meal or some corn oil, usually for 6 weeks, but at least until 2 weeks beyond apparent clinical cure. The drug has an unpleasant taste and may cause vomiting in many animals. The product should never be given to pregnant animals, since it causes birth defects. More potent antifungals, such as ketoconazole, may be helpful in unresponsive patients.

Recently, hyperthermia using electrodes to generate a temperature of 50 C at the skin surface by means of radiofrequency current has also been successfully used to treat dermatophytosis. Immunotherapy for fungal infections (Mycotrin: Willamette) has recently also become available, but significant clinical trials have yet to be done.

Environmental decontamination is essential, since such fungi as *Microsporum canis* may persist in the environment for over a year. All grooming utensils should be disinfected with a dilute solution of household bleach or formaldehyde (*eg*, Formacide), all bedding laundered, and carpets and furniture thoroughly vacuumed. Disinfectants that contain chlorine, iodine or quaternary ammonium compounds are suitable for cleansing runs and cages. Environmental decontamination is the most difficult component of dermatophyte eradication.

Additional Reading

1. Chester, DK: Superficial fungal infection of the skin. *Comp Cont Ed Pract Vet* 1:910-916, 1979.

2. Carroll, HF: Evaluation of dermatophyte test medium for diagnosis of dermatophytosis. *JAVMA* 165:192-195, 1974.

3. Burke, WA and Hones, BE: A simple stain for rapid office diagnosis of fungous infection of the skin. *Arch Dermatol* 120:1519-1520, 1984.

4. Lueker, DC and Kainer, RA: Hyperthermia for the treatment of dermatomycosis in dogs and cats. *VM/SAC* 75:.658-659, 1981.

5. Angarano, DW and Scott, DW: Use of ketoconazole in treatment of dermatophytosis in a dog. *JAVMA* 190:1433-1434, 1987.

Intermediate Mycoses

These fungi, for the most part, are common soil-dwelling microbes usually contracted by penetration of the skin with foreign objects (*eg*, thorns, sticks, etc). They are usually harmless but may produce disease under certain circumstances, such as incompetence of the immune system due to deficiency, suppression, or debilitating diseases.

Chapter 3

There are no ways to easily categorize the intermediate mycoses, but Table 1 attempts to make generalizations where appropriate.

Eumycotic Mycetoma

Eumycotic mycetomas are caused by several different fungi (eg, *Curvularia geniculata*, *Pseudoallescheria boydii*, *Acremonium hyalinum* and *Madurella* spp) that gain entry to the body via injury to the skin. The classic triad of clinical signs includes formation of a lump (tumefaction), with draining tracts, in which are found "grains" of fungal mycelia. The condition may resemble a chronic abscess that does not respond to antibiotic therapy.

Diagnosis is by direct microscopic examination of pus, fungal culture and biopsy. Direct examination of pus occasionally reveals fungal hyphae and spores. Fungal culture produces colonies with single conidia borne at the tips and sides of simple conidiophores. Histologically, the lesions appear as purulent granulomas surrounding masses of hyphae and chlamydospores. The fungi are best demostrated with PAS, methenamine silver and Gridley's stains.

Table 1. Major intermediate mycoses and their causative agents.

Condition	Characteristics	Genus
Eumycotic mycetoma	Septate pigmented mycelia with "grains"	*Pseudoallescheria* *Acremonium* *Curvularia* *Madurella*
Hyalohyphomycosis	Septate nonpigmented mycelia	*Aspergillus* *Penicillium* *Paecilomyces* *Chrysosporium*
Phaeohyphomycosis	Septate pigmented mycelia	*Phialophora* *Drechslera* *Cladosporium*
Phycomycosis	Broad nonseptate hyphae	*Mucor* *Rhizopus* *Absidia*
Pythiosis	Broad nonseptate hyphae	*Pythium*
Rhinosporidiosis	Sporangia in tissue	*Rhinosporidium*

The treatment of choice for mycetoma is complete excision, since medical therapy is usually ineffective. Parenteral miconazole may offer benefit in some cases, but most are resistant to ketoconazole. If left without treatment, the infection usually becomes deeper and may involve muscle and bone.

Additional Reading

1. Coyle, V et al: Canine mycetoma: A case report and review of the literature. *J Small Anim Pract* 25:261-268, 1984.

2. Walker, RL et al: Eumycotic mycetoma caused by *Pseudoallescheria boydii* in the abdominal cavity of a dog. *JAVMA* 192:67-70, 1988.

3. Allison, N et al: Eumycotic mycetoma caused by *Pseudoallescheria boydii* in a dog. *JAVMA* 194:797-799, 1989.

Hyalohyphomycosis

Hyalohyphomycosis describes intermediate mycoses due to such organisms as *Aspergillus*, *Penicillium* and *Paecilomyces*.

Aspergillosis is a rare cause of fungal infection in the dog. Two species, *Aspergillus fumigatus* and *Aspergillus flavus*, are among the most common fungi found in the environment and are considered to be opportunistic invaders, only colonizing traumatized skin or patients with defective immune systems.

Aspergillus spores are common in dust and organic debris, and are not uncommon causes of rhinitis and inhalant allergy (see Chapter 4). The most common site at which the fungi invade the body is around the nose. Occasionally they cause digestive signs if the fungi invade the gastrointestinal tract. When *Aspergillus* organisms affect the skin or mucous membranes of the nose, they normally appear as nodules or ulcers. This usually represents a form of the disease where internal spread may have already occurred.

Penicillinosis is caused by the related organism, *Penicillium*. It has similar clinical manifestations, and is diagnosed and treated in a similar fashion.

Since *Aspergillus* organisms are so common in the environment, definitive diagnosis of aspergillosis requires not only a positive fungal culture but supportive histopathologic findings as well. Fungal cultures should normally be grown on Sabouraud's agar rather than dermatophyte test medium since *Aspergillus* is sensitive to cycloheximide. Biopsies normally show tissue invasion by *Aspergillus*, usually apparent with hematoxylin-eosin but best visualized with Gridley's stain or Gomori's methenamine silver. Cytologic evaluation of purulohemorrhagic exudate with or without new methylene blue may reveal the thick (4-6 μ) septate hyphae. Skull radiographs may show decreased turbinate density and increased soft tissue density in affected nasal cavities and maxillary or frontal sinuses. Serologic examination may have some use with nasal aspergillosis but has not been well documented.

Treatment should be aimed at eliminating fungi and correcting any underlying defects. If the underlying problems can be corrected, prognosis is good. If the inciting cause cannot be identified or treated, prognosis is poor. Treatment is often attempted with a number of antifungal agents, such as ketoconazole (20 mg/kg daily for 6 weeks), nystatin, flucytosine (60 mg/kg TID for 6-8 weeks), or thiabendazole (10 mg/kg BID for 6 weeks). Surgical therapy includes trephination of affected sinuses, rhinotomy, drain placement and flushing with antiseptics.

Additional Reading

1. Sharp, N et al: Canine nasal aspergillosis: Serology and treatment with ketoconazole. *J Small Anim Pract* 25:149-158, 1984.

2. Weitkamp, RA: Aspergilloma in two dogs. *JAAHA* 18:503-506, 1982.

3. Sharp, NJH and Sullivan, M: Use of ketoconazole in the treatment of canine nasal aspergillosis. *JAVMA* 194:782-786, 1989.

Phaeohyphomycosis

Phaeohyphomycosis is caused by several different fungi (*eg, Drechslera spicifera, Phialophora verrucosa*) that normally invade the subcutaneous tissue without damage to the epidermis and dermis. The only difference between phaeohyphomycosis and pigmented eumycotic mycetoma is the presence of discernible grains in the latter.

The condition often is manifested as a solitary lump that is painless to the touch and may exude pus.

Diagnosis is by fungal culture and biopsy. Since these fungi are pigmented, they are easily visualized in routine tissue sections stained with hematoxylin-eosin, methenamine silver, PAS or Gridley's. The lesion appears as a pyogranuloma with giant cells and large number of septate, branching hyphae with chlamydospores, and frequently pigmented.

Treatment of phaeohyphomycosis is disappointing if not all of the material can be removed by surgery. To date, medical intervention has done little to control the condition, though amphotericin B would be the drug of choice.

Additional Reading

1. Kwochka, KW *et al*: Canine phaeohyphomycosis caused by *Drechslera spicifera*: A case report and literature review. *JAAHA* 20:625-633, 1984.

Phycomycosis (Zygomycosis)

Phycomycosis is caused by several fungi of the order Mucorales (*eg, Rhizopus, Mucor, Absidia, Mortierella*) and Entomophthorales (*Conidiobolus, Basidiobolus*). They may enter the system through injury to skin or via the digestive tract. A number of patients previously thought to have phycomycosis have instead been affected by a species of *Pythium*, thus really having (for lack of a better term) pythiosis. Depending on the route of infection, affected animals may have cutaneous and/or gastrointestinal symptoms. With skin or oral involvement, lesions are often ulcerated and draining, with associated regional lymphadenomegaly, while vomiting, diarrhea and weight loss accompany GI lesions.

Diagnosis is by direct microscopic examination, biopsy and fungal culture. Many animals have nonresponsive anemia and neutrophilia. Diagnosis is confirmed by finding broad, nonseptate hyphae in tissue samples. Visualization of the organism may be enhanced by an indirect perioxidase technique. Absolute identification requires fungal culture. A barium series may reveal thickened bowel wall and frequently strictures with gastrointestinal involvement.

To date, all forms of therapy for this condition have been disappointing, though amphotericin B would probably be the drug of choice.

Additional Reading

1. Troy, GC: Canine phycomycosis: A review of twenty-four cases. *California Vet* 39(2):8-11, 1985.

2. O'Neill Foil, CS *et al*: A report of subcutaneous pythiosis in five dogs and a review of the etiologic agent *Pythium* spp. *JAAHA* 20:959-966, 1984.

3. Alder, PL: Phycomycosis in fifteen dogs and two cats. *JAAHA* 174:1216-1221, 1979.

Rhinosporidiosis

Rhinosporidiosis is a rare fungal disorder caused by *Rhinosporidium seeberi*. Most cases have been reported in the southeastern United States.

Clinical signs are more respiratory than dermatologic and include sneezing, unilateral nasal discharge and occasionally a polypoid vegetative to nodular mass.

Diagnosis is based on cytologic and histopathologic examinations, and fungal culture. Serologic and immunofluorescent studies, rhinoscopy and radiography are additional tests that may be used. On cytologic preparations, 6- to 8-μ organisms may be apparent. Some organisms contain aggregates of deeply basophilic spherules. On tissue sections, the large sporangia (up to 400 μ in diameter) are visualized in a fibrous stroma. The organisms do not grow on conventional fungal culture media and must be propagated in tissue culture.

Treatment options include excision and medical therapy with dapsone.

Additional Reading

1. Wilson, RB et al: Canine rhinosporidiosis. *Comp Cont Ed Pract Vet* 11:730-732, 1989.

2. Easley, JR et al: Nasal rhinosporidiosis in the dog. *Vet Pathol* 23:50-56, 1986.

Sporotrichosis

Sporotrichosis is caused by *Sporothrix schenckii*, a dimorphic soil microbe usually contracted through abraded skin. Infection may also result from ingestion or inhalation. It is generally regarded as a noncontagious, though people have contracted the fungus from infected cats.

Clinical Signs: The clinical picture is one of cutaneous nodules and ulcers with associated crusting, though many other syndromes have been described (Fig 13). The infection may then spread internally, especially to the lungs and liver.

Diagnosis: Diagnosis is by fungal culture, biopsy for histopathologic examinations and immunologic tests. Aspirates of unopened lesions should be used for fungal culture, plated on Sabouraud's agar, and kept at room temperature and 37 C. Direct microscopic examination of pus is usually insufficient to confirm a diagnosis. Gram's stain may facilitate visualization of the organism, which is pleomorphic and 2-3 μ x 3-6 μ with 1-2 buds. Biopsies may reveal the fungi, and several special stains (*eg*, periodic acid-Schiff or Gomori's methenamine silver) often highlight the organisms.

Management: Treatment of sporotrichosis varies with the extent of the infection. When the infection has spread to the lungs and liver, the outlook is not very bright. Infections limited to the skin usually respond to such drugs as sodium iodide, amphotericin B or some of the newer antifungal medications as ketoconazole at 15 mg/kg BID and itraconazole at 10 mg/kg/day. Treatment with sodium iodide 20% commences with 0.22 ml/kg TID (40 mg/kg) and must be continued at least one month past disappearance of all clinical signs. When treating with sodium iodide, one must always be alert to the possibility of iodine toxicity, which is usually manifested by a dry coat, discharge from the nose and mouth, vomiting, depression and occasionally cardiac collapse. These signs can be easily treated by discontinuation of therapy if recognized immediately. Potassium iodide can also be given orally as a form of therapy

Additional Reading

1. Urabe, H and Honbo, S: Sporotrichosis. *Intl J Dermatol* 25:255-257, 1986.

2. Restrepo, A *et al*: Itraconazole therapy in lymphatic and cutaneous sporotrichosis. *Arch Dermatol* 122:413-417, 1986.

3. Stowe, CM: Iodine, iodides, and iodism. *JAVMA* 179:334-336, 1981.

4. Moriello, KA *et al*: Cutaneous-lymphatic and nasal sporotrichosis in a dog. *JAAHA* 24:621-626, 1988.

Systemic Mycoses

Systemic fungal infections are normally acquired by inhaling infectious spores and are therefore not considered contagious, though blastomycosis has been transmitted from dogs via bite wounds. Systemic mycoses typically are characterized by a primary respiratory infection, with spread to other organs including the skin. Therefore, respiratory signs, such as coughing, normally precede other symptoms. Three fungi, *Blastomyces dermatitidis*, *Coccidioides immitis* and *Histoplasma capsulatum*, exist in a hyphal or spore stage in nature and grow as budding yeasts in tissues. *Cryptococcus neoformans* exists in only one form, as a budding yeast.

In most cases, animals that contract the infection often resolve it on their own without incident. Only the exceptional animal, usually one with a less than optimal immune system, manifest the full clinical disease.

Blastomycosis

Blastomycosis is caused by the soil organism *Blastomyces dermatitidis*, which normally resides in areas drained by rivers in the eastern United States and parts of southern Canada. Dogs (and people) become infected by inhalation of conidia from colonies of the mold growing as saprophytes in soil or similar substrate. Most cases of blastomycosis are chronic and of insidious onset. It is also more commonly seen in younger dogs, especially of the hunting breeds.

Clinical Signs: The principal clinical signs observed are respiratory, with possible spread to a number of different organ systems, but most commonly the skin, eyes and bone. Lymphadenomegaly is a common finding. Cutaneous lesions include abscesses, ulcers and draining tracts (Fig 14). Blastomycotic contamination of sputum may occur as a direct extension of bronchial airway consolidation and thus pose a potential zoonotic concern.

Diagnosis: Diagnosis of blastomycosis is based on the history, clinical signs, ancillary laboratory tests, radiography, cytologic and histopathologic examinations, complement fixation and agar gel immunodiffusion. A complete blood count may reveal leukocytosis with neutrophilia and monocytosis. Thyroid levels are frequently depressed. Hypercalcemia is occasionally noted.

Radiographic findings vary with the severity of the condition, from mild to severe interstitial, bronchial and peribronchial pneumonitis and hilar lymphadenomegaly.

An impression smear or fine-needle aspirate from skin lesions or a lymph node frequently reveals the characteristic budding organisms. Enhanced cytologic preparation can make the yeasts more easily recognized. Using Diff-Quik, dip the air-dried slide in fixative as directed, omit the red eosin dye, then allow the slide to set for at least 10 minutes in the azure/methylene blue dye to ensure staining of the yeast cell wall. The inflammatory infiltrate should then be scanned for *Blastomyces* organisms. In the yeast form, the organisms are round and 5-20 μ in diameter, with a thick cell wall but no capsule. Biopsies of cutaneous granulomas, abscesses or lymph nodes may also reveal the causative organisms. GMS or PAS stains may facilitate localization of the fungi.

When direct visualization of the organism is not possible, a tentative diagnosis can be based on clinical findings, radiography and a positive agar gel immunodiffusion test. This immunologic test has a sensitivity and specificity of over 90% in canine blastomycosis. Older antibody tests were subject to more false-positive reactions from past exposure and false-negative reactions from poor antigenicity of blastomycin or the host's inability to mount an antibody response. Complement-fixation titers of >1:16 are considered positive, while titers of 1:16 are suspect. However, complement-fixation titers are less useful because canine serum is often anticomplementary and cross-reactions exist with histoplasmosis. In-house fungal culture is usually not recommended because of the public health concern.

Management: Treatment is most often attempted with ketoconazole or amphotericin B. This is more completely covered in Appendix 1.

Additional Reading

1. Pyle, RL *et al:* Canine blastomycosis. *Comp Cont Ed Pract Vet* 3:963-974, 1981.

2. Legendre, AM *et al:* Canine blastomycosis: A review of 47 clinical cases. *JAVMA* 178:1163-1168, 1981.

3. Harasen, GLG and Randall, JW: Canine blastomycosis in southern Saskatchewan. *Can Vet J* 27:375-378, 1986.

4. McGee, ED: Diagnosing blastomycosis with aspirates. *MVP* 67:664, 1986.

Coccidioidomycosis

Coccidioidomycosis (valley fever, oidiomycosis) is caused by the organism *Coccidioides immitis*, which normally resides in the lower Sonoran life zone of the southwestern United States (California, Arizona, New Mexico, Texas, Nevada, Utah), Mexico and some parts of Central and South America. The Sonoran zone is characterized by sandy, alkaline soils, high environmental temperature, low rainfall and low elevation. Apart from the respiratory signs, affected dogs may have cutaneous ulcers, abscesses and draining tracts.

Clinical Signs: It is presumed that most dogs with coccidioidomycosis have inapparent infections, recover spontaneously and develop lifelong immunity. The fungus usually infects the respiratory tract, though the viscera, bones, skin, lymph nodes, eyes, urogenital tract and heart may be involved. The skin is rarely involved alone; draining tracts are usually associated with underlying osteomyelitis. Disseminated infection is usually manifested as a cough, dyspnea, lymphadenopathy, fever unresponsive to antibacterials, lameness and such skin lesions as ulcers, abscesses and draining tracts.

Diagnosis: The diagnosis is usually based on the history, clinical signs, radiographs, and cytologic, histopathologic and serologic examinations. Mild nonregenerative anemia and neutrophilic leukocytosis are common. Azotemia, isosthenuria and proteinuria may herald renal involvement. Thoracic radiographs may show a diffuse interstitial pattern often mixed with a bronchovesicular pattern. Hilar lymphadenopathy is a common finding. Transtracheal aspirates, bronchial washes, lymph node aspirates and impression smears provide samples for cytologic evaluation. Double-walled spherules containing endospores are diagnostic. Tissue sections may be enhanced with silver, periodic acid-Schiff (PAS) or fluorescent antibody stains. Fungal cultures are diagnostic but pose a health hazard to personnel, so they should not be performed in veterinary clinics.

Serologic testing is an important diagnostic and prognostic procedure for coccidioidomycosis. The humoral responses of precipitin (IgM) and complement-fixation (IgG) antibodies provide a proportionate measure of the severity of the disease. The precipitin test detects IgM early in the infection, typically beginning 10-14 days after infection. The response wanes by 4-6 weeks after infection. In contrast, complement-fixation antibodies usually appear 8-10 weeks after infection. Titers of 1:16 likely indicate primary pulmonary coccidioidomycosis, while higher titers usually indicate disseminated disease. Complement-fixation titers usually remain elevated for many months, in contrast to precipitin titers. Thus, early in the course of the disease, the precipitin test is usually positive and the complement-fixation test negative. With early active infection, both tests are positive. Later in the disease, the precipitin test is negative and the complement-fixation test remains positive for many months.

About 25% of serum samples are anticomplementary; in these cases, double electroimmunodiffusion or quantitative immunodiffusion can also be used as a rapid qualitative screening test. Some cross reactivity occurs with histoplasmosis and blastomycosis in CF tests. Apparently, circulating immune complexes (CIC) are also elevated in these cases.

Management: Treatment may be attempted with ketoconazole given with the food at 5-10 mg/kg BID. Dosages may need to be doubled when therapeutic levels are required in the brain, testes or possibly even the digits. Addition of vitamin C or tetracycline to the regimen may enhance the antifungal effect. Therapy is often administered until the titer drops to $\leq 1:4$; this often requires 4-12 months.

Additional Reading

1. Armstrong, PJ and DiBartola, SP: Canine coccidioidomycosis: A literature review and report of eight cases. *JAAHA* 19:937-946, 1983.

2. Wolf, AM: Cutaneous coccidioidomycosis in a dog and a cat. *JAVMA* 174:504-506, 1979.

3. Bartsch, R: Diagnosis and management of coccidioidomycosis and ehrlichiosis. *Proc 54th Ann Mtg AAHA*, 1987. pp 346-349.

Cryptococcosis

Cryptococcosis is caused by *Cryptococcus neoformans*. The disease is universal in its distribution and believed to be spread by pigeon droppings, in which the infective form can survive for up to 5 years. In addition to the respiratory tract, the fungi may spread to the skin, central nervous system, bone and other organs. Skin lesions are normally found around the head or in the mouth or nose.

Clinical Signs: The diagnosis is usually based on the history, clinical signs, and cytologic, pathologic and serologic examinations. The large mucoid capsule of the cryptococcal organisms is often visible on impression smears. Gram staining or addition of a few drops of diluted India ink to an air-dried slide facilitates visualization of the organisms. The capsule appears red with Gram staining. The organism remains unstained with India ink, and is silhouetted against a dark background.

Diagnosis: The diagnosis can be confirmed by identifying the 5- to 15-μ organisms surrounded by their characteristic clear capsule. Budding is a useful identifying feature but is not always apparent. The organisms may be found within multinucleated histiocytes and extracellularly among inflammatory cells. Gram staining is not very helpful, but new methylene blue, methenamine silver, Mayer's mucicarmine or periodic acid-Schiff stains are useful. The histopathologic appearance of cryptococcosis varies, but characteristically there is nodular to diffuse granulomatous dermatitis and panniculitis, with many cryptococcal organisms.

Management: Ketoconazole, amphotericin B with flucytosine or itraconazole is the treatment of choice.

Additional Reading

1. Willard, MD: Cryptococcosis. *California Vet* 12(2):13-16, 1982.

2. MacDonald, DW and Stretch, HC: Canine cryptococcosis associated with prolonged corticosteroid therapy. *Can Vet J* 23:200-202, 1982.

3. Noxon, JO *et al:* Ketoconazole therapy in canine and feline cryptococcosis. *JAAHA* 22:179-183, 1986.

4. Stampley, AR and Barsanti, JA: Disseminated cryptococcosis in a dog. *JAAHA* 24:17-21, 1988.

Histoplasmosis

Histoplasmosis is caused by *Histoplasma capsulatum* var *capsulatum* and is most prevalent around the Great Lakes and the Mississippi, St. Lawrence and Ohio River valleys. Fungal spores may be deposited in the soil by contaminated droppings of birds and bats. Inhalation of microaleurospores is the primary route of infection. Most infections are inapparent.

Clinical Signs: There are apparently 2 forms of the disease: pulmonary and disseminated. Chronic large bowel diarrhea is the most usual manifestation of chronic disseminated histoplasmosis. Chronic pulmonary histoplasmosis is clinically and radiographically indistinguishable from blastomycosis. Dermatologic signs are not an important feature of histoplasmosis. When they occur, dermatologic lesions include ulcers, abscesses and draining tracts (Fig 15).

Diagnosis: The diagnosis is usually based on the history, clinical signs, and cytologic, histopathologic and serologic examinations. A CBC usually shows anemia and leukocytosis with neutrophilia and monocytosis. Blood chemistry assays may reveal cholestatic liver disease, with increased serum alkaline phosphatase activity, elevated serum bilirubin levels, hypoalbuminemia and increased BSP retention. Radiographs may reveal hepatosplenomegaly, thickened bowel walls, diffuse interstitial pneumonitis and hilar lymphadenopathy.

Romanowsky, Wright's or Giemsa staining of impression smears may reveal 2- to 4-μ *Histoplasma* organisms within cells of the mononuclear phagocyte series. Occasionally organisms are found in peripheral blood cells. On biopsy specimens, periodic acid-Schiff stains the organism's cell wall red.

Complement fixation and agar gel immunodiffusion are the most reliable diagnostic tests. Complement fixation is often used (considered positive at titers $\geq 1:32$ and suspect at 1:16), but canine serum samples may be anticomplementary. A 4-fold rise in titers from paired serum samples confirms the diagnosis. Blastomycosis may cause cross reactivity. A precipitin line on agar gel immunodiffusion also indicates infection.

Management: Treatment is usually attempted with ketoconazole or amphotericin B.

Additional Reading

1. Ford, RB: Canine histoplasmosis. *Comp Cont Ed Pract Vet* 2:637-642, 1980.

2. Mitchell, M and Stark, DR: Disseminated canine histoplasmosis: A clinical survey of 24 cases in Texas. *Can Vet J* 21:95-100, 1980.

3. Clinkenbeard, KD *et al:* Disseminated histoplasmosis in dogs: 12 cases (1981-1986). *JAVMA* 193:1443-1447, 1988.

Diagnosis of Systemic Mycoses

Diagnosis of all of the systemic mycoses is approached in a similar manner. Patient history, clinical signs, direct microscopic examination, biopsy, skin tests and blood tests are all part of the diagnostic regimen. Direct microscopic examination of material removed from nodules or lymph nodes, to which special stains have been added, may reveal the causative organism. Otherwise, samples may be sent to the laboratory for histopathologic examination or blood tests. Nowadays it is unusual to perform skin tests using fungal antigen (*eg,* histoplasmin, coccidioidin) to arrive at a diagnosis. The complement-fixation test on serum is frequently used in diagnosis of blastomycosis, histoplasmosis, and coccidioidomycosis, though canine serum may contain interfering substances, and cross reactions occur between blastomycosis and histoplasmosis. Immunodiffusion (AGID) testing has less cross reaction than does complement fixation, and positive reactions may correlate better with the clinical form of the disease. The latex-agglutination test is a rapid and sensitive test for coccidioidomycosis and cryptococcosis, and is best suited to detection of fungal antigen in body fluids (including blood), rather than detection of antifungal antibodies.

Additional Reading

1. Carakostas, MC *et al:* Clinical laboratory evaluation of deep mycotic diseases in dogs. *J Small Anim Pract* 25:687-693, 1984.

2. Jackson, JA: Immunodiagnosis of systemic mycoses in animals: A review. *JAVMA* 188:702-705, 1986.

Chapter 4
Allergic Skin Disorders

INHALANT ALLERGIES

Allergic inhalant dermatitis, or atopy, the canine variant of hayfever, represents one of the most common dermatologic problems presented to veterinarians. Most affected animals react to a variety of inhaled substances, such as tree, grass and weed pollens, molds, house dust, house dust mites, feathers and dander.

Clinical signs may be seasonal or year-round, depending on the allergen. Whereas people with allergies often sneeze, allergic pets develop pruritus. They lick, chew and scratch, and have decreased resistance to infection. The most common sign is chewing at the feet. The constant licking may stain the haircoat with a rust-like hue.

Other pruritic areas include the flanks, groin and axillae. Many animals rub their faces on the carpet, furniture or other convenient surfaces. Self-traumatized areas may develop recurrent bacterial infections.

Atopic dogs usually first begin to show signs between 4 months and 3 years of age. In time, such chronic and secondary changes as infections, thickening of the skin and increased pigmentation may become prominent.

Though the mechanics of developing allergies are not well understood, it is clear that susceptibility to inhalant allergies is an inherited trait. Breeds with a particularly high incidence of allergies include terriers (especially the West Highland White Terrier, Skye Terrier, Scottish Terrier, Boston Terrier), Golden Retrievers, Poodles, Dalmatians, German Shepherds, Shar Peis, Shih Tzus,

Pugs, Irish Setters and Miniature Schnauzers. Any animal, however, purebred or mutt, may be affected by inhalant allergies.

Diagnosis

Allergies are diagnosed by a combination of the history, clinical signs, skin tests and possibly blood tests.

In 1967, 2 research groups working independently discovered that "reaginic" antibodies (previously thought to be responsible for causing allergic symptoms in people) were actually members of a new immunoglobulin class, IgE. IgE-producing plasma cells are distributed primarily in lymphoid tissue near the site of antigen encounter, but IgE is eventually spread throughout the whole body. Synthesis of IgE is stimulated by allergen exposure, but ultimately production is under the control of T-helper and T-suppressor lymphocytes that are IgE and antigen specific. The antibody has an affinity for mast cells in tissue and basophils in the blood. "Bridge" formation between 2 IgE molecules is necessary for degranulation of mast cells. The half-life of IgE in the bloodstream is only 2-3 days (the shortest of all the immunoglobulins) but its persistence in the system is a reflection of its high affinity for receptors on mast cells and its low dissociation constant.

Inhalant allergies in dogs may be mediated by IgE or IgG, which yield an immediate hypersensitivity reaction when allergen contacts antibody on the surface of a mast cell in tissue or basophil in the blood. The short half-life of free IgE (2-3 days), along with its being present only in minute quantities, greatly complicates *in-vitro* assay procedures. *In-vitro* tests purportedly measure levels of free allergen-specific IgE in the bloodstream, while *in-vivo* (intradermal) tests measure the ability of allergen-specific IgE antibody to bind to effector mast cells in the dermis and initiate mast-cell degranulation with an associated inflammatory response (wheal).

Intradermal Allergy Testing: Intradermal allergy testing has been helpful in diagnosis and management of inhalant allergies in dogs for over 2 decades. The disadvantages of skin testing are that it requires some expertise to perform, is variable in its determinations, and is unstandardized on the basis of examiner, source of allergen or reproducibility.

Once a skin test is completed, the information acquired by the testing should be compared to the clinical history of the patient.

Table 1. Minimum withdrawal times for some drugs before skin testing.

Drug	Minimum Withdrawal Time
Anesthetics	2-7 days
Astemizole	4 weeks
Classic antihistamines	2 days
Methylprednisolone acetate	4-8 weeks
Prednisone	2 weeks
Sedatives	2 days
Terfenadine	1 week

Positive reactions on a skin test only indicate sensitivity to a particular allergen. It is up to the pet owner and veterinarian to decipher this information so that it is relevant to the particular animal tested.

Skin testing for inhalant allergies is accomplished in a procedure modified from that used in people (Fig 16). Candidates for skin testing should be chosen on the following basis:

- The diagnosis of allergic inhalant dermatitis is fairly certain from the history and clinical signs.
- Corticosteroid doses needed to control pruritus are unsafe, cause undesirable side effects or are unacceptable to the owner.
- Other forms of symptomatic therapy are unsuccessful, too expensive or unacceptable to the owner.
- The owner thoroughly understands the concept of testing and immunotherapy, and is prepared to invest the required time and money.

The patient can be readied by withdrawing all medication that could inhibit formation of a diagnostic wheal. Table 1 presents minimum withdrawal times for some commonly used antipruritics. Note that these withdrawal times are minimum intervals. It is often necessary to allow longer intervals between discontinuing use of a drug and initiating skin testing. For example, the ideal withdrawal time for prednisone is 1 week for every consecutive month the drug was used. Hydroxyzine (Atarax) use should be discontinued at least 10 days before skin testing.

The patient can then be adequately prepared for testing as follows:

1. Fast the patient for 12 hours before testing.

2. Clip the hair with a #40 blade.

3. As an option, flood the test site with alcohol 5 minutes before testing.

4. Do not apply soaps or disinfectants to the area before testing.

5. If sedation is necessary, use xylazine (2 mg/kg SC or 0.1-0.2 mg/kg IV) with atropine (0.04 mg/kg).

Allergy testing should be done by someone who performs it regularly enough to reliably identify potential allergens. Many practitioners refer patients to clinics equipped to perform such procedures. Also, false-negative and false-positive reactions may occur; therefore, skin testing should be performed by a clinician familiar with the limitations of the procedure (Table 2).

Proper selection of testing and treatment allergens is very important. Allergens are standardized according to 2 different systems: weight to volume (w/v) and protein nitrogen units (PNU). The w/v system measures the weight of defatted allergen in a given volume of diluent. For example, 10 g of allergen in 100 ml of diluent is a 10% or 1:10 solution. The second system involves the amount of protein precipitated by phosphotungstic acid, with 1 mg of protein nitrogen equivalent to 100,000 PNU. This should not be construed, however, as a direct measure of allergen protein.

Aqueous solutions of allergens should be used for testing. Many human test solutions are preserved with glycerin and are unsuitable for veterinary use, since as little as 2% glycerin can

Table 2. Causes of false-positive and false-negative skin test results.

False-Positive	False-Negative
Allergens too concentrated	Interfering substances present
Allergens contaminated	Extracts not concentrated enough due to lack of potency groupings or being outdated
Irritants included with allergens	
Patients sensitized	Off season
Dermographism	Patient hyporeactive: estrus, stress, parasitism, anergy
Poor technique	

cause irritant reactions in animals. Once they have been diluted, allergens lose potency relatively quickly. I recommend mixing a new batch of allergens each month, though a batch may remain useful for up to 2 months if refrigerated and stored in glass containers. Allergens refrigerated for 3 months retain about 50-60% of potency. Whether that is sufficient to render good skin test results has not been determined.

Ideally, the list of test substances should include at least 25 allergens to be considered comprehensive. Very few of these should be mixes (tree mix, weed mix, etc), since this greatly reduces the accuracy of the test. Be aware also that even though a number of potential allergens are being tested, there are still hundreds or thousands of potentially allergenic materials that have not been included in the test. To keep tests practical and affordable, the injections should be limited to substances that have a fair to good chance of evoking a reaction. Such information is available from companies that manufacture allergens and from allergists in your geographic region. We must realize then that allergy tests are not complete but statistically should uncover the most common allergies.

Note that the 2 systems are not interchangeable. One cannot reliably convert PNUs to w/v, and *vice versa*. For convenience (but not accuracy), however, a 1:1000 w/v solution for intradermal testing is roughly equivalent to 1000 PNU. Bulk extracts of 1:10 are roughly equivalent to 40,000 PNU for pollens and 20,000 PNU for molds. Most dermatologists use concentrations of 1000-1500 PNU (1:1000 w/v) for testing with pollens and mold spores, and 500 PNU (1:2000 w/v) with house dust mites and epidermals. Nonglycerinated flea antigen is used at a 1:1000 concentration. The PNU system is more commonly used in the United States, while w/v is more common in Canada and Europe.

Selecting Allergens for Skin Testing: The fact that not all plants that pollinate cause clinical allergies must be considered in selection of allergens for testing. The allergen must be buoyant to become airborne, be of a certain size and weight (5000-60,000 daltons and 2-60 μ) to reach the proper level in the respiratory tract, and be present in significant quantities. For instance, since most flower pollens are heavy and evolved to be insect pollinated, they cause relatively few clinical allergies in animals unless there is direct contact.

Each allergen molecule has several antigenic determinants (epitopes) that offer distinct specificity for antibody production.

The allergenic molecules represent only a small proportion of the crude material (about 1% of the total weight). There are 1-4 major allergens in each allergen extract. Allergen E in ragweed was the first major allergen recognized. Though major allergens have been identified in many grasses, trees, mites and molds, many more remain yet undetermined.

Trees commonly pollinate profusely but for relatively short periods. Members of the birch (Betulaceae), oak (Quercaceae), elm (Ulmaceae), maple-boxelder (Aceraceae), walnut-hickory-pecan (Juglandaceae) and mulberry (Moraceae) families are the most significant pollinators.

Birch trees produce copious amounts of pollen; the gray, white, yellow, sweet, spring, paperbark and river varieties are of allergenic significance. The related alders (*Alnus rhombifolia, A rugosa*) produce much pollen from February through April, and commonly cause allergic reactions. Hornbeams (*Carpinus carolineana*), hophornbeams (*Ostrya virginiana*) and hazels (*Corylus americana* and *C cornuta*) cross react antigenically.

Oaks (*Quercus* spp) shed more pollen than most other trees and are allergenically important where the trees are abundant. The different species tend to hybridize and many cross react, but it is still important to test for species that predominate regionally.

The American elm (*Ulmus americana*), slippery elm (*U fulva*), rock elm (*U thomasii*) and winged elm (*U alata*) pollinate in the spring, while such southern varieties as the cedar elm (*U crassifolia*), Chinese elm (*U parvifolia*) and September elm (*U serotina*) pollinate in the fall. The related hackberries (*Celtis occidentalis*) and sugarberries (*Celtis* spp) are important allergens in Texas and Oklahoma but rarely achieve large populations elsewhere.

Of the maple-boxelder family, the box elder (*Acer negundo*) is the most potent member from an allergenic standpoint. The other maples cause fewer allergy problems.

Walnut, hickory and pecan are related trees within the family Juglandaceae. The pecan (*Carya pecan*) blooms from March to May and causes allergy problems where prevalent. Walnut (*Juglans regia*), butternut (*Juglans cinerea*) and hickory (*Carya ovata, C laciniosa, C tomentosa*) bloom from April to June. The pollen of all of these trees is large and does not travel far.

The Moraceae family consists of the white (*Morus alba*), red (*M rubra*), black (*M tatarica*) and paper (*Broussonetia papyrifera*) mulberry, and the hedge plant or osage orange (*Maclura pomifera*). They are important southern allergenic plants that pollinate in April and May.

Among the olive family, ash (*Fraxinus* spp) are most often found in low moist or wet areas and are entirely wind pollinated; their pollen is moderately allergenic. The related olives (*Olea europaea*) are partly wind pollinated and strongly allergenic where prominent. The privet (*Ligustrum* spp) is insect pollinated and therefore not an important allergenic plant, though some pollen is carried by the air for short distances.

Conifers produce immense quantities of pollen but most (pine, spruce) are of questionable allergenic significance. The spruce, fir, larch and cedars have large nonallergenic pollen. Juniper (mountain cedar, white cedar, red cedar), Arizona, Monterey and Italian cypresses (*Cupressus* spp) and bald cypress (*Taxodium distichum*) have buoyant small pollen with much interspecies cross reactivity. Junipers with berries do not produce pollen. The allergenic components of pine pollen do not evoke a strong allergic response, though a few rare cases of pine pollen allergy have been documented.

Willows are mainly insect pollinated but also somewhat wind pollinated. The pussy willow (*Salix discolor*) is of limited allergenic significance, its catkins (spike-like clusters of tiny flowers) being produced long before the leaves appear. The black willow (*Salix nigra*), found predominantly in the eastern states, opens its catkins after its leaves are fully extended. The related poplars (*Populus* spp), aspens (*Populus tremuloides*) and cottonwoods (*Populus trichocarpa, P deltoides, P fremontii*) are entirely wind pollinated and pollinate from March through May, but are only mildly allergenic.

Other trees of some significance include the sycamore, mesquite, citrus and palm. Sycamores (*Platanus* spp) have small pollen that is windborne and moderately allergenic. Mesquite (*Prosopis juliflora*) is partially insect pollinated but has reportedly caused allergy problems, especially in the southwestern United States. The wood is popular for barbeques but allergy to the smoke has not been reported. Citrus trees are insect pollinated and virtually no pollen gets into the air. They do not cause inhalant allergies, though food allergies and contact allergies (to their sap) are well known. The date (*Phoenix* spp), queen (*Cocos plumosa*) and dwarf (*Chamearops humilus*) palms are wind

Table 3. Degree of importance of allergenic trees in geographic regions of the United States.

Common Name and Genus	Some Important Species	Northeast	Mid-Atlantic	Southeast/South Central	Midwest	Great Plains	Central Texas/Oklahoma	Desert Southwest	Intermountain	Southern California	West Coast/Alaska	Southern Florida/Hawaii/Caribbean
Ash *Fraxinus* spp	White, Arizona, Green Ash	**	**	**	**	*	*	***	*	*	*	
Birch *Betula* spp	White, Paper, Red, Sweet, Spring Birch	***	**	**	**	*	*		**	*	*	
Cedar *Juniperus* spp	Mountain, Red, Rocky Mountain Cedar, Western Juniper	*	*	**	*	*	***	**	**	*	**	**
Elm *Ulmus* spp	American, Chinese, Fall Blooming Elm	**	**	**	***	**	***	*	*	*	**	
Maple *Acer* spp	Sugar, Red, Silver Maple, Box Elder	**	**	*	*	**	*		**	*	*	
Oak *Quercus* spp	White, Red, Black, Scrub, Live, Post, California Live Oak	***	***	***	***	***	***	**	**	**	**	**
Pecan *Carya* spp	Pecan, White Hickory, Shagbark Hickory	**	**	***	*	*	**	*		*	*	**
Walnut *Juglans* spp	Black, English, Hinds, California Black Walnut	*	**	**	**	*	*	*	*	**	***	
Sycamore *Platanus* spp	Eastern, Western Sycamore, Plane Tree	**	***	**	***	**	**	*	*	**	**	

Table 4. Degree of importance of allergenic grasses in geographic regions of the United States.

Common Name and Genus	Some Important Species	Northeast	Mid-Atlantic	Southeast/South Central	Midwest	Great Plains	Central Texas/Oklahoma	Desert Southwest	Intermountain	Southern California	West Coast/Alaska	Southern Florida/Hawaii/Caribbean
Bermuda grass *Cynodon dactylon*		*	**	***	*	*	***	***		***	*	***
Bluegrass *Pao* spp	Kentucky (June), Canadian, Annual Bluegrass	***	***	***	***	***	***	**	**	***	**	*
Johnson grass *Sorghum halepense*		*	*	**	*	*	***	**	*	**		**
Orchard grass *Dactylis glomerata*		***	***	**	***	**	*		*		*	
Rye grass *Lolium* spp	Perennial, Italian Rye Grass	***	***	***	***	***	***	**	**	***	***	*
Timothy grass *Phleum pratense*		***	***	**	***	***	**	**	**	**	**	*

Degree of importance: * Minor, ** Moderate, *** Major

Source: *Veterinary Medicine,* Lenexa, KS and Center Laboratories, Port Washington, NY.

pollinated and produce copious pollen locally but are only mildly allergenic. Many other palms are insect pollinated.

The melaleuca (cajeput or punk tree), which is native to Australia, is frequently blamed for allergies, yet there is mounting evidence that it is rarely a significant allergen. Similarly, the eucalyptus appears to be mainly insect pollinated and not a major cause of allergies, though its pollen is sometimes recovered in air surveys.

Grasses (Gramineae) represent the most abundant sources of pollen. The start of the pollen season is correlated to soil temperature. The actual amount of pollen in the area correlates with the weather. Pollen is only liberated during the day, mostly in the morning, and counts are low on cold, rainy days, and high on hot, dry days. Wind conditions have a profound effect on pollen release and distribution.

The most important summer grasses from an allergenic standpoint include Kentucky (*Poa* spp), orchard or cocksfoot (*Dactylis glomerata*), timothy (*Phleum* spp), rye (*Elymus* and *Lolium* spp), redtop (*Agrostis* spp), sweet vernal (*Anthoxanthum odoratum*), canarygrass (*Phalaris* spp), velvet grass (*Holcus lanatus*), brome grass (*Bromus inermis*), broncho grass (*Bromus rigidus*), western wheatgrass (*Agropyron smithii*) and meadow fescue (*Festuca* spp).

In the southern United States., Bermuda grass (*Cynodon* spp), Johnson grass (*Sorghum* spp) and saltgrass (*Distichlis* spp) have prolonged pollinating seasons. Grass pollens other than that of Bermuda grass are considered to be antigenically cross reactive.

There may be as many as 20 active components in the pollen of a single species of grass. Rye, blue, fescue, orchard and timothy have very similar allergenic components. Johnson (*Sorghum halepense*), Sudan (*Sorghum sudanense*) and grama grasses (*Bouteloua* spp) are closely related botanically and allergenically. Brome, broncho, sweet vernal and Bahia (*Paspalum notatum*) grasses are also closely related. Quack grass (*Agropyron repens*), western wheatgrass, saltgrass and Bermuda grass are somewhat related. St. Augustine grass (*Stenotaphrum secundatum*) has heavy pollen, of which little becomes airborne. It does, however, harbor *Helminthosporium* molds, which are released into the environment when a lawn is mowed.

Weeds are also common sources of allergenic pollen. The most important families are the Compositae, Chenopodiaceae, Amaranthaceae, Plantaginaceae and Polygonaceae.

The Compositae family is large, and ragweed is probably its most important allergen, though regional distribution is an important consideration. A single ragweed plant may produce 1 billion pollen grains, and a 1-square-mile plot of ragweed plants produces 16 tons of pollen. A ragweed-allergic person only needs to inhale 1 μg of pollen (10 ng of allergen) per day to experience hay fever symptoms.

The giant ragweed (*Ambrosia trifida*), short ragweed (*A artemisiifolia*) and western ragweed (*A psilostachya*) are important ragweed species. There are multiple antigens in ragweed pollens but the most significant is antigen E, present in *Ambrosia* and *Franseria* spp (rabbitbush, beachbur, canyon ragweed, desert ragweed, false ragweed, slender ragweed). Sagebrush (*Artemisia tridentata*), the related wormwoods (*A biennis, A annua, A absinthium*) and mugworts (*A douglasiana, A heterophylla*) share similar antigens and may cause clinical allergy. The related sagebrushes (*Artemisia* spp) and marshelders (*Iva* spp) share similar antigens but do not include antigen E. Burweed and rough marsh elder (povertyweed) are significant relatives, while other members of the Compositae family (cocklebur, goldenrod, dandelion, burrobrush, plus a number of flowers) are of secondary importance unless regionally prominent.

The Chenopodiaceae include goosefoot (*Chenopodium murale*), Russian thistle (*Salsola kali*), greasewood (*Sarcobatus vermiculatus*), pickleweed (*Salicornia ambigua*), summer cypress/burning bush (*Kochia scoparia*), lamb's quarters (*Chenopodium album*), smother weed or 5-hook bassia (*Bassia hyssopifolia*), Mexican tea (*Chenopodium album*) and saltbush (*Atriplex wrightii*). These have variable clinical relevance, depending on region. Saltbush, shadscale, spearscale and orach (*Atriplex* spp) are found on dry, alkaline soils in the western U.S. and pollinate in late summer and early fall. The sugar beet (*Beta vulgaris*) blooms in May and though newer hybrids have diminished pollination, significant allergies can be seen on a regional basis.

Antigenically similar to the Chenopodiaceae are the Amaranthaceae, which include rough redroot pigweed (*Amaranthus retroflexus*), common pigweed (*A hybridus*), careless weed/Palmer's amaranth (*A palmeri*), and western water hemp (*A tamaris-*

cina). The pollens of pigweed and goosefoot cross react quite extensively.

Of the Plantaginaceae, English plantain (*Plantago lanceolata*) is the most allergenic and pollinates from May to November. Of the Polygonaceae, sheep sorrel (*Rumex acetosella*) and curly dock (*R crispus*) bloom and provoke allergies from May to September. Buckwheat is a related plant that may also cause allergies.

Molds often cause allergies and occur all year round, though some are more prevalent in the spring and fall. The most important molds from an allergenic standpoint are *Alternaria, Hormodendrum (Cladosporium), Aspergillus, Penicillium, Helminthosporium, Mucor* and *Rhizopus*. Most molds flourish at high relative humidities and temperatures above 10 C. They produce vast numbers of small spores (3-10 μ) that outnumber pollen grains in the air. Pets are exposed to varying concentrations of mold particles both indoors and outdoors, which may result in the sensitization of atopic individuals.

Alternaria alternata (*tenuis*), of the class Fungi Imperfecti, order Moniliales, family Dematiaceae, is considered to be predominantly an outdoor mold commonly found in soil, damp hay, grain and other vegetation. The spores are easily made airborne. Sporulation follows warm and humid weather. It has been implicated as a cause of baker's asthma and possibly wood pulp worker's lung in people.

Aspergillus fumigatus, of the class Fungi Imperfecti, order Moniliales, family Moniliaceae, has a worldwide distribution and grows well in a wide variety of temperatures. It is commonly recovered from houses, bedding, house dust, raw textiles, soil, swimming pools and vegetation. Inhalation of conidia and mycelia can lead to several diseases, including allergic inhalant dermatitis, aspergilloma and an intermediate mycosis (see Chapter 3). Since the organism is so ubiquitous, isolating it on culture does not establish it as the cause of an allergy.

Cladosporium (Hormodendrum) herbarum, of the class Fungi Imperfecti, order Moniliales, family Dematiaceae, is the most abundant mold spore identified in air samples. It often occurs as heavy showers of spores, frequently after rains and damp weather. The dry conidia are carried easily through the air and reach very high concentrations (up to 35,000 conidia/sq meter) both indoors and out. *Cladosporium* is frequently found in uncleaned refrigerators, on moist window frames, in houses with poor ventilation, in

Chapter 4

Table 5. Degree of importance of allergenic weeds in geographic regions of the United States.

Common Name and Genus	Some Important Species	Northeast	Mid-Atlantic	Southeast/South Central	Midwest	Great Plains	Central Texas/Oklahoma	Desert Southwest	Intermountain	Southern California	West Coast/Alaska	Southern Florida/Hawaii/Caribbean
Cocklebur *Xanthium* spp	Common, Spiny Cocklebur	*	**	***	***	***	***	**	**	*	*	*
English plantain *Plantago lacelolata*		**	**	***	**	**	**	**	*	**	*	*
Kochia *Kochia scoparia*					**	***	**	*	***	*	*	
Lamb's-quarters *Chenopodium* spp	Mexican Tea	**	**	**	**	**	**	**	*	*	*	*
Pigweed *Amaranthus* spp	Redroot, Spiny Pigweed	*	**	***	***	***	***	**	**	*	*	**
Ragweed, tall *Ambrosia trifida*		***	***	***	***	**	***		*			
Ragweed, short *Ambrosia artemisifolia*	Western, Southern Ragweed	***	***	***	***	***	***	**	**	*	*	**
Russian thistle *Salsola kali*			*	*	*	***	***	***	***	*	**	*
Sage *Artemisia* spp	Mugwort, Wormwood Sagebrush, Carpet Sage, Pasture Sage	**	**	*	*	***	**	***	***	**	**	*

Degree of importance: *Minor, **Moderate, ***Major

Source: *Veterinary Medicine*, Lenexa, KS and Center Laboratories, Port Washington, NY.

houses situated in low, damp environments, in various soil types, and on most vegetation.

Penicillium notatum, of the class Fungi Imperfecti, order Moniliales, family Moniliaceae, is a major cause of indoor mold allergy. It has no real seasonal variation, though peaks occur in the winter and spring. This is the familiar blue-green mold found on stale bread, cheese, citrus fruits and apples, in wine cellars, and as a contaminant in rye flour in bakeries. It is also a frequent soil inhabitant. Penicillin is produced from only a few strains of *Penicillium*. The highly purified antibiotics manufactured today do not cross react significantly with the allergens of the spores and mycelia.

Helminthosporium halodes, of the class Fungi Imperfecti, order Moniliales, family Dematiaceae, is predominantly a seasonal mold. Spores are released on dry, hot days. They are best known as parasites of cereals and grasses, and are commonly recovered from soil and textiles. Together with other members of the family Dematiaceae, *Helminthosporium* is considered a common cause of inhalant allergies.

Mucor racemosus, of the class Phycomycetes, order Mucorales, family Mucoraceae, is called a "sugar fungus" because it attacks carbohydrates and can be found in decaying vegetable material, manure and soil. It is a dominant mold in house dust and in soft fruits, fruit juices, sour milk and marmelade. Sporulation requires high humidity (95%), and optimum temperatures are 22-25 C.

Rhizopus nigricans, of the class Phycomycetes, order Mucorales, family Mucoraceae, is widespread in nature and grows readily on bread, cured meats and root vegetables indoors, and outdoors in forest and cultivated soils. The optimal temperature for growth is around 25 C. Because of the high numbers of positive reactors on skin testing, it is likely that *Rhizopus* has some irritant effects in addition to its allergenicity.

Phoma betae, of the class Fungi Imperfecti, order Spheropsidales, family Sphaeriodaceae, is a very common soil fungus found in damaged plants and on paper products, such as books and magazines. It is also found frequently indoors as a contaminant of moist surfaces, especially in association with painted walls. It also has been isolated from mildewed shower curtains.

Other molds that may cause inhalant allergies include *Botrytis cinerea, Chaetomium, Curvularia lunata, Epicoccum purpurascens, Fusarium moniliforme, Gliocladium, Monilia sitophila, Paecilomyces, Pullularia, Spondylocladium, Stemphylium botryosum* and *Trichoderma viride*.

A classic question in mold allergy is whether spores/conidia or mycelia are the greater source of allergens. The problem is complicated by the complexity of fungal antigens. For *Cladosporium (Hormodendrum) herbarum*, 60 antigens have been demonstrated, of which at least 36 are allergens. Its major allergen exists in 5 molecular variants that are antigenically and allergenically identical. The cross reactivity of different genera of molds has been implied but not documented.

House dust is a common cause of allergies. The actual allergenic culprit is a minute mite that feeds on materials of animal origin in house dust. Two species of *Dermatophagoides* (*D farinae, D pteronysinus*) are implicated. Their fecal debris probably is the actual allergenic substance.

About 50% of nonallergic people and animals show some reaction to intradermal injection of house dust mite solution. These mites cannot survive on disinfected surfaces and cannot reproduce at relative humidities of <60%. It is important to appreciate these concepts, since the relative significance of house dust mite allergy can then be determined by hospitalizing a patient in a disinfected stainless-steel cage for 4-5 days. Animals with house dust mite allergy improve significantly during this interval. This is not specific for house dust mite sensitivity, however, since caging is also an excellent means of screening for contact allergies.

Other allergens, such as cat, dog, goat, horse and human hair and dander, often evoke positive responses on skin tests yet must be considered of relatively minor significance and of questionable specificity. For example, dogs often react to intradermal injections of a variety of cat allergens including cat-allergen I (CA-1) but do not distinguish between sensitization from prior exposure to cats and actual allergy. Testing with wool, cotton, silk and other fabrics is of questionable significance, since contact allergies cannot be diagnosed by intradermal allergy tests. Testing with feather and kapok are likely only to mimic house dust mite reactions.

Blood Tests: Blood tests have been developed to measure the amount of circulating allergen-specific antibody. Unfortunately, most allergy antibodies (IgE) are bound to mast cells in the skin or basophils in the blood, and are not floating free in the bloodstream to be easily harvested and measured.

Enzyme-linked immunosorbent assay (ELISA) and the radioallergosorbent test (RAST) are commercially available. Blood tests appear to have about 50% agreement with skin test results. Unfortunately, documentation is unavailable supporting the sensitivity, specificity or reproducibility of these tests. It appears that conditions other than allergy can cause elevations of serum IgE and that elevated levels of allergen-specific IgE do not necessarily mean the animal is allergic. Serum levels of IgE specific for house dust mites and fungi are frequently elevated above normal (?) levels, even in clinically normal dogs. In fact, the whole question of what constitutes normal and elevated levels of serum IgE has never been addressed. Elevated serum levels of IgE also do not imply that these immunoglobulins will fix to mast cells in the dermis and result in degranulation on exposure to allergen. The ultimate role of IgE is also in question, since dogs that are responding well to immunotherapy do not demonstrate reduced serum IgE levels. Also, animals with elevated levels of IgE for other reasons (*eg,* parasitism) get clinically better with specific (*eg,* antiparasitic) therapy despite the fact that their IgE levels remain elevated on testing.

The potential value of *in-vitro* testing should not be lost in the shuffle, however. Clearly, the assay is not an "allergy test" at all but a set of laboratory values. Similarly, SGPT (ALT) is not a "liver" test and amylase is not a "pancreas" test but rather both are tools with which veterinarians may ultimately make a diagnosis. And, like any test, we get in trouble when we diagnose and treat laboratory values rather than patients. Allergic pets are no different. One should not be surprised that normal nonallergic pets, and pets with conditions other than allergy, may have elevated levels of IgE to one or more allergens on testing.

It is my firm belief (until convinced otherwise) that grouping of allergens (tree, weed or mold mixes) adversely affects these blood tests, as it does with skin testing. When possible, individual allergens should be used for testing. This problem of grouping is further compounded by new in-house *in-vitro* allergy test kits used to confirm allergies by a quick method before more comprehensive evaluation.

We all look forward to the day when skin testing becomes obsolete and an accurate and reproducible blood test provides definitive information. In the meantime, skin testing is still the only practical means of identifying allergens, though there is no doubt that a significant percentage of animals tested with a blood assay and properly managed with immunotherapy will benefit. This success rate is bound to increase as the technologies evolve and more individual allergens are used.

Additional Reading

1. Ackerman, L: Recognizing the signs and sources of canine inhalant allergies. *Vet Med* 83:770-776, 1988.

2. Ackerman, L: Diagnosing inhalant allergies: Intradermal or in vitro testing? *Vet Med* 83:779-788, 1988.

2. Scott, DW: Observations on canine atopy. *JAAHA* 17:91-100, 1981.

3. Nesbitt, GH *et al*: Aeroallergens. *Comp Cont Ed Pract Vet* 6:63-68, 1984.

4. Nesbitt, GH *et al*: Canine atopy. Part I. Etiology and diagnosis. *Comp Cont Ed Pract Vet* 6:73-84, 1984.

5. Schick, RO and Fadok, VA: Responses of atopic dogs to regional allergens: 268 cases (1981-1984). *JAVMA* 189:1493-1496, 1986.

6. Helton-Rhodes, K *et al*: Investigation into the immunopathogenesis of canine atopy. *Sem Vet Med Surg* 2:199-201, 1987

7. Jelks, M: *Allergy Plants*. World-Wide Printing, Tampa, Florida.

8. White, SD and Ohman, Jr, JL: Response to intradermal skin testing with four cat allergen preparations in healthy and allergic dogs. *Am J Vet Res* 49:1873-1875, 1988.

9. Barbet, JL and Halliwell, REW: Duration of inhibition of immediate skin test reactivity by hydroxyzine hydrochloride in dogs. *JAVMA* 194:1565-1569, 1989.

Allergy Therapy

Why all of the concern about diagnosis? Why not just treat the allergies symptomatically? The answer to this question is both simple and complex, and revolves around the issue that allergies are chronic, life-long conditions. Palliative treatment (usually with corticosteroids) may be convenient in the short term but potentially dangerous over the long term.

Environmental Control

Having the dog avoid inhaling allergens is the ideal solution but is rarely practical. Avoidance is much more likely with contact allergies involving substances that can be removed from the animal's environment, such as plastic food bowls and wool. Unless the allergy is to cats, furniture stuffing, houseplants or other removable items, environmental control is usually aimed at limiting exposure to the offending allergens.

For pollen allergies, keeping the animal indoors most of the day is partially effective. Though air conditioners do little to remove airborne allergens, they limit pollen exposure because the doors and windows are kept closed. Humidifiers, vaporizers, dehumidifiers and air conditioners may develop growths of mold and should be periodically cleaned.

Molds occur year round, though some are more prevalent in the spring and fall. Depending on the type of mold, spores may be dispersed by rainfall, humidity or winds. When the sun warms the air during the day, most airborne spores are carried high into the atmosphere, only to descend again with the cool night air. Thus, many mold-allergic patients have worse clinical signs at night, unless they also spend their days in such mold-rich environments as damp basements or outside with their nose to the ground.

Usually there are just as many molds inside a home as outside. A crude method of detecting problem mold areas is to put saucers containing potato slices, just covered by water, in various places around the home. Comparing the rate and amount of mold growth roughly indicates problem areas.

Low-lying properties or those near lakes or marshes have high mold counts, as do old homes with damp, dark basements. Adequate ventilation is essential to prevent mold growth in attics or roof crawl spaces. Venting is insufficient if there are ice crystals in the attic in the winter.

Basements should be well lit and well ventilated. Basement floors and walls should be treated with mold-resistant paint. Fungicides can be sprayed in problem areas to limit mold growth.

Pillows and mattresses are also a source of molds. Pillows ideally should be made of synthetic fibers or chipped foam, and mattresses encased in zippered protectors that can be removed and laundered. Bedding should be cleaned frequently.

Houseplants should be removed because they harbor large numbers of molds. If they cannot be removed, their mold content can be reduced by covering the soil surface with aquarium tank filter charcoal bits. The resin from Christmas trees traps pollen and mold spores, and eventually releases it into the air.

An aquarium can also be a source of mold. An algacide should be added to tank water and any immersed items periodically cleaned with chlorine bleach and detergent. Obviously, all objects need be thoroughly rinsed before being replaced in the tank.

It is impossible to completely eradicate house dust and house dust mites from a home, but these can be controlled. Control measures should be most stringent in areas where the allergic dog spends most of its time. The stuffing of any pet bedding should be of a synthetic material. Kapok, feathers, wool and horsehair should be avoided. Cotton is good but not as hypoallergenic as synthetics. Bedding should be frequently washed.

Rooms with carpet, kapok-stuffed furniture or houseplants cause severe reactions in dust-allergic pets. Animal hair and dander attract dust, so rooms frequented by pets are often dusty. Therefore, keeping pets well groomed is an important consideration. Dust-allergic animals are also likely to be more affected when they share a home with other animals.

Control of house dust and house dust mites is an important component of therapy for dust allergy. Immunotherapy (allergy shots) cannot be relied upon as the entire answer. Because a home heating and cooling system can trap much dust, ducts and filters should be periodically cleaned. Activated charcoal filters are best at clearing odors from cooking, foods, smoke and pets but are less helpful for pollens and molds; they are very helpful when installed with other types of filters, in tandem. Electrostatic filters help reduce the amount of dust in the air by about 80% but cannot produce a dust-free environment. In addition, they produce ozone, which may cause headaches in some individuals. High-efficiency particulate air (HEPA) filters can clear over 95% of pollens, molds, yeasts, bacteria, and viruses in the air, and when coupled with a charcoal filter can remove most of the dust. This is the best choice for treating the household environment.

Relative humidity between 30-50% is best. (House dust mites cannot reproduce at humidity <60%.) A hygrometer, available from most hardware stores, allows easy monitoring. Humidifiers and dehumidifiers allow control of the relative humidity.

Household vacuuming should be done with a canister or cylindric type of vacuum cleaner, as the upright bag types return much dust to room air as it passes through the bag. Water-trap vacuum cleaners collect dust in water instead of an air bag, so dust is not continually recirculated into the air. Central vacuum systems are also beneficial if they are properly vented to the outside. Furniture should be dusted with a vacuum attachment or a damp paper towel that is thrown away after use.

Finally, scented, perfumed or strong-smelling products should be avoided. Tobacco smoke and smoke from fireplaces also aggravate allergies.

Additional Reading

1. Ackerman, L: Medical and immunotherapeutic options for treating atopic dogs. *Vet Med* 83:790-797, 1988.

Corticosteroids

Corticosteroids (glucocorticoids), along with antibacterials, are the most widely used (and abused) class of drugs in veterinary medicine. Cortisol is an endogenous corticosteroid produced by the adrenal glands. The amount of cortisol produced by a normal dog is equivalent to 1 mg of hydrocortisone or 0.2 mg of prednisone per kilogram body weight per day. Thus, a 10-kg dog (22 lb) on an average day produces an equivalent of 2 mg of prednisone. Slightly larger than physiologic dosages of prednisone (0.25-1.5 mg/kg/day) are considered antiinflammatory and antiallergic, while dosages >2.2 mg/kg/day are considered immunosuppressive.

When greater than physiologic doses of exogenous corticosteroids are given, especially for long periods, the adrenal glands stop producing their own cortisol and may atrophy. Simultaneously, the other tissues of the body are subjected to the abnormally high levels of exogenous corticosteroids. This usually is first manifested by polydipsia, polyuria and polyphagia.

Long-term use may result in diabetes mellitus, since corticosteroids are antagonistic to the effects of insulin. It may also decrease resistance to infection, decrease thyroid and growth hormone levels, decrease the threshold for seizure activity, cause fluid retention, and cause deposition of fat in the liver. Chronic elevation of corticosteroid levels results in iatrogenic hyperadrenocorticism or Cushing's disease. Because of all of these potential side effects, corticosteroids should be cautiously used, especially in diabetes mellitus, pregnancy, young animals, epilepsy, heart or kidney disease, infectious diseases, osteoporosis or GI ulcers.

Why, then, are corticosteroids so commonly prescribed? Properly used, corticosteroids are an important tool in management of many dermatologic conditions. If the allergic season is short or the amount of prednisone required to control clinical signs is small (0.5 mg/kg every other day), there is probably not much danger to corticosteroid therapy apart from some transient side effects.

Start off with a dosage of prednisone that controls the pruritus (1-1.5 mg/kg/day), then gradually reduce the dosage until signs recur. This represents the lowest dosage that will control the problem at that time (Table 6).

When possible, alternate-day therapy should be instituted so that the adrenal glands have an opportunity during the "off" day to produce some cortisol, thus making adrenal atrophy a less likely possibility. Only certain corticosteroids may be used on an alternate-day basis; these should always be the first choice of therapy (Table 7). Repository forms of corticosteroids (Depo-Medrol, Depocoid 40) are a much less desirable alternative and have little or no place in maintenance therapy unless the pet owner is completely unprepared to administer safer medications in tablet form, or in some other extenuating circumstances. Though corticosteroids can be used safely, alternatives should always be considered.

Additional Reading

1. Ferguson, DC: Rational glucocorticoid therapy in small animals. Part 1. *MVP* 66: 101-105, 1985.

2. Ferguson, DC: Rational glucocorticoid therapy in small animals. Part II. *MVP* 66:175-179, 1985.

3. Scott, DW: Dermatologic use of glucocorticoids. *Vet Clin No Am* 12:19-32, 1983.

4. Dillon, AR *et al*: Prednisolone-induced hematologic, biochemical, and histologic changes in the dog. *JAAHA* 16:831-837, 1980.

5. Gallant, C and Kenny, P: Oral glucocorticoids and their complications. *J Am Acad Dermatol* 14:161-177, 1986.

6. Claman, HN: Anti-inflammatory effects of corticosteroids. *Clin Immunol Allergy* 4:317-329, 1984.

Antihistamines

Most mammalian tissues contain histamine. The highest concentrations are found in the skin, lungs and intestines. Mast cells in the tissues and circulating basophils may bind allergic antibodies (IgE) on their surfaces. When triggered by allergens (pollens, molds, house dust), they release their contents of his-

Table 6. Sample schedule for use of corticosteroids.

Drug _____ Strength_____
Give _____ tablet(s) daily for _____ days (___ total tablets)
Then _____ tablet(s) daily for _____ days (___ total tablets)
Then _____ tablet(s) daily for _____ days (___ total tablets)
Then _____ tablet(s) every other day for ____ days (___ total tablets)
Then _____ tablet(s) every other day for ____ days (___ total tablets)
Then _____ tablet(s) every other day for ____ days (___ total tablets)
Total tablets dispensed _____

Table 7. Corticosteroids and their suitability for alternate-day therapy.

Drug	Relative Potency	Equivalent Dose (mg)	Suitable for Alternate-Day Therapy
Hydrocortisone	1	25	no
Prednisone	4	5	yes
Methylprednisolone	5	4	yes
Triamcinolone	5	4	yes
Flumethasone	15	1.5	no
Dexamethasone	30	0.75	no
Betamethasone	30	0.60	no

tamine, which causes an inflammatory reaction. It is this reaction that is blocked by administration of antihistamines.

In dogs it appears that substances other than histamine may be responsible for some pruritus, such as proteolytic enzymes, leukotrienes, serotonin and kinins. Therefore, antihistamines have never been regarded as very effective in this species. The major disadvantage of most of the classic antihistamines is that the large doses required to diminish pruritus in dogs can cause sedation.

Table 8 lists the different classes of antihistamines available and some generic members of those classes. This knowledge has

Table 8. Classes of antihistamines.

Class	Generic Name	Example
Alkylamines	Chlorpheniramine maleate	Chlortripolon
	Brompheniramine maleate	Dimetapp
Ethanolamines	Diphenhydramine HCl	Benadryl
	Clemastine	Tavist
	Doxylamine	Cremacoat 4
Ethylenediamines	Pyrilamine maleate	Triaminic
Phenothiazines	Trimeprazine tartrate	Temaril
	Promethazine	Phenergan
Piperazine	Hydroxyzine HCl	Atarax
Piperidines	Astemizole	Hismanal
	Cyproheptadine HCl	Periactin
	Loratadine	Claritine
	Terfenadine	Seldane

some practical applications in that if an animal does not respond to one antihistamine, it is probably advisable not to attempt therapy with another member of that same class. Administration of an unrelated antihistamine is more productive in this instance. More information on antihistamines is provided in Appendix 1.

The newer antihistamines, such as terfenadine (Seldane, Trilu-dan), loratadine (Claritine) and astemizole (Hismanal), are nonsedative and in fairly large doses can minimize the pruritus of inhalant allergies in many dogs. These antihistamines do not relieve pruritus to the same extent as corticosteroids but nor do they have the problem of side effects. Doxepin is a tricyclic antidepressant with strong antihistaminic activity. It has been used in dogs at 0.5-1 mg/kg BID, but its safety and efficacy have not been investigated.

Table 9 lists antihistamines and their recommended dosages. Please note that these products have not been approved for use, and standardized dosages have not been calculated. These products should only be used with this express understanding. Clinicians prescribing these products do so at their own risk.

Additional Reading

1. Ackerman L: Antihistamines in the treatment of canine allergic skin diseases. *Vet Allergist* 1:1-2, 1986.

2. Flowers, FP *et al*: Antihistamines. *Intl J Dermatol* 25:224-231, 1986.

3. Rosser, Jr EJ: Antipruritic drugs. *Vet Clin No Am* 18:1093-1099, 1988.

Table 9. Antihistamines and recommended dosages for dogs.

Drug	Trade Name	Suggested Dosage
Astemizole	Hismanal	0.1-1 mg/kg SID-BID
Brompheniramine maleate	Dimetane	0.25-0.5 mg/kg BID-TID
Chlorpheniramine maleate	Chlortripolon	0.25-1.0 mg/kg BID-TID
Clemastine	Tavist	0.25-1.0 mg/kg BID
Cyproheptadine	Periactin	0.1 mg/kg BID-TID
Diphenhydramine HCl	Benadryl	1-2 mg/kg BID-TID
Hydroxyzine HCl	Atarax	2.2-4.4 mg/kg TID
Pyrilamine maleate	Triaminic	1-2 mg/kg BID-TID
Terfenadine	Seldane	1-5 mg/kg BID
Trimeprazine tartrate	Temaril	1-2 mg/kg BID

4. Girard, JP *et al*: Double-blind comparison of astemizole, terfenadine and placebo in hay fever with special regard to onset of action. *J Int Med Res* 13:102-108, 1985.

Omega 3 and Omega 6 Fatty Acids

The omega 3 fatty acids include eicosapentanoic acid (EPA), docosapentanoic acid (DPA) and docosahexanoic acid (DHA). Eicosapentanoic acid is chemically similar to arachadonic acid and interferes with formation of leukotrienes, which are important mediators of inflammation. As such, they also block some of the inflammation that causes pruritus in allergic dogs. Products suitable for veterinary use include Derm Caps (DVM), OFA-Plus (NutriSpecialties), EFA-Z Plus (Allerderm), Pet-F.A. Liquid (Beecham), Opticoat II (Natural Animal Nutrition) and EfaVet (Efamol). These products are also discussed in Chapter 7 and Appendix 1.

The omega 6 fatty acids include gamma linolenic acid (GLA). Evening primrose oil, which contains 9% GLA, appears to be the most commonly used source though other products (*eg*, black currant seed oil, borage oil, fungal oil) may contain GLA in higher concentrations.

The positive effects of omega 3 and 6 fatty acids are likely due to enzyme bypass rather than correction of any immune defect.

Most veterinary products (Derm Caps, OFA-Plus, EFA-Z Plus, EfaVet) contain both omega 3 and 6 fatty acids.

Additional Reading

1. Ackerman, L: Omega 3 fatty acids. *Bull Can Acad Vet Dermatol* 3(2):2, 1986.

2. Somer, E: The Omega 3 fatty acids: A review. *Nutrit Rept* 4(6):42-48, 1986.

3. Ackerman, L: Fatty acid supplementation in the treatment of allergic inhalant dermatitis. *Vet Allergist* Fall:4, 1987.

4. Radha, E *et al:* Krill as a dietary source of EPA and DHA in the prevention of cardiovascular disease. *Fed Proc* 45:353, 1986.

5. Miller, Jr WH *et al:* Clinical trial of DVM Derm Caps in the treatment of allergic disease in dogs: A nonblinded study. *JAAHA* 25:163-168, 1989.

Miscellaneous Drugs

Though they may not control signs as well as the corticosteroids, they also do not have harmful side effects. Vitamin C (250-750 mg BID-TID) and aspirin (20 mg/kg TID) may have some minor beneficial effects in relieving pruritus.

Immunotherapy

A long-term alternative is immunotherapy ("allergy shots"), which involves serial injections of progressively larger amounts of the offending allergen(s). The major advantage is that the majority of treated animals respond and have a decreased need for antipruritics. The major disadvantage is that it is a slow process sometimes taking up to a year before improvement is noted in animals that do eventually respond. Symptomatic therapy, preferably with nonsteroidal antipruritics or small alternate-day doses of corticosteroids, may be required to keep an animal comfortable while waiting for immunotherapy to take effect.

"Allergy shots" are given as SC injections in gradually increasing doses to minimize the possibility of anaphylactic reactions. Adverse reactions are very rare in dogs given allergy shots; but to be on the safe side, the animal should be monitored closely for 1-2 hours after each injection.

Any adverse reaction encountered should be treated as a potential emergency but does not necessitate discontinuation of therapy. Mild to moderate reactions can be controlled with a fast-acting injectable antihistamine. Severe reactions should be treated as for shock. Epinephrine (0.2-0.5 ml of 1:10,000 solution) may be given IV every 20-30 minutes as needed. A rapid-acting corticosteroid (hydrocortisone sodium succinate) and oxygen therapy may also be beneficial. If a reaction is noted, the next injection should be reduced 50% in volume and given under strict veterinary supervision.

Immunotherapy solutions may contain aqueous antigens, alum-precipitated antigens or aqueous allergens in a base such as propylene glycol. Alum-precipitated products require fewer injections but are more expensive and have fewer allergens from which to select. Aqueous allergens are fairly inexpensive and include a broad range of allergens but must be given frequently. Adding aqueous allergens to a propylene glycol base (15% of total volume) extends the duration between injections. At this low concentration, propylene glycol appears to cause no pain or postinjection lumps.

There has been no real standardization of immunotherapy schedules. It is best to adhere to the schedule recommended by the dermatologist doing the testing or the manufacturer of the allergen solution. As a general rule, an animal should receive no more than 20,000 PNU per injection.

It is not unusual for animals to require 6-12 months before deriving benefit from immunotherapy. The ultimate success rate of immunotherapy depends on many variables, the most important being proper selection of allergens. The response cannot be objectively measured (IgE levels and skin test results are not altered by immunotherapy); therefore, the client or veterinarian must make a subjective judgment of the success of therapy.

About one-quarter of treated dogs have excellent results, one-quarter have good results, one-quarter have fair results, and one-quarter have poor results. Therefore, if success is defined as some benefit from immunotherapy, 75% is a realistic rate of success. Examiners defining successful treatment as that with excellent or good results can expect a 50% success rate.

What can be done if the allergy shots do not appear to be working? The most common reasons for apparent failure of immunotherapy are parasitic infestations (especially fleas), infections, undiagnosed allergies (foods, untested pollens) and newly developed allergies. Flea infestation and some bacterial infections can be very pruritic and mimic the signs of allergy. Be sure these are not implicated by carefully examining the animal if you suspect that allergic signs are recurring. Also, the dog may not respond completely to allergy shots if some allergens were not initially identified. If the problem is nonseasonal, be sure to evaluate the animal for food allergy.

If allergy shots worked well initially but then became less effective, the animal may have acquired some new allergies. This is particularly true of young animals. Allergy-prone animals may continue to develop new allergies throughout their lives. Allergy testing should be repeated in these cases to identify the new allergens and include them in the immunotherapy. Long-term corticosteroid administration to control pruritus should be considered as a last resort.

Additional Reading

1. Nesbitt, GH et al: Canine atopy—Part II: Management. *Comp Cont Ed Pract Vet* 6:264-278, 1984.

2. Willemse, A et al: Effect of hyposensitization on atopic dermatitis in dogs. *JAVMA* 184:1277-1280, 1984.

ADVERSE REACTIONS TO FOODS

The nomenclature regarding adverse reactions to food has been confusing at best, with many disorders classified as allergy or hypersensitivity without supporting documentation. The preferred term "adverse reaction to a food" refers to any clinically abnormal response attributed to the ingestion of a food or food additive and does not presuppose an etiology.

Adverse reactions to foods may be due to food hypersensitivity or food intolerance. Food hypersensitivity refers to an immunologically mediated adverse reaction to food unrelated to any physiologic effect of the food or food additive. This hypersensitivity reaction may be mediated by IgE (Type-I hypersensitivity) but alternatively may be due to Type-III or Type-IV hypersensitivity reactions. Though IgE may be the principal immunoglobulin capable of sensitizing mast cells and basophils to food antigens, a short-term sensitizing IgG antibody has also been reported in allergic patients.

Food intolerance refers to any abnormal physiologic response to a food not immunologic in nature, and can be further designated as idiosyncrasy, food toxicity (poisoning), pharmacologic reaction or metabolic reaction. Egg whites, strawberries, shellfish, tomatoes and citrus fruits can cause nonimmunologic mast-cell degranulation in certain individuals. Other foods that can cause pharmacologic adverse food reactions contain such vasoactive amines as tyramine, tryptamine (cheese), phenylethylamine (chocolate), caffeine, dopamine (bananas), norepinephrine (tomatoes, avocados), serotonin (cheeses, pineapples) and histamine (fish such as tuna and mackerel can contain large amounts of histamine and saurine if spoiled or stored at high temperatures). Lectins, found in a series of vegetables, fruits and cereals, can cause histamine release by nonspecific binding to mast-cell-fixed IgE.

Toxicities may result from food contaminants, such as bacterial toxins (botulism), endogenous toxins (certain mushrooms, shellfish poisoning), insect parts, molds and mold products (*eg*, in fermented foods such as dried fruits, cheeses, yogurts), and antibiotics. Additives, such as dyes (tartrazine), flavorings and preservatives (nitrites, nitrates, monosodium glutamate, matabisulfites) can also be problematic.

Metabolic reactions may be seen in association with primary gastrointestinal diseases, such that acute clinical signs are evidenced following food ingestion. Examples might be hiatal hernia, gastrointestinal ulceration, cholelithiasis, pancreatic insufficiency and neoplasia. In addition, vascular diseases, such as systemic lupus erythematosus and enzyme deficiencies (*eg*, lactase, glucose-6-phosphate dehydrogenase), may be confused with food hypersensitivity.

Food allergies are an uncommon hypersensitivity, constituting perhaps less than 10% of all allergic disorders. We pursue so strongly the possible diagnosis of this relatively rare disorder because food-allergic pets can be effectively "cured" without medication by simply avoiding the offending foodstuffs. Most other allergies are controlled only by medical intervention.

The most common causes of food allergies are beef, pork, chicken, milk, whey, eggs, fish, corn, soy and preservatives. Since at least some of these ingredients are present in most commercial pet foods, merely changing brands or types of food does not alleviate signs and is therefore useless in trying to confirm a diagnosis of food allergy. Several studies in people have shown that the allergenic fractions of food allergens are usually glycoproteins with a molecular weight of 18,000-36,000 daltons and are generally heat and acid stable.

Hypersensitivity responses to ingested antigens are precise. Any factors that alter the antigenicity of dietary components, such as cooking, processing or digestion, can significantly alter a substance's ability to evoke a specific hypersensitivity response in a sensitized animal.

Much remains unknown about the antigenic properties of foods. Only a few specific food antigens responsible for IgE-mediated reactions have been isolated and characterized; among them are the allergens from codfish, shrimp, peanuts and soybeans. Though more than 20 different proteins are present in cow's milk, only 5 (beta-lactoglobulin, casein, bovine serum albumin, bovine gamma globulin, alpha-lactalbumin) appear to be allergenic. Beta-lactoglobulin, the principal protein of whey, appears to be the most allergenic of the milk proteins. Individuals allergic to beef are not usually sensitive to milk proteins but should avoid veal, liver and gelatin. Individuals hypersensitive to eggs are usually sensitive to proteins in the egg white, which include ovomucoid, lysozyme, ovalbumin and ovotransferrin. Patients allergic to egg usually tolerate chicken meat but not vaccines grown on egg. Fish contains very potent allergens and Allergen M, the major allergen in cod muscle, was the first food allergen isolated. Soy protein is a weak allergen and its allergenicity can be further reduced by heating. Soy protein may cause adverse reactions from the contained lectin. Gluten is the elastic protein in wheat, rye, oat and barley. Gliadin, a component of gluten, has been shown to elicit IgE-mediated allergic reactions in people. About 20 wheat proteins are potentially allergenic, and digestion with proteolytic enzymes markedly reduces the allergenicity of wheat protein.

Clinical Signs

There is no age, sex or breed predisposition reported for adverse reactions to foods though the Shar Pei appears to be overrepresented. Many affected animals have been fed the offending antigen for 2 or more years before development of clinical signs. A high index of suspicion for food hypersensitivity is warranted when a pruritic dermatosis is seen in a very young (<6 months) or very old (>8 years) animal.

Clinical signs of food hypersensitivities may relate to the skin, digestive tract, nervous system and/or respiratory system. The most consistent cutaneous manifestation is a nonseasonal pruritic maculopapular dermatitis, with associated erythema and/or exfoliative dermatitis (Fig 17). The pruritus may be generalized or limited to the head, feet, axillae, inguinal region, or ears. Pruritus may be partially or poorly corticosteroid responsive.

The otitis may be exudative, and is rarely the only clinical sign present. Urticaria and angioedema are also seen in a small percentage of cases. Superficial recurrent pyoderma and/or pyotraumatic dermatitis (hot spots) may also have food hypersensitivity as the underlying cause.

Noncutaneous manifestations in dogs are less common but include gastrointestinal, respiratory and neurologic disorders. This may include vomiting, diarrhea, pruritus ani, flatulence, sneezing, asthma-like conditions, behavioral changes and seizures.

Diagnosis

To diagnose food hypersensitivity, one must identify the antigen, demonstrate a relationship between antigen exposure and a reaction in the patient, and discover the immunologic mechanism involved. Unfortunately, there is no single test to confirm or refute the presence of food hypersensitivity.

The definitive way to diagnose an adverse reaction to food is with a hypoallergenic diet trial. This, however, does not necessarily distinguish a true hypersensitivity reaction from food intolerance. The food used should include a protein and carbohydrate source to which the animal has not been previously exposed. Lamb and rabbit are common hypoallergenic protein sources, since they are not commonly found in commercial diets. Unfortunately, lamb has begun showing up in a variety of new diets (eg, Nature's Recipe, NutroMax, Avoderm, Condition, Wysong) available to pet owners, so it is questionable for how much longer lamb will be a suitable test diet. Chicken, fish, pork and beef are all commonly used in many commercial foods and are therefore not helpful in a hypoallergenic diet trial.

Any of the above suitable protein sources may be mixed with a carbohydrate, such as rice and/or potatoes. The rice should be long grain and not of an "instant" variety. The meal is prepared by mixing 1 part lamb or rabbit to 2 parts rice and/or potatoes. All ingredients should be served boiled and fed in the same total volume as the pet's normal diet. Once cooked, the meal can be packaged in individual portions, frozen and then thawed as needed, greatly decreasing the need for cooking daily. During the trial, hypoallergenic foods and fresh, preferably distilled water must be fed exclusively of all else.

Suitable but less desirable commercial alternatives include canned d/d (Hill's), dry d/d (Hill's), Nature's Recipe, Avoderm,

Nutro Max, Condition and Wysong. A good hypoallergenic diet for small dogs is lamb baby food. These hypoallergenic foodstuffs, together with fresh (preferably distilled) water, must be fed exclusive of all else. Absolutely nothing else must be fed, such as treats, snacks, vitamins, chew toys and even flavored heartworm preventive tablets.

The hypoallergenic food trial must be conducted for at least 3 and preferably 4 weeks to provide useful information. Some authors advocate enemas and a 2-day fast before initiating a food trial. If an adverse reaction to food is the cause of the problem, a noticeable improvement should be seen by the end of the trial. If so, the animal should then be fed its regular diet to see if the problem recurs, confirming that the problem is indeed food related and that remission was not just coincidental.

Allergists in human medicine routinely use intradermal injections of a variety of food antigens to test for food hypersensitivity, but this technique has not gained favor in the veterinary field. For this procedure, dilute aqueous-based allergens are injected intradermally, much like inhalant allergens, and the patient is monitored for immediate and delayed reactions. In people, the negative predictive accuracy is quite good, though the positive predictive accuracy is lower. The sensitivity of this test in dogs is believed to be less than 20%.

In-vitro tests for food hypersensitivity using ELISA and RAST technologies have recently become available for dogs. These tests, as offered, can be very misleading because use of an IgE assay for detecting food allergens has never been validated in dogs. Both tests are of little value as a diagnostic screen. This is not surprising because not all adverse food reactions are immunologic in nature, and those that are may not necessarily be mediated by IgE. Therefore, RAST and ELISA testing should never replace a hypoallergenic food trial as a screening test for food hypersensitivities in pets. More often than not, the results supplied will not prove helpful and can be misleading.

Measurement of circulating IgG and IgE food-immune complexes (in serum samples from human patients) has recently become available from several commercial laboratories. Preliminary evaluation suggests that current evidence could not support the validity of the assay.

In cytotoxicity testing, a specific allergen is added to whole blood or serum leukocyte suspensions and the sample is observed for a reduction in the white blood cell count or death of leukocytes. This procedure has also never been scientifically validated for use in dogs.

Management

Once an adverse reaction to food has been confirmed, numerous alternatives are available. Commercial hypoallergenic diets not only contain few allergenic foodstuffs but are also nutritionally balanced. A balanced homemade hypoallergenic diet can be concocted by mixing 4 oz cooked lamb, 1 cup cooked rice (not instant), 1 tsp vegetable oil and 1.5 tsp dicalcium phosphate. This portion is fed for each 10 kg body weight, providing about 550 kcal of energy. A good vitamin-mineral supplement should also be added if it does not cause a reaction. One can also do further testing to find out which foodstuffs are actually causing the problem, and then feed a commercial dog food that does not contain these ingredients. This can be accomplished by adding 1 new food item each week to the hypoallergenic diet. Fortunately, people and animals with food hypersensitivities usually have reactions to only one or a few substances. Individual foodstuffs (*eg,* beef, liver, pork, chicken, veal, lamb, fish, corn, soy, wheat, milk, egg) can be added to the hypoallergenic diet for 5-7 days, and if they fail to initiate an adverse reaction, it can be assumed that they are tolerated by the pet. For example, if an animal responds well to the hypoallergenic diet trial, one might consider adding some chicken to the diet for a week. If the dog tolerates this, identify some chicken-based dog foods and note their other ingredients. By introducing other chicken-based commercial foods for a week or so each, one can determine which commercial food will be hypoallergenic for that particular animal.

Additional Reading

1. Ackerman, L: Food hypersensitivity: A rare, but manageable disorder. *Vet Med* 83:1142-1148, 1988.

2. Ackerman, L and Lewis, T: Adverse reactions to food. *Vet Allergist* Spring: 2-4, 1989.

3. August, JR: Dietary hypersensitivity in dogs: Cutaneous manifestations, diagnosis, and management. *Comp Cont Ed Pract Vet* 7:469-477, 1985.

4. White, SD: Food hypersensitivity in 30 dogs. *JAVMA* 188:695-698, 1986.

5. White, SD: Food hypersensitivity. *Vet Clin No Am* 18:1043-1048, 1988.

ALLERGIC CONTACT DERMATITIS

Allergic contact dermatitis is a rare form of hypersensitivity in dogs, probably because their dense haircoat largely prevents contact with potential contact allergens. The substances responsible for allergic contact dermatitis are small particles that, on their own, are nonallergenic. When applied to the skin, however, they penetrate the epidermis and bind to carrier proteins in the epidermal cells, forming an allergenic complex. Substances that can cause contact sensitivity in dogs include plants, medications (neomycin, local anesthetics, tar shampoos, flea products), fibers (wool, synthetics), leather, disinfectants, carpet deodorizers and plastics.

Clinical signs of contact sensitivity include inflammation limited predominantly to the sparsely haired regions of the body. With reactions to topical medication, the distribution is confined to the area of application. Reactions to plastic food bowls and chew toys are usually confined to the lips and muzzle.

Diagnostic testing is complicated by the fact that contact sensitivity is common in people but the tests used for confirmation have not been standardized for use in dogs. The history, clinical findings and biopsies for histopathologic examination may be suggestive, but patch testing can confirm the diagnosis.

Biopsies are nonspecific and normally demonstrate epidermal hyperplasia with intercellular edema and a superficial perivascular infiltrate of mononuclear cells, with lymphocytes predominating.

Patch testing is performed by applying test substances to the shaved skin and covering the area with gauze or cloth secured with tape. The sites are then evaluated at 24, 48 and/or 72 hours. One can appreciate the logistic problems in performing this test in dogs.

Commercial contact allergens that may be important in dogs incude carba rubber mix, thiuram mix, epoxy resin, mercapto rubber mix, nickel sulfate and colophony. A commercial patch test kit used with Finn chambers is available from Hermal Pharmaceutical Laboratories.

If the contact allergen is identified, avoidance is the best way to control the problem. Allergy shots (immunotherapy) are not successful in controlling contact allergies, since contact allergies stem from a very different mechanism than inhalant allergies. Oral or topical corticosteroids ease clinical signs but do little to cure the problem.

Allergic contact dermatitis and irritant contact dermatitis may be clinically indistinguishable. Irritant contact dermatitis is due to contact with irritating substances, such that any dog would be affected, not just allergic ones. Animals with sensitive skin especially may be adversely affected by many products that do not cause allergic reactions but rather inflammation due to irritation. Such things as shampoos, detergents, disinfectants, and salt on roadways in winter may be irritating to the skin of dogs. Treatment requires gentle cleansing of the skin with mild shampoos and avoiding contact with the offending substances. Topical corticosteroids may be necessary initially to help reduce inflammation.

Additional Reading

1. Ahmed, AR and Blose, DA: Delayed-type hypersensitivity skin testing. *Arch Dermatol* 119:934-945, 1983.

2. Nesbitt, GH and Schmitz, JA: Contact dermatitis in the dog: A review of 35 cases. *JAAHA* 13:155-163, 1977.

3. Nishioka, K: Allergic contact dermatitis. *Intl J Dermatol* 24:1-8, 1985.

4. Adams, RM and Fisher, AA: Contact allergen alternatives. *J Am Acad Dermatol* 14:951-969, 1986.

5. Bajaj, AK and Gupta, SC: Contact hypersensitivity to topical antibacterial agents. *Intl J Dermatol* 25:103-105, 1986.

6. Comer, KM: Carpet deodorizer as a contact allergen in a dog. *JAVMA* 193:1553-1554, 1988.

7. Kunkle, GA: Contact dermatitis. *Vet Clin No Am* 18:1061-1068, 1988.

DRUG ERUPTION

Drug eruption, an immune-mediated reaction to medication, occurs rarely in dogs. Any drug may be involved. The eruption may be seen after the drug has been given for days or years, or even after the drug has been withdrawn for a few days. Affected dogs have reacted to antibacterials (ampicillin, chloramphenicol, trimethoprim-sulfas), antifungals (griseofulvin, ketoconazole), antiparasitics (thiabendazole, levamisole, diethylcarbamazine), vaccines, topicals, hormones (thyroid hormones, estrogens, progestogens), tranquilizers (acepromazine), antineoplastic agents (etoposide) and other drugs. In fact, any product can result in a drug eruption.

Fixed drug eruptions are quite rare in dogs and are manifested as uniformly well-circumscribed erythematous lesions that may progress to bullae and ulcerations. Hyperpigmentation is a frequent sequel and readministration of the offending substance results in recurrence of the lesion at the same location. Diethylcarbamazine, the heartworm prophylactic drug, has recently been implicated as a potential cause of fixed drug eruption.

Diagnosis is not easy, since a drug eruption can mimic any skin condition except hormonal disorders and cancer (Fig 18). The reaction noted can be confused with parasitism, bacterial or fungal infections, allergies, autoimmune disorders and nutritionally related disorders. Even some skin cancers, especially T-cell lymphoma, which appears as a generalized scaly rash, can be confused with drug eruption.

The history is the most important clue in diagnosing drug eruption. Therefore, one should always obtain a complete history, including use of nutritional supplements, treats and nondermatologic medication, plus any other applicable information. Biopsies may support a diagnosis but are never specific for drug eruption. Palliative treatment usually is successful if use of the offending substance is discontinued, though occasionally the eruption may persist for weeks or months after use of the product has been stopped.

Additional Reading

1. Davis, LE: Hypersensitivity reactions induced by antimicrobial drugs. *JAVMA* 185:1131-1136, 1984.

2. Giger, U *et al:* Sulfadiazine-induced allergy in six Doberman Pinschers. *JAVMA* 186:479-484, 1985.

3. Van Hees, J *et al:* Levamisole-induced drug eruptions in the dog. *JAAHA* 21:255-260, 1985.

4. Mason, KV: Fixed drug eruption in two dogs caused by diethylcarbamazine. *JAAHA* 24:301-303, 1988.

HORMONAL HYPERSENSITIVITY

Hormonal hypersensitivity is a rare maculopapular pruritic dermatosis presumed to be a Type-I or -IV hypersensitivity reaction to endogenous progesterone, estrogen or testosterone. This condition remains speculative until it can be better defined.

Most cases have been reported in intact females, often with a history of false pregnancy or irregular estrous cycles. The condition tends to involve the perineal and caudal thigh areas in a bilaterally symmetric inflammatory pattern. The feet, face, ears, vulva and nipples may also become involved.

Diagnosis is equivocal and based on intradermal testing with aqueous progesterone (0.025 mg), estrogen (0.0125 mg) and testosterone (0.05 mg) and observed for immediate and delayed reactions. Confirmation relies on response to therapy, which involves either ovariohysterectomy or periodic injections of repository testosterone (0.5 mg/kg) or HCG (500 IU IM on alternate days for a total of 4 treatments). Assay of sex hormones has not been helpful and not all affected dogs have demonstrable cystic ovaries.

Additional Reading

1. Chamberlain, KW: Hormonal hypersensitivity in canines. *Canine Pract* 2(5):18-25, 1974.

Chapter 5
Immune-Mediated Skin Disorders

The body's ability to discriminate between its own tissues (self) and foreign material (nonself) is fundamental to the existence of living organisms. The body's immune system is designed to react against nonself and reject foreign material; this is not only normal but essential in most circumstances. Occasionally, however, the body creates autoantibodies and directs its defenses against one or many of its own tissues.

If the target tissue is not very critical to the animal, the process may go unnoticed. If, however, the target organ becomes compromised in its function, adversely affecting the individual, then we are confronted with a clinical picture recognizable as autoimmune disease. In this chapter we will discuss a number of known and suspected autoimmune skin diseases, including lupus erythematosus, pemphigus, pemphigoid, alopecia areata, uveodermatologic syndrome (Vogt-Koyanagi-Harada-like syndrome) and scleroderma.

Lupus Erythematosus

Lupus erythematosus is characterized by multiple circulating autoantibodies that participate in immune-mediated tissue injury directed against the animal's own system. Two forms of the condition have been recognized in animals and people: systemic lupus erythematosus and cutaneous (discoid) lupus erythematosus.

Systemic Lupus Erythematosus

Systemic lupus erythematosus (SLE) appears to result from hyperactivity of the immune system, with a great number of autoantibodies appearing in the bloodstream. These antibodies may be directed against nuclear or cytoplasmic constituents, red blood cells, white blood cells, clotting cells and factors, and ribonucleic acids. There is some evidence to suggest that the disorder may be associated with interaction of a C-type virus with a disturbed immune system in a genetically predisposed host. Collies, Shetland Sheepdogs and Doberman Pinschers are some of the breeds most commonly affected.

The most common clinical findings in dogs with SLE are arthritis, fever unresponsive to antibiotics, kidney disease (glomerulonephritis) with protein loss in the urine, anemia and skin disease. Many other syndromes have been reported in association with this disorder, such as muscle disease (polymyositis), heart disease (myocarditis/pericarditis) and lung disease (pleuritis/pneumonitis). The diversity of clinical presentations and the fact that affected dogs may only have a few signs cause SLE to mimic other syndromes. The skin disorders seen with SLE are also diverse and may include scaling (dandruff), red rashes, scarring, exfoliative dermatoses, pyoderma, lymphedema, rheumatoid-like nodules, hair loss, panniculitis, purpura, loss of pigment and erosive-ulcerative lesions of the mucous membranes (mouth, nose, anus, vulva, penis, nail beds) (Fig 19).

Specific diagnostic testing for SLE includes the lupus erythematosus cell test, the antinuclear antibody test, and biopsy for histopathologic examination, with or without immunopathologic assay.

The antinuclear antibody (ANA) test, performed on serum, detects antibodies directed against cell nuclei. Though it is used as a screening test for lupus erythematosus, it has been reported positive (false positive?) in such diseases as pemphigus erythematosus, thrombocytopenia, endocarditis, heartworm disease, generalized demodicosis, cholangiohepatitis, various neoplasms, autoimmune hemolytic anemia, rheumatoid arthritis, myeloma, autoimmune thyroiditis, atopy, aural hematoma and glomerulonephritis. The test may also be positive in some normal dogs. However, it is a good screening test, and detects up to 90% of affected dogs. Titers of 1:20 or greater are usually considered significant, though each diagnostic laboratory establishes its own reference ranges.

The lupus erythematosus (LE) cell test is performed on clotted or heparinized blood. The tube containing the sample should be slightly shaken to damage the WBC to expose their nuclei to the antibodies used in the test. The WBC that engulf these nuclei are called LE cells. About 60% of affected dogs have LE cells. The LE cell test may also be positive in dogs with autoimmune hemolytic anemia, rheumatoid arthritis, lymphosarcoma, lymphoblastic leukemia, pulmonary granulomatosis and warfarin poisoning. The test is too subjective and not sensitive enough to be recommended as a screening test for LE.

Biopsies taken for histopathologic examination may show changes as variable as the clinical presentation but characteristic changes at the junction between the dermis and epidermis (interface dermatitis) are highly suggestive. Skin biopsies may not be diagnostic and confirmation of the diagnosis may be quite difficult when not all diagnostic criteria are met. Biopsies taken for immunopathologic tests may reveal a positive "lupus band" at the dermal-epidermal junction. The sensitivity of this test in dogs has not yet been determined.

In people, definite criteria established by the American Rheumatism Association must be met before a diagnosis of systemic lupus erythematosus can be made. Following are suggested criteria necessary to establish a diagnosis of systemic lupus erythematosus in dogs. A diagnosis is justified if the dog exhibits 4 or more of these criteria.

Criteria for Diagnosis of SLE

1. Dermatologic presentation as described above, including maculopapular eruptions, scarring alopecia or exfoliative dermatosis.

2. Erosive-ulcerative mucocutaneous lesions.

3. Nonerosive polyarthritis without deformity.

4. Hemolytic anemia, leukopenia and/or thrombocytopenia.

5. Profuse proteinuria with renal casts and characteristic renal biopsy.

6. Generalized lymphadenomegaly.

7. Fever of unknown origin and not responsive to antibiotics.

8. Pleuritis, pericarditis, pneumonitis or myocarditis.

9. Polymyositis or polymyalgia.

10. Vascular lesions such as petechiae, purpura or vasculitis.

11. Positive ANA, LE cell and/or Coombs' tests.

12. Characteristic histopathologic findings of interface dermatitis (either hydropic or lichenoid) or a sterile nodular panniculitis (lobular and/or septal).

13. Positive direct immunofluorescence testing at basement membrane zone.

Treatment of SLE must be individualized for each patient. In general, immunosuppressive doses of corticosteroids are used, with or without chemotherapy (eg, azathioprine, cyclophosphamide), or plasmapheresis (Appendix 1). Chrysotherapy (gold salt therapy) is usually not used because the signs of toxicity with gold are very similar to the clinical presentations of lupus. Therefore, exacerbation of clinical signs while on therapy create a difficult dilemma: is the dosage too low and the disease is not being controlled, or is the dosage too high and the clinical signs manifestations of toxicity? A Chinese herb, tripterygium (leigongteng), is currently being evaluated for its antiinflammatory actions in cases of systemic lupus erythematosus.

Cutaneous (Discoid) Lupus Erythematosus

Cutaneous (discoid) lupus erythematosus (CLE or DLE) is generally regarded as a less harmful variant of SLE, wherein systemic involvement is absent and autoantibodies are rarely found. The most common presenting sign is red, scaling dermatitis of the face (Fig 20).

Histopathologic and immunopathologic findings are identical to those of SLE, but positive ANAs are seen in less than 5% of cases. Increased amounts of mucin in the dermis and/or epidermis in animals with interface dermatitis further support the diagnosis of DLE.

Treatment of DLE differs from that of SLE in that immunosuppressive therapy is usually not warranted. Generally, antiinflammatory dosages of corticosteroids (1.0-1.5 mg/kg daily then tapered to alternate-day therapy), together with vitamin E at 400 IU twice daily, are sufficient to control the condition. Limited exposure to sunlight or use of sunblockers also is likely to benefit patients with DLE.

Additional Reading

1. Ackerman, L and Bargman, H: Postvaccinal signs suggestive of systemic lupus erythematosus in a dog. *MVP* 66:867-870, 1985.

2. Scott, DW et al: Canine lupus erythematosus. I. Systemic lupus erythematosus. *JAAHA* 19:461-479, 1983.

3. Drazner, FH: Systemic lupus erythematosus in the dog. *Comp Cont Ed Pract Vet* 2:243-254, 1980.

4. Grindem, CB and Johnson, KH: Systemic lupus erythematosus: Literature review and report of 42 new canine cases. *JAAHA* 19:489-503, 1983.

5. Monier, JC et al: Systemic lupus erythematosus in a colony of dogs. *Am J Vet Res* 49:46-51, 1988.

6. Scott, DW et al: Canine lupus erythematosus. II. Discoid lupus erythematosus. *JAAHA* 19:481-488, 1983.

7. Walton, DK et al: Canine discoid lupus erythematosus. *JAAHA* 17:851-858, 1981.

8. Wenyan, X et al: Tripterygium in dermatologic therapy. *Intl J Dermatol* 24:152-157, 1985.

Pemphigus

Pemphigus (Greek for blister) describes a complex of disorders characterized by autoantibody deposition within the epidermis, which causes separation of epidermal cells from one another such that spaces are created. Four variants of pemphigus are recognized in animals. Pemphigus vulgaris was first described in 1975, pemphigus foliaceus and pemphigus vegetans in 1977,

Table 1. Diagnostic criteria for pemphigus and pemphigoid.

Disorder	Clinical Signs	Morphologic Findings	Location of Immunoglobulin Deposition
Pemphigus vulgaris	Vesiculobullous, erosive to ulcerative dermatitis, usually involving oral cavity, mucocutaneous junctions, axillae and groin	Suprabasilar acantholysis with cleft and vesicle formation	Intercellular spaces of stratified squamous epithelium
Pemphigus vegetans	Vesiculopustular dermatitis that evolves into verrucous vegetations and papillomatous proliferations, often studded with pustules	Epidermal hyperplasia, papillomatosis, intra-epidermal microabscesses	Intercellular spaces of stratified squamous epithelium
Pemphigus foliaceus	Generalized vesiculobullous, pustular or exfoliative dermatitis, usually beginning on the face and commonly involving the feet, footpads or groin	Subcorneal or intragranular acantholysis, with cleft, vesicle or pustule formation	Intercellular spaces of stratified squamous epithelium
Pemphigus erythematosus	More localized form of pemphigus foliaceus involving the head and ears	Subcorneal or intragranular acantholysis, with cleft, vesicle or pustule formation	Intercellular spaces of stratified squamous epithelium $\pm$ dermal-epidermal junction of stratified squamous epithelium
Bullous pemphigoid	Vesiculobullous, ulcerative dermatitis, with a distribution similar to that of pemphigus vulgaris	Subepidermal cleft and vesicle formation, without acantholysis	Dermal-epidermal junction of stratified squamous epithelium
Cicatricial pemphigoid	More localized form of pemphigoid, usually confined to the oral cavity and mucous membranes	Subepidermal cleft and vesicle formation, without acantholysis	Dermal-epidermal junction of stratified squamous epithelium

and pemphigus erythematosus in 1980. Each differs from the other in terms of clinical presentation and histopathologic and immunopathologic characteristics.

The lesions of pemphigus in people result from binding of an autoantibody to an antigen (or antigens) in or near the epidermal cell membrane. Autoantibodies can be found in the circulation and deposited in the epithelium. The autoantibodies described occur almost exclusively in patients with pemphigus. Autoantibodies are detectable in areas before histologic lesions apear. Autoantibody titers can correspond with disease severity. Plasmapheresis, which reduces the concentration of circulating antibodies, is an effective adjunct to treatment. Pemphigus responds only to immunosuppressive forms of therapy. Pemphigus often is found in association with other autoimmune diseases. Passive autoimmunity has been documented in which neonates born to mothers with pemphigus are affected, presumably transplacentally, but recover completely within weeks. Pemphigus in dogs bears many similarities to its human counterpart and, therefore, the pathomechanisms are presumed to be similar.

Pemphigus Vulgaris

Pemphigus vulgaris (PV) is an ulcerating disease primarily involving nonhaired mucous membranes (*eg,* mouth, anus, conjunctiva, nasal mucosa, vagina, prepuce) and their junctions with the skin, before becoming generalized (Fig 21). Approximately 60% of pemphigus vulgaris patients initially show oral lesions, such as glossitis, stomatitis and gingivitis. These lesions eventually appear in about 90% of cases. Other areas predominantly affected include the groin, axillae, footpads, eyelids and nail beds. Mucous membrane lesions rarely occur as intact blisters because of the fragility of the blister roof. They instead appear as irregularly shaped erosions that bleed easily and heal slowly. Additional findings include epidermal collarettes and a positive Nikolsky's sign. Impression smears may reveal acantholytic keratinocytes with enlarged nuclei and pleomorphic nucleoli. Secondary bacterial complications develop, and severely affected individuals can be anorectic, depressed and febrile. Differential diagnoses include bullous pemphigoid, systemic lupus erythematosus, toxic epidermal necrolysis, drug eruption, cutaneous T-cell-like lymphoma, lymphoreticular neoplasia and ulcerative stomatitis.

Pemphigus Vegetans

Pemphigus vegetans (PVe) is the least common form of pemphigus and is currently believed to be a less harmful variant of PV in individuals with increased resistance to the disease. A combined disorder of B-cell and T-cell systems might be involved in the pathogenesis. In people, pemphigus vegetans is subdivided into Hallopeau and Neumann types, but the Neumann type has not been documented in dogs. In the Hallopeau variety, groups of pustules evolve into eruptive papillomatous lesions and verrucous vegetative masses, often studded with pustules and erosions exuding serum (Fig 22).

Pemphigus Foliaceus

Pemphigus foliaceus (PF) is probably the most common variant in animals and is characterized by a scaling and/or pustular dermatitis that often originates on the head and ears before becoming generalized (Fig 23). Unlike pemphigus vulgaris, mucosal and mucocutaneous involvement is not a prominent feature with this condition. The footpads often become hyperkeratotic. Predominating lesions include crusts, scales, alopecia, erythema, erosions, pustules and epidermal collarettes. Nikolsky's sign can be present. Intact vesicles can appear transiently, but because of their superficial position in the epidermis they are even shorter-lived than the vesicles of pemphigus vulgaris. Vesicles rapidly become purulent but usually are sterile on culture. Secondary infection is less common than expected and animals usually do not become systemically ill. The differential diagnosis includes bacterial folliculitis, dermatophytosis, dermatophilosis, demodicosis, candidiasis, keratinization disorders, systemic lupus erythematosus, pemphigus erythematosus, subcorneal pustular dermatosis, drug eruption, zinc-responsive dermatitis, dermatomyositis, tyrosinemia, cutaneous T-cell-like lymphoma, and lymphoreticular malignancy. Impression smears made from pustules usually reveal numerous detached epidermal cells (acantholytic keratinocytes) mixed with inflammatory cells.

Pemphigus Erythematosus

Pemphigus erythematosus (PE) is indistinguishable from PF clinically and histopathologically but usually remains localized to the head and face. Lesions include erythema, crusting, scaling, oozing, alopecia and erosions bordered by epidermal collarettes. Oral involvement is not a feature of pemphigus erythematosus. Commonly, the nose loses some of its pigment, making it susceptible to sun damage. Differential diagnoses include pemphigus foliaceus, systemic lupus erythematosus, discoid lupus erythematosus, bacterial nasal pyoderma, demodicosis, dermatophytosis, actinic dermatosis, dermatomyositis, epidermolysis bullosa simplex and Vogt-Koyanagi-Harada-like syndrome. It is possible that PE actually represents a crossover or overlap syndrome between lupus erythematosus and pemphigus. This has been suggested because with immunofluorescence testing, there often is immunofluorescence at both the dermal-epidermal junction and in the intercellular spaces.

Diagnosis: Diagnosis of pemphigus relies on clinical examination and biopsies for histopathologic examination, with or without immunopathologic assay. Blister formation within the epidermis is classic but infrequently seen due to the thinness of the epidermis in animals. Multiple, carefully chosen biopsies and careful examination by a competent and patient pathologist may reveal diagnostic changes in about 80% of cases. The characteristic histologic feature of pemphigus vulgaris is suprabasal acantholysis. Clefts and bullae occur between the stratum spinosum and stratum germinativum. The basal cells separate from the overlying epidermal cells and from one another yet remain attached to the basement membrane zone resembling a "row of tombstones." Pemphigus vegetans in characterized by papillomatous epidermal hyperplasia and intraepidermal microabscesses consisting of acantholytic keratinocytes admixed with eosinophils and neutrophils. Clefting can vary in location from suprabasilar to subcorneal. Both pemphigus foliaceus and pemphigus erythematosus are characterized by acantholysis and clefting just beneath the stratum corneum. Marked dyskeratotic changes of the granular layer also help distinguish these from pemphigus vulgaris. Important diagnostic features include numerous acantholytic cells and neutrophils in the blister, hair follicle involvement, and stratum granulosum cells adhering to the roof of the blister.

Direct immunofluorescence testing (immunopathologic examination) may reveal autoantibodies in the intercellular spaces in about 65% of cases. Pemphigus erythematosus may occasionally also show autoantibody deposition at the dermal-epidermal junction. Both kappa and lambda light-chain immunoglobulins have been found in the intercellular spaces of the epithelium in people with pemphigus vulgaris and pemphigus vegetans, while either immunoglobulin light-chain but not both were found in patients with pemphigus foliaceus or erythematosus, the subcorneal variants. It is important to remember that biopsies intended for direct immunofluorescence should be taken from normal-appearing skin adjacent to lesions, since inflammation quickly destroys immunoglobulins in tissue. The sample must then be preserved in Michel's solution and forwarded to laboratories that run this specialized test (see Introduction).

Indirect immunofluorescence is very helpful in diagnosis of pemphigus in people but is unproductive in animals and cannot be relied on at this time.

Cytologic examination is helpful in evaluation of pemphigus patients in that many acantholytic cells admixed with granulocytes is a frequent characteristic finding.

Nikolsky's sign is characteristic of pemphigus, though it may also be seen in toxic epidermal necrolysis and sometimes, in pemphigoid. A positive Nikolsky sign is obtained when finger pressure applied laterally to an erosion or to normal-appearing skin dislodges the epidermis from the dermis and creates a new erosion.

Management: Treatment of all forms of pemphigus is similar but differs in degree, depending on the particular variant involved, the individual susceptibility, and the initial response to therapy. PV is the most aggressive form, followed by PF, with PE and PVe representing the least harmful variants.

Prednisone remains the initial treatment of choice because of its rapid onset of action, low cost and ready availability. Unfortunately, corticosteroids alone are unsatisfactory in most cases, either because of side effects or inability to induce remission. By combining them with other chemotherapeutic agents, such as azathioprine, cyclophosphamide or gold salts, improved efficacy and diminution of side effects can be realized (Appendix 1).

Long-term remissions requiring no additional therapy occur more frequently with gold salts than with any other form of therapy. Thus, corticosteroids, coupled with either azathioprine or gold salts, represent the best long-term choice in treatment of pemphigus. Animals with nasal dermatitis and depigmentation also benefit from application of commercial sunscreens and confinement during peak periods of sunshine.

Chapter 5

Pemphigoid

Pemphigoid (Greek for pemphigus-like) refers to a complex of blistering conditions characterized by autoantibody deposition at the junction between the epidermis and dermis, with blister formation immediately deep to the epidermis. Pemphigoid differs from pemphigus in that cleft formation is subepidermal rather than within the epidermis. Current evidence suggests that bullous pemphigoid in people is an autoimmune inflammatory disorder in which autoantibodies are directed against an antigen found in the lamina lucida of the basement membrane zone of squamous epithelium. Evidence indicates that circulating bullous pemphigoid autoantibodies alone are pathogenic but that both antibody and complement must be present to initiate dermal-epidermal separation.

Of the 3 variants of pemphigoid recognized in people, only bullous pemphigoid has been well documented in animals. A suspected case of cicatricial pemphigoid has been reported.

Bullous Pemphigoid

Bullous pemphigoid (BP) has a similar distribution to pemphigus vulgaris, the principal lesions being transient blisters, crusts, epidermal collarettes and ulcerations (Fig 24). The blisters are more apparent than in pemphigus because of their deeper, subepidermal location. The mucous membranes, head, neck, axillae, ventral abdomen and footpads are particularly susceptible regions. There is an apparent breed predilection for Collies, Shetland Sheepdogs, and perhaps Doberman Pinschers. Differential diagnoses include pemphigus vulgaris, systemic lupus erythematosus, toxic epidermal necrolysis, drug eruption, cutaneous T-cell-like lymphoma, lymphoreticular neoplasia, ulcerative stomatitis and hidradenitis suppurativa.

Impression smears made from these blisters may reveal inflammatory cells but few or no detached epidermal cells.

Characteristic biopsies display subepidermal clefting without acantholysis, but regeneration of the epithelium at the floor of the bullae can occur quickly enough to give the impression of an intraepidermal bulla. The bullae can contain proteinaceous material admixed with a few neutrophils, eosinophils and mononuclear cells.

With direct immunofluorescence, a linear or globular deposit of immunoglobulin and/or complement often appears at the dermal-epidermal junction. A linear pattern of immunofluorescence in this region also can be compatible with several other diagnoses, including lupus erythematosus, cicatricial pemphigoid, linear IgA disease, dermatitis herpetiformis, vesicular pemphigoid and epidermolysis bullosa acquisita.

The indirect immunofluorescent test, performed on serum, is frequently positive in people with pemphigoid but has proven unreliable in animals.

Cicatricial Pemphigoid

Cicatricial or mucous membrane pemphigoid is a chronic blistering disease affecting primarily the mucous membranes of the mouth and eyes. No cases have been well documented in animals, though suspect cases have been recognized.

Like bullous pemphigoid, cicatricial pemphigoid is diagnosed by clinical, histopathologic and immunopathologic examinations. The classic biopsy changes include blister formation deep to the epidermis. On immunopathologic examination, autoantibody and/or complement deposition is seen at the dermal-epidermal junction.

Management: Treatment of pemphigoid is identical to that of pemphigus and includes corticosteroids, adjuvant chemotherapy with azathioprine, 6-mercaptopurine, cyclophosphamide and chrysotherapy. Cicatricial pemphigoid usually does not require such drastic therapy and may respond to topical corticosteroids. Topical cyclosporine A (1-2%) may also be effective in cicatricial pemphigoid involving the ocular mucous membranes.

Additional Reading

1. Ackerman, LJ: Pemphigus and pemphigoid in the dog and cat. Part I. Pemphigus. *Comp Cont Ed Pract Vet* 7:89-97, 1985.

2. Ackerman, LJ: Pemphigus and pemphigoid in the dog and cat. Part II. Pemphigoid. *Comp Cont Ed Pract Vet* 7:281-286, 1985.

3. Ackerman, LJ: Pemphigus and pemphigoid in domestic animals: An overview. *Can Vet J* 26:185-189, 1985.

4. Ackerman, L: Pemphigus and pemphigoid in dogs and cats. Part I: Clinical signs, diagnosis and treatment. *MVP* 67:260-265, 1986.

5. Ackerman, L: Pemphigus and pemphigoid in dogs and cats. Part II: A clinical survey. *MVP* 67:358-360, 1986.

Chapter 5

Uveodermatologic Syndrome
(Vogt-Koyanagi-Harada-like Syndrome)

The cause of uveodermatologic syndrome, or Vogt-Koyanagi-Harada-like (VKH) syndrome, is unknown, but it may represent an autoimmune attack against pigment-producing cells, the melanocytes, or possibly an abnormal response to a viral infection. The condition is characterized by a serious eye disorder (granulomatous panuveitis) and concurrent loss of pigment from the nose, lips, eyelids and occasionally the entire body (Fig 25). Unlike affected people, dogs appear to rarely have any neurologic involvement. Most affected individuals are young adults. The acute blindness that accompanies the syndrome is usually more alarming than the loss in pigment.

Diagnosis of uveodermatologic syndrome relies on biopsies of affected tissues for histopathologic evaluation. There is a pronounced inflammatory reaction at the dermal-epidermal junction. Melanocyte numbers within the epidermis are markedly reduced. The inflammatory component is strongly histiocytic, unlike the condition in people.

The mainstay of therapy is topical and/or systemic corticosteroids. Once blindness has occurred, return of sight is unlikely, but early therapeutic intervention is usually successful. Repigmentation may be complete, partial or unsubstantial.

Additional Reading

1. Bussanich, MN et al: Granulomatous panuveitis and dermal depigmentation in dogs. JAAHA 18:131-138, 1982.

2. Kern, TJ et al: Uveitis associated with poliosis and vitiligo in six dogs. JAVMA 187:408-414, 1985.

3. Romatowski, J: A uveodermatological syndrome in an Akita dog. JAAHA 21:777-780, 1985.

4. Cottrell, BD and Barnett, HC: Harada's disease in the Japanese Akita. J Small Anim Pract 28:517-521, 1987.

5. Kaswan, RL et al: Topically applied cyclosporin for modulation of induced immunogenic uveitis in rabbits. Am J Vet Res 49:1757-1759, 1988.

Alopecia Areata

Alopecia areata literally means "an area of hair loss." The lesion in alopecia areata is a well-circumscribed smooth patch of nonscarring hair loss that may persist, remit or expand (Fig 26). It is usually not accompanied by any significant inflammatory reaction. The exact pathogenesis in people is unknown, but there is some circumstantial evidence that autoimmunity is involved, including an association with other autoimmune disorders. Furthermore, direct immunofluorescence testing may reveal deposits of C_3 and occasionally IgG or IgM along the basement membrane zone of hair follicles or the intercellular spaces of the external root sheath. Also noted are an increased frequency of a variety of circulating organ-specific autoantibodies, a decrease in the number of circulating T-cells, and a favorable response to topical, intralesional and systemic corticosteroids.

Diagnosis of alopecia areata is confirmed by the characteristic biopsy finding of an inflammatory infiltrate that surrounds the lower half of the growing hair follicle. In the later stages, when the inflammation has passed, there is an absence of growing hairs, much like that seen with hormonal disorders. Direct immunofluorescence testing may be of some benefit.

Therapy in people may include intralesional, topical or systemic corticosteroids, topical irritants (eg, phenol, benzyl benzoate, UV light), contact allergens (eg, DCNB, squaric acid dibutyl ester), photochemotherapy (PUVA), vasodilators (eg, minoxidil) or immunostimulants (eg, inosiplex), while other cases undergo spontaneous remission. Since the animal's health is usually not affected and the problem is more of a cosmetic concern, if any treatment is indicated at all, probably topical or intralesional corticosteroids should be considered the treatment of choice.

An interesting form of therapy in people is minoxidil, a potent vasodilator used in treatment of severe hypertension. In a 1-2% topical solution in a vehicle of ethanol, propylene glycol and water, it is used to grow hair not only in patients with alopecia areata but with male pattern baldness as well. I have done some work with the product Rogaine (Upjohn) in dogs but I cannot yet recommend its use, pending further assessment.

Additional Reading

1. Nelson, DA and Spielvogel, RL: Alopecia areata. *Intl J Dermatol* 24:26-34, 1985.

2. Mitchell, AJ and Krull, EA: Alopecia areata: Pathogenesis and treatment. *J Am Acad Dermatol* 11:763-778, 1984.

Scleroderma

Scleroderma is a connective tissue disease characterized by thickening and firmness of the skin. It can occur as a localized phenomenon (morphea) or as a systemic and often fatal variant (progressive systemic sclerosis). Only the localized form has been documented in dogs. The systemic disorder, characterized by fibrotic and degenerative changes of the skin, muscles, joints and viscera, has been further subdivided into 2 forms: diffuse and the CREST syndrome (calcinosis, Raynaud's, esophageal dysfunction, sclerodactyly, telangiectasia). In people, autoimmunity may play a role in the condition; ANAs of diffuse scleroderma are present, directed against a 4-6S RNA, in 40-50% of cases. Anticentromere antibodies are found in 80-90% of CREST patients. Immunoglobulin deposits may be found at the dermal-epidermal junction and in perivascular patterns in some patients. Circulating immune complexes are demonstrable in almost 50% of cases. Rheumatoid factor may also be present.

Diagnosis is made by physical and histopathologic examination. The lesions evolve from an inflammatory infiltrate in the deep dermis and panniculus to a fibrous, scarring end-stage. On biopsy alone it is impossible to distinguish between the localized and systemic forms. Early scleroderma shows a lymphocytic inflammatory infiltrate in the deep dermis and subcutaneous fat. Hyalinized or sclerotic collagen later dominates the dermis and subcutis. The localized morphea-like form of scleroderma has recently been recognized in dogs.

Treatment is often attempted with topical or systemic corticosteroids. While the localized forms are often relatively benign, the systemic forms often eventuate in degenerative and scarring changes of the muscles, joints and internal organs.

Additional Reading

1. Doyle, JA *et al*: Cutaneous and subcutaneous inflammatory sclerosis syndromes. *Arch Dermatol* 118: 886-890, 1984.

2. Lee, EB *et al*: Pathogenesis of scleroderma. *Intl J Dermatol* 23:85-89, 1984.

3. Scott, DW: Localized scleroderma (morphea) in two dogs. *JAAHA* 22:207-211, 1986.

Sjogren's Syndrome

Sjogren's syndrome is a sicca complex characterized by dry eyes (keratoconjunctivitis sicca) and a dry mouth (xerostomia), coupled with an autoimmune connective tissue disease. This syndrome may overlap with rheumatoid arthritis and SLE. Lymph node and parotid gland enlargement, myositis, arthritis and kidney disease may also be seen.

Sjogren's syndrome should be considered in dogs with the signs described above. Biopsy of the lacrimal glands shows periductal or diffuse mononuclear-cell invasion, fibrocytic replacement of acinar elements, and lymphoid nodules. Of dogs with keratoconjunctivitis sicca, 42% have a positive ANA test and 34% are positive for rheumatoid factor.

Treatment may be attempted with topical or systemic corticosteroids.

Additional Reading

1. Kaswan, RL *et al*: Keratoconjunctivitis sicca: Histopathological study of nictitating membrane and lacrimal glands from 28 dogs. *Am J Vet Res* 45:112-118, 1984.

2. Kaswan, HL *et al*: Rheumatoid factor determination in 50 dogs with keratoconjunctivitis sicca. *JAVMA* 183:1073-1075, 1983.

Chapter 6

Endocrine Skin Disorders

A number of disorders of the endocrine system can cause cutaneous manifestations. The most common are hypothyroidism, hyperadrenocorticism and growth hormone-responsive dermatosis. Most hormones are regulated by a negative-feedback mechanism much like the thermostat in a house. As the blood level of a hormone drops, a stimulus is given to secrete more hormone. When the blood value is too high, the stimulus is eliminated and the value drops once again. The thermostat-like regulator for most hormones is found in the brain, usually in the pituitary gland or hypothalamus.

Additional Reading

1. Kemppainen, RJ and Sartin, JL: Evidence for episodic but not circadian activity in plasma concentrations of adrenocorticotrophin, cortisol and thyroxine in dogs. *Endocrin* 103:219-226, 1984.

2. Reimers, TJ: Radioimmunoassays and diagnostic tests for thyroid and adrenal disorders. *Comp Cont Ed Pract Vet* 4:65-75, 1982.

Hypothyroidism

Hypothyroidism is the most commonly diagnosed endocrine disorder in dogs and reflects a low level of thyroid hormones in the blood. The thyroid gland produces 2 hormones, thyroxine (T_4) and 3,5,3-triiodothyronine (T_3). Thyroid-stimulating hormone (TSH) released from the pituitary gland stimulates the thyroid gland to secrete these hormones, predominantly T_4. In turn, thyrotropin-releasing hormone (TRH) from the hypothalamus stimulates the pituitary gland to secrete TSH. At least one-third of all T_4 produced by the thyroid gland is converted to T_3, principally in the liver and kidney. T_3 is 3-4 times more potent than T_4. More than 99% of T_3 and T_4 circulates in the blood tightly bound to proteins. Only the free, unbound hormone circulating in the blood is actually available to tissues. Hypothyroidism may be due to low circulating blood levels of either T_3 or T_4.

Clinical Signs

The clinical presentation of hypothyroid dogs is quite diverse, and affected dogs may have one or more of the following characteristics: noninflammatory hair loss equally distributed along both sides of the back (bilaterally symmetric alopecia); dull, dry, lusterless haircoat; increased pigmentation of the skin; secondary scaling and oiliness of the skin; chronic bacterial infections on the skin surface; tendency towards obesity; lethargy; inability to tolerate cold; a "tragic" facial expression; and puffiness under the skin (myxedema). In the most extreme form of hypothyroidism, animals may become comatose. Other affected animals may appear clinically normal. A great many breeds are prone to developing hypothyroidism, including Akitas, Chow Chows, Great Danes, Irish Wolfhounds, Boxers, English Bulldogs, Dachshunds, Afghans, Newfoundlands, Malamutes, Doberman Pinschers, Brittany Spaniels, Poodles, Golden Retrievers, Irish Setters, Shar Peis and Schnauzers.

Diagnosis

Hypothyroidism may be suspected on the basis of the history, clinical signs, blood test results and skin biopsy (Fig 27). Nonspecific findings include anemia in about one-quarter of cases, high circulating levels of cholesterol in about one-third of cases and elevated levels of creatine phosphokinase in about half of cases. Skin biopsies may suggest a hormonal disorder (telogen follicles predominating, adnexal atrophy, orthokeratotic hyperkeratosis, etc) but are usually not specific for hypothyroidism.

The diagnosis must be confirmed by evaluating thyroid hormone levels in the blood. The best method of detection is still a matter of great controversy, as thyroid function testing is a continuously evolving science.

Baseline Levels: A test measuring simply T_3 and T_4 levels is easy to perform and inexpensive but quite unreliable, since thyroid hormone levels fluctuate greatly throughout the day. There is thus a great interpretative problem, since at any one time, thyroid levels may be normal in 30-60% of hypothyroid dogs and abnormal in 20% of normal dogs.

TSH Stimulation: The classic diagnostic test has been the TSH stimulation test, in which baseline blood T_3 and T_4 levels are determined, 2.5-5.0 IU TSH are injected IV and a second blood sample is obtained in 4-6 hours. This measures the ability of the thyroid gland to respond to maximal stimulation and is a useful test, though TSH is expensive and difficult to obtain. It may be purchased commercially as a veterinary product (Dermathycin: Wellcome) or as a human product (Thytropar: Harris) available from pharmacies. Levels of T_3 double earlier than those of T_4, perhaps by 1-2 hours poststimulation. The TSH stimulation test is less helpful in evaluating secondary (pituitary) or tertiary (hypothalamic) hypothyroidism caused by inadequate secretions of TSH or TRH, respectively. Reconstituted TSH can be safely refrigerated for 3 weeks. Freezing may extend its usefulness further (months), though this has not been conclusively demonstrated.

TSH Assay: A TSH assay (Canadian Bioclinical) is currently being evaluated. This test measures endogenous blood TSH levels, making it a potentially useful test for pituitary- and thyroid-dependent hypothyroidism. The results of these investigations are pending but do not appear to be as optimistic as originally hoped.

TRH Stimulation: The TRH stimulation test is another alternative currently being evaluated. TRH is given IV at 0.1 mg/kg and serum is collected 4-6 hours later. An increase of 1.5 times over basal T_4 levels is considered normal. Apparently, short-term freezing does not adversely affect the potency of TRH but post-injection levels may not be as high as those seen with TSH. Potential side effects of TRH administration include salivation, vomiting, tachycardia, tachypnea, pupillary dilation, urination and defecation.

Free Thyroxine and Triiodothyronine Levels: A recently developed test measures not only the total T_3 and T_4 values but also the free levels available to the tissues. This test requires only 1.5 ml of serum and is relatively inexpensive. It appears to be reliable but has not been used long enough to be extensively evaluated. It is available through the Animal Health Diagnostic Laboratory, Michigan State University (address may be found in Appendix 3). The test not only measures thyroid hormone levels but also may indirectly predict circulating T_3 autoantibodies.

Abnormal triiodothyronine-binding factor may interfere with the radioimmunoassay for total T_3. Spuriously low or high results are due to interference from the autoantibody with the RIA antibody.

Predictive Formulas: Recently, K values have been proposed to enhance the accuracy of diagnosis of primary hypothyroidism. The K value is obtained using the linear discriminant formula K = 0.5 x basal T_4 (in nmol/L) plus the increase in T_4 following TSH stimulation. Animals with K values of <15 may be hypothyroid, while those with a K value of >30 are normal or treatment nonresponsive. Time and continued research will tell. Similarly, if free levels of thyroxine were determined, a K value could be obtained with the linear discriminant formula K = 0.7 x free T_4 (in pmol/L) minus cholesterol (in mmol/L). Dogs with a K-value of ≤-4 are considered hypothyroid, while those with values >+1 are considered normal or nonresponsive to treatment. I am cautious using this formula, since cholesterol is highly variable in both hypothyroid and euthyroid dogs and I am not convinced it will significantly improve predictive value. Clinical trials are warranted.

Thyroid Autoantibodies: Autoantibody to thyroglobulin can be detected by specialty laboratories but such assays are generally not available to most practitioners. Thyroglobulin autoantibodies occur with greater frequency in dogs with clinical hypothyroidism or other endocrine diseases than in normal dogs. There appears to be a genetic predilection; Great Danes, Irish Setters and Old English Sheepdogs have an increased occurrence of autoantibodies. In some dogs, autoantibody may indicate impending thyroid failure.

Antithyroid autoantibodies can interfere with RIA of thyroid hormones if the titer is high enough to bind a considerable fraction of the radiolabeled hormone used in the RIA procedure.

The endocrinology laboratory at Michigan State University is now measuring for actual T_3 and T_4 autoantibodies, with normal ranges of 0-10% for the former and 0-25% for the latter. Continued evaluation is necessary.

Nonthyroidal Illness

Many dogs evaluated for thyroid function have values only considered borderline normal. Some of these dogs are actually hypothyroid, but probably many more have nonthyroidal illness. Many medications, especially corticosteroids, profoundly influence the levels of thyroid hormones in circulation. Marked decreases may be seen with any disease causing anorexia for more than 2 days. These animals could be put on a 6-week trial course of thyroid supplementation, but an alternative is to measure the circulating levels of reverse T_3 (rT_3). Elevated serum levels of rT_3 provide supportive evidence that the disorder is in fact a nonthyroidal illness so that you can begin further patient assessment, rather than wasting time and money on thyroid supplementation unlikely to benefit the patient.

Management

Treatment of hypothyroid dogs is easy and relatively inexpensive, and involves supplementing the dog with either T_4 (eg, Synthroid or Eltroxin) at 20 μg/kg BID (0.1 mg/10 lb BID) or at dosages of 0.5 mg per square meter of body surface area. T_3 (Cytobin or Cytomel) is usually given at 4.4 μg/kg TID daily for life. Supplementation with T_3 alone may provide sufficient hormone for most organs, but the brain and pituitary gland derive most of their T_3 from T_4 and may still manifest a deficiency. Thyroid levels should be monitored periodically to ensure that values remain within normal limits. Patients should be reevaluated 6 weeks after commencing twice-daily therapy with thyroxine. If levels are well into normal range, once daily dosing should be considered. If levels remain normal in another 6 weeks, reevaluation only need be done on an annual basis unless problems arise.

Additional Reading

1. Ferguson, DC: Thyroid function tests in the dog: Recent concepts. *Vet Clin No Am* 14:783-808, 1984.

2. Nesbitt, GH et al: Canine hypothyroidism: A retrospective study of 108 cases. *JAVMA* 177:1117-1122, 1980.

3. Lorenz, MD and Stiff, ME: Serum thyroxine content before and after thyrotropin stimulation in dogs with suspected hypothyroidism. *JAVMA* 177:78-81, 1980.

4. Oliver, JW and Held, JP: Thyrotropin stimulation test-new perspective on value of monitoring triiodothyronine. *JAVMA* 187:931-934, 1985.

5. Lothrop, CD Jr et al: Canine and feline thyroid function assessment with the thyrotropin-releasing hormone response test. *Am J Vet Res* 45:2310-2313, 1984.

6. Haines, DM et al: Survey of thyroglobulin autoantibodies in dogs. *Am J Vet Res* 45:1493-1497, 1984.

7. Oliver, JW and Waldrop, V: Sampling protocol for thyrotropin stimulation test in the dog. *JAVMA* 182:486-489, 1983.

8. Young, DW et al: Abnormal canine triiodothyronine binding factor characterized as a possible triiodothyronine autoantibody. *Am J Vet Res* 46:1346-1350, 1985.

9. Rosychuk, RAW et al: Serum concentrations of thyroxine and 3,5,3-triiodothyronine in dogs before and after administration of freshly reconstituted or previously frozen thyrotropin-releasing hormone. *Am J Vet Res* 49:1722-1725, 1988.

10. Larsson, MG: Determination of free thyroxine and cholesterol as a new screening test for canine hypothyroidism. *JAAHA* 24:209-217, 1988.

11. Ferguson, DC: The effect of nonthyroidal factors on thyroid function tests in dogs. *Comp Cont Ed Pract Vet* 10:1365-1377, 1988.

12. Chastain, CB *et al*: Anti-triiodothyronine antibodies associated with hypothyroidism and lymphocytic thyroiditis in a dog. *JAVMA* 194:531-534, 1989.

13. Rachofsky, MA *et al*. Clinical relevance of results from the new canine specific endogenous thyroid stimulating hormone assay: A review of 79 cases. *Southwestern Vet* 38:30-33, 1988.

Hyperadrenocorticism (Cushing's Disease)

Hyperadrenocorticism is due to high circulating blood levels of cortisol. Corticotropin-releasing factor (CRF) is produced in the hypothalamus, causing production of adrenocorticotropic hormone (ACTH) by the pituitary gland. ACTH then stimulates the adrenal gland to produce cortisol. This thermostat-like negative-feedback mechanism is very similar to that of thyroid hormones. Blood cortisol levels do not follow a circadian rhythm as was once thought, but are released in periodic bursts. Because of this phenomenon, it is usually impossible to arrive at a diagnosis from a single determination of the blood cortisol level.

Cortisol exerts an effect on many organs of the body. A high circulating level of cortisol may be caused by diseases of the pituitary or adrenal glands, a defective feedback mechanism or use of corticosteroids to treat various medical conditions. Animals stressed by such chronic conditions as diabetes mellitus, liver disease and kidney disease may have abnormal cortisol levels supposedly related to an adaptive change in the hypothalamic-pituitary-adrenal axis.

Clinical Signs

The clinical signs of cortisol excess may include one or more of the following: increased thirst (polydipsia); increased urination (polyuria); increased hunger (polyphagia); noninflammatory hair loss equally distributed along both sides of the back (bilaterally symmetric alopecia); thinning of the skin; plugging of the hair follicles on the abdomen with blackheads (comedones); vascular dilatations (phlebectasias); increased susceptibility to infection; pot-bellied appearance; muscle atrophy; an enlarged liver due to fatty deposits; and abnormal behavior. In addition, animals may have neurologic signs (*eg*, rotary nystagmus, symmetric tetraparesis) as a result of large, compressive pituitary tumors. Hypertension is seen in a considerable number of cases (perhaps 60%). Various breeds are prone to hyperadrenocorticism, especially the Boxer, Boston Terrier, Poodle and Dachshund.

Diagnosis

Hyperadrenocorticism may be suspected on the basis of the history, clinical signs, blood and urine test results, and skin biopsy (Fig 28). Nonspecific findings include abnormal urinalysis results (eg, low specific gravity, concurrent urinary tract infection with bacteriuria, concurrent diabetes mellitus with glucosuria), increased serum alkaline phosphatase activity (in about 80% of cases), hypercholesterolemia, hyperglycemia and elevated activity of serum alanine transaminase (SALT, formerly SGPT). Blood counts may reveal a stress leukogram. Radiography may reveal hepatomegaly, osteoporosis, dystrophic mineralization or even calcified adrenal tumors.

The diagnosis must be confirmed by measuring adrenal hormone levels in the blood. The best way to do this is a matter of much controversy. Because cortisol is released from the adrenal glands in periodic bursts, assays of single samples alone are rarely diagnostic and not of much practical value. Hyperadrenocorticism is most accurately diagnosed by either the ACTH stimulation test or a low-dose dexamethasone suppression test.

ACTH Stimulation Test: The ACTH stimulation test is accomplished by taking a blood sample for baseline cortisol level, injecting ACTH IM at 2.2 IU/kg to a maximum of 40 IU and taking a second blood sample for cortisol assay in 2 hours. The diagnostic premise is that although cortisol is secreted in periodic bursts and blood cortisol levels vary considerably throughout the day, an injection of ACTH stimulates the adrenal glands maximally to release cortisol at the highest rate possible. Since normal animals with normal adrenal mass cannot respond to ACTH stimulation with blood cortisol levels above the normal range, animals that respond with blood cortisol levels significantly above normal levels are likely to have increased adrenal size. This does not mean that the poststimulation cortisol levels must be 2-5 times normal, since these determinations depend on the resting cortisol values. Thus, a dog with a resting cortisol level of 40 nmol/L (1.3 μg/dl) and a poststimulation cortisol level of 300 nmol/L (10 μg/dl) would still be considered normal, whereas a dog with a resting cortisol level of 300 nmol/L and poststimulation level of 500 nmol/L (20 μg/dl) is in the diagnostic range of Cushing's disease.

ACTH is inexpensive and may be purchased commercially as a veterinary product (*eg*, Austin or Quantum) or as a human product (*eg*, Acthar: Harris or Cosyntropin: Organon). The test is 85% diagnostic and the adrenal glands of animals with hyperadrenocorticism are usually stimulated to secrete cortisol well above normal levels. Some drawbacks are that dogs with iatrogenic Cushing's disease often have low-normal cortisol levels due to exogenous corticosteroid administration, and up to half of dogs with adrenal tumors fail to hyperrespond. The adrenal carcinoma patients tend to hyperrespond more frequently and have a higher response than do dogs with adenomas. The test also fails to differentiate adrenal- from pituitary-related disease. Its advantages are that ACTH is inexpensive, the test can be performed in as little as 2 hours, it is diagnostic about 85% of the time, and if animals go on medical therapy, the ACTH stimulation test is the one used to monitor patients.

Low-Dose Dexamethasone Suppression Test: The low-dose dexamethasone suppression test is accomplished by taking a blood sample for a baseline cortisol value, injecting dexamethasone IV at 0.015 mg/kg and measuring cortisol levels at intervals over an 8-hour period. The most important time interval is 6-8 hours, but a sample taken at 3-4 hours is sometimes also helpful. The test is based on the premise that administration of corticosteroids decreases secretion of ACTH through CNS and pituitary negative-feedback inhibition in normal animals.

In hyperadrenocorticism, the pituitary-adrenal axis controlling ACTH and/or cortisol secretion is abnormally resistant to suppression by dexamethasone. The test is considered about 90% diagnostic, and normal dogs show postinjection levels less than 30 nmol/L (1.0 μg/dl) cortisol by 8 hours. Most dogs with Cushing's disease due to either pituitary or adrenal disease fail to respond at all, have values not below 30 nmol/L (1.0 μg/dl) or do not have suppressed levels by 8 hours. Once again, it is not necessary that cortisol levels are suppressed by 50% to be diagnostic, since it does not take into consideration the presuppression cortisol value. The low-dose dexamethasone suppression test does not distinguish between adrenal-dependent and pituitary-dependent Cushing's disease.

over the first week, then gradually reduced while the remaining adrenal gland takes over cortisol production).

About half of all dogs surviving surgery succumb to postoperative complications, such as acute renal failure, pneumonia and thromboembolism. If the diagnosis was adrenal carcinoma, hyperadrenocorticism will likely recur at some point, despite surgery. With an adrenal carcinoma and liver metastasis, o'p'DDD at 50-150 mg/kg/day may postpone the inevitable.

Additional Reading

1. Chastain, et al: Evaluation of the hypothalamic-pituitary-adrenal axis in clinically stressed dogs. *JAAHA* 22:435-442, 1986.

2. Emms, SB et al: Adrenalectomy in the management of canine hyperadrenocorticism. *JAAHA* 23:557-564, 1987.

3. Feldman, EC: Comparison of ACTH response and dexamethasone suppression as screening tests in canine hyperadrenocorticism. *JAVMA* 182:506-510, 1983.

4. Feldman, EC: Distinguishing dogs with functioning adrenocortical tumours from dogs with pituitary-dependent hyperadrenocorticism. *JAVMA* 182:195-199, 1983.

5. Feldman, EC: Effect of functional adrenocortical tumors on plasma cortisol and corticotropin concentrations in dogs. *JAVMA* 178:823-826, 1981.

6. Lester, SJ et al: A rapid radioimmunoassay method for the evaluation of plasma cortisol levels and adrenal function in the dog. *JAAHA* 17:121-128, 1981.

7. Peterson, ME: Hyperadrenocorticism. *Vet Clin No Am* 14:731-750,1984.

8. Scavelli, TD et al: Results of surgical treatment for hyperadrenocorticism caused by adrenocortical neoplasia in the dog: 25 cases (1980-1984). *JAVMA* 189:1360-1364, 1986.

9. Voorhout, G et al: Computed tomography in the diagnosis of canine hyperadrenocorticism not suppressible with dexamethasone. *JAVMA* 192:641-646, 1988.

10. Sarfaty, D et al: Neurologic, endocrinologic, and pathologic findings associated with large pituitary tumors in dogs: Eight cases (1976-1984). *JAVMA* 193:854-856, 1988.

11. Bruyette, DS and Feldman, EC: Ketoconazole and its use in the management of canine Cushing's disease. *Comp Cont Ed Pract Vet* 10:1379-1386, 1988.

12. White, SD et al: Cutaneous markers of canine hyperadrenocorticism. *Comp Cont Ed Pract Vet* 11:446-464, 1989.

Growth Hormone-Responsive Dermatosis

Growth hormone-responsive dermatosis has only been recognized in recent years and has been presumed due to decreased growth hormone levels in the blood. If an animal is deficient in growth hormone since birth, it becomes a dwarf. A unique adult-onset acquired condition probably related to the hormone has been reported, but evidence is circumstantial. Growth hormone is not regulated by the same thermostat-like negative feedback as are the thyroid and adrenal hormones, but rather by intermediate insulin-like growth factors called somatomedins.

O'p'DDD (mitotane) destroys much of the adrenal tissue responsible for the increased cortisol levels. Overtreatment is not recommended, however, because cortisol in normal levels is essential to the body. The medication is carefully administered at 15-50 mg/kg daily for 5-7 days, and then 15-50 mg/kg weekly to keep the condition under control. Corticosteroids, such as prednisone at 0.2 mg/kg or cortisone at 1 mg/kg, given on the day of o'p'DDD administration often relieve the side effects of vomiting, diarrhea and ataxia. ACTH stimulation tests should be performed after 3 months initially (earlier if warranted), and then every 6-12 months to monitor the condition.

Ketoconazole may be an adequate form of therapy for presurgical stabilization of dogs with operable adrenal tumors, primary therapy when surgery is declined, primary medical therapy in dogs with resistance to mitotane, or in patients that experience severe side effects with mitotane administration. Ketoconazole administration results in rapid but transient reduction in plasma cortisol concentration and clinical signs of hyperadrenocorticism. Ketoconazole is given PO with food at 10 mg/kg body weight twice daily for 7-10 days, at which time an ACTH stimulation test is done and the dosage adjusted as necessary. If dosages ≥30 mg/kg are required, then either ketoconazole is not a sufficient therapy or poor absorption is a potential cause. If poor absorption is confirmed with blood levels of ketoconazole 3-4 hours after administration, the product can be administered as a solution by dissolving 400 mg ketoconazole in 10 ml of 0.1-M hydrochloric acid and administered with 30 ml of distilled deionized water. Mineralocorticoid deficiency is apparently not a concern with ketoconazole therapy. Once adequate control has been achieved, the maintenance dosage is administered twice daily and the patient monitored by ACTH stimulation testing every 3-6 months.

Adrenal tumors account for less than 15% of cases. About half of those are malignant and many are metastatic, often with spread to the liver, caudal vena cava or renal vein. Surgery to remove the tumor is the treatment of choice but requires much intraoperative and postoperative care, since shock is a common sequel to rebounding low cortisol levels once the gland is removed. To combat this, corticosteroids must be administered during (3-5 mg of dexamethasone or 25-50 mg of prednisone sodium succinate) and after surgery (prednisone at 0.5 mg/kg BID on the first postoperative day, tapered to 0.2 mg/kg daily tisol (11-DOC) to cortisol. The protocol is as follows: Collect a blood sample for baseline cortisol and 11-DOC levels. Administer metyrapone (Metopirone) at 25 mg/kg PO every 6 hours for 4 doses. Postsuppression blood samples are collected for cortisol and 11-DOC assay 6 hours after the last dose of metyrapone.

A marked increase in 11-DOC levels suggests that cortisol synthesis is ACTH driven and that the patient has pituitary-dependent hyperadrenocorticism. Conversely, little or no change in 11-DOC levels suggests adrenal tumor.

Insulin Tolerance Test: The insulin tolerance test is another proposed method of identifying cushingoid patients, especially in those with equivocal dexamethasone suppression tests. High levels of circulating cortisol induce insulin resistance. The test is based on the assumption that large IV doses of regular insulin (>0.3 U/kg) are necessary to induce hypoglycemia (glucose <40 mg/dl). The patient is fasted for 8 or more hours and then given an injection of 0.4 U regular (crystalline) insulin/kg body weight and a blood glucose curve determined for samples taken before the test and 15, 30, 45, 60 and 90 minutes after the test. Most normal animals suppress their glucose by 50% by 30 minutes and rebound to normal by 60-90 minutes. The merit of this test has yet to be determined. Also, this test appears to be a lot of work for such a qualitative assessment.

Glucagon Tolerance Test: A glucagon tolerance test has also been proposed for diagnosis of Cushing's disease in dogs. Blood is collected before and 30 minutes after administration of 0.14 mg glucagon/kg body weight. Dogs with Cushing's disease have prolonged hyperglycemia (often >300 mg/dl) by the second test. Patients that are already hyperglycemic are poor candidates for this test.

Computed Tomography: If the specialized facilities are available, bilateral adrenal hyperplasia can be differentiated from unilateral hyperplasia by computed tomography. In some instances, contrast-enhanced computed tomography has even discerned masses in the pituitary fossa. It is unlikely, however, that this diagnostic option will be readily available to most veterinary practitioners.

Treatment

Pituitary-dependent hyperadrenocorticism accounts for about 85% of all cases and is amenable to medical treatment.

Combined Dexamethasone Suppression-ACTH Stimulation Test: Combinations of the dexamethasone suppression test and the ACTH stimulation test have been evaluated, but results are ambiguous and offer no real advantage over the individual tests. The combined test also does not suitably do what it was intended to, which is both diagnose Cushing's disease and differentiate between adrenal- and pituitary-related disease.

High-Dose Dexamethasone Suppression Test: If a diagnosis of hyperadrenocorticism has been confirmed, a high-dose dexamethasone suppression test may be warranted to help localize the disease to the adrenal gland or the pituitary gland. The test is very similar to the low-dose test but the higher levels of dexamethasone administered (1.0 mg/kg IV) suppress cortisol levels in animals with pituitary-related disease to levels less than 45 nmol/L (1.5 μg/dl) but not in dogs with adrenal tumors. Animals with pituitary tumors normally have postsuppression cortisols of 10-45 nmol/L (0.3-1.5 μg/dl), while normal animals normally suppress well below 10 nmol/L (0.3 μg/dl). The test should only be cautiously used in diabetic animals, since ketoacidosis can result from the high dosages of corticosteroids being administered.

Plasma ACTH Assay: A test that measures the actual plasma concentration of ACTH is being evaluated to discriminate between pituitary- and adrenal-related disease and may eventually prove quite useful. Optimal sample handling includes prompt cooling of blood after collection in plastic tubes and shipment on dry ice or with a freeze pack via overnight delivery service. This test is available from the Endocrine Diagnostic Service at Auburn University, and at University of California, Davis, Michigan State University and Tufts University (Appendix 3). Low plasma ACTH levels suggest adrenal neoplasia, while high values suggest pituitary-dependent disease. Michigan State recommends that though VacuTainers are adequate to collect blood, samples should be quickly transferred to plastic tubes, cooled on ice, centrifuged at room temperature for 5 minutes and then the plasma frozen and shipped by Express Mail or courier service in well-insulated containers with 2-3 frozen gel packs. Lipemic samples may not be valid. Further controlled studies must be completed before this assay becomes widely available.

Metyrapone Suppression Test: The metyrapone suppression test is based on the premise that metyrapone causes specific inhibition of 11B-hydroxylase, an enzyme that converts 11-desoxycor-

Clinical Signs

The condition is typically manifested as generalized noninflammatory hair loss that spares the head and legs and is accompanied by intense darkening of the skin (Fig 29). Males are much more commonly affected than females, and most affected animals are quite young, often 1-3 years of age. Various breeds are affected, but those predisposed include the Chow Chow, Pomeranian, Poodle, Airedale, Samoyed, American Water Spaniel and Keeshond.

Diagnosis

Growth hormone-responsive dermatosis may be suspected on the basis of the history, clinical signs, blood test results and skin biopsy. Blood tests measuring growth hormone or somatomedin levels are the only way to confirm a diagnosis. These tests are expensive and performed by very few laboratories, and may be difficult to interpret. A growth hormone stimulation test can be performed by taking blood samples for growth hormone levels before and 15, 30, 45 and 60 minutes after injection of a measured amount of xylazine (100-300 μg/kg IV), clonidine hydrochloride (10 mg/kg) or human growth hormone-releasing factor (1-5 μg/kg). These assays can be performed by the University of Tennessee and the University of Pennsylvania. The addresses for these laboratories may be found in Appendix 3.

Blood levels of somatomedin C, a growth hormone intermediary, are supposedly reduced in growth hormone-responsive dermatosis, but this has not been convincingly demonstrated. Somatomedin C can be assayed at the Animal Health Diagnostic Laboratory of Michigan State University (Appendix 3). Biopsies from dogs with growth hormone-responsive dermatosis cannot be readily differentiated from those from dogs with other endocrinopathies. These specimens may have decreased dermal elastin levels when stained with Verhoeff's elastin stain, but this interpretation is subjective at best, requiring age-, breed- and site-matched controls, and should definitely not be relied on for a diagnosis.

Treatment

Therapy of growth hormone-responsive dermatosis requires deliberation. Since the condition does not affect the health of the animal, I strongly recommend conscientious neglect as the first line of action in confirmed cases. Additionally, I recommend neutering affected dogs, a percentage of which improve within 3-6 months from this alone. Growth hormone is in short supply and relatively expensive. Modern technology using monoclonal antibody techniques should soon provide a useful supply of the hormone. In the meantime, the hormone is difficult to acquire. It is usually administered in doses of 1-10 units SC every other day for 10 treatments. Alternatively, it can be given at 0.1 IU/kg 3 times weekly for 4-6 weeks. A side effect of treatment is transient or permanent diabetes mellitus; therefore, blood glucose levels should be monitored. Affected male dogs often benefit significantly from castration, whether or not growth hormone is administered. In addition, some dogs benefit from testosterone administration. Supplementation with methyltestosterone at 1 mg/kg PO every other day for 2-3 weeks, then reduced to twice weekly is recommended. The maximum should not exceed 30 mg. The CBC and liver function should be monitored closely in patients receiving testosterone supplementation. Growth-hormone responsive dermatosis deserves further scrutiny, since the hormonal aberration involved is the subject of much controversy.

Additional Reading

1. Eigenmann, JE and Patterson, DF: Growth hormone deficiency in the mature dog. *JAAHA* 20:741-746, 1984.

2. Morrison, WB *et al*: Growth hormone response to oral clonidine in young and middle-aged dogs. *Proc Ann Mtg Soc Comp Endocrinol*, 1987. p 73.

3. Scott, DW and Walton, DK: Hyposomatotropism in the mature dog: A discussion of 22 cases. *JAAHA* 22:467-473, 1986.

4. Smith, EK: Diagnosing growth hormone reponsive alopecia in adult dogs. *Vet Med* 78:48-52, 1985.

5. Lothrop, CD Jr: Pathophysiology of canine growth hormone-responsive alopecia. *Comp Cont Ed Pract Vet* 10:1346-1352, 1988.

Sex Hormone Disorders

Hyperestrogenism, formerly known as ovarian imbalance type I, is a rare disorder mainly due to formation of cysts on the ovaries or occasionally due to development of ovarian tumors. A similar syndrome can be induced by administration of estrogens used to treat such conditions as urinary incontinence, mismating and male aggression. The disorder is characterized by noninflammatory hair loss equally distributed along both sides of the genital area and down the hind legs. Often the vulva and nipples are swollen due to the high circulating levels of female sex hormones. Pruritus, waxy ears and a greasy, scaly haircoat are frequent secondary features of the disorder (See also hormonal hypersensitivity in Chapter 4). Often heat cycles are irregular, prolonged or suppressed.

Diagnosis is on the basis of the history, physical examination and response to therapy. The treatment of choice is ovariohysterectomy. Medical therapy with products that destroy the cysts has been successful in a limited number of cases, but the problem frequently recurs with the next heat. There may be a hereditary component to developing cystic ovaries. Chronic elevation of estrogens in the blood may make the animal more susceptible to bone marrow suppression, inflammatory reactions in the uterus and possibly mammary cancers.

Estrogen-responsive dermatosis, presumably due to low circulating levels of estrogens in the blood, was formerly known as ovarian imbalance type II. It has never been documented, however, that these animals are really deficient in estrogen. The condition is usually seen in older females spayed at an early age. The condition is very similar to hyperestrogenism, except that the nipples and vulva are infantile in appearance. Dribbling of urine (urinary incontinence) is common. Diagnosis is based on the history, clinical examination and response to estrogen supplementation. Estrogens should be used cautiously because of possible suppression of the bone marrow. As for all conditions that do not affect the health of the patient, conscientious neglect is preferable to administering medications with potential side effects.

Testicular tumors, usually Sertoli-cell tumors but occasionally interstitial-cell tumors and seminomas, can secrete female sex hormones and result in hyperestrogenism in male dogs. The incidence is much higher in dogs whose testicles have not descended completely from the abdominal cavity into the scrotum. The syndrome is characterized by noninflammatory hair loss about the rear end, enlargement of the mammary glands (gynecomastia), drooping of the prepuce, and other signs of feminization (Fig 30). Affected male dogs may squat to urinate, attract other male dogs, have a decreased sex drive and even produce milk from the enlarged mammary glands. Diseases of the prostate gland and estrogen-induced bone marrow suppression are possible consequences of the disorder. Diagnosis is based on the history, physical examination and response to castration. Since about 10% of these tumors are malignant and may metastasize, chest radiographs and blood tests should be considered before castration.

Chapter 6

Additional Reading

1. Barsanti, JA *et al*: Diethylstilbestrol-induced alopecia in a dog. *JAVMA* 182:64-65, 1983.

2. Carlson, RA: Endocrine alopecia in a dog showing response to FSH administration. *JAAHA* 21:735-739, 1985.

3. Dorn, AS *et al*: Sex hormone-related diseases treated surgically in bitches. *MVP* 66:621-625, 1985.

4. Dorn, AS *et al*: Sex hormone-related diseases treated surgically in male dogs. *MVP* 66:727-733, 1985.

5. Eilts, BE *et al*: Use of ultrasonography to diagnose Sertoli-cell neoplasia and cryptorchidism in a dog. *JAVMA* 192:533-534, 1988.

6. Fadok, VA *et al*: Hyperprogesteronemia associated with Sertoli cell tumor and alopecia in a dog. *JAVMA* 188:1058-1059, 1986.

7. Smith, EK: Canine ovarian imbalance. *Canine Pract* 8(5):41-44, 1981.

8. Cain, JL *et al*: Use of pulsatile intravenous administration of gonadotropin-releasing hormone to induce fertile estrus in bitches. *Am J Vet Res* 49:1993-1996, 1988.

Chapter 7
Nutritionally Related Skin Disorders

Nutritionally related skin disorders have received much attention in the past few years, most of it centered on the role of zinc and vitamin A. Canine dietary needs include a protein content of 20-25% of caloric intake (18-30% of dry matter) and a fat content providing 25-50% of the calories (7-9% of dry matter), with 2% of the total caloric intake in the form of linoleic acid. Dr. L.D. Lewis of Mark Morris Associates, Topeka, Kansas, suggests that adding the following supplemental formula daily to the diet of a 10- to 15-kg dog will provide the fat, protein, vitamins A and E, biotin, riboflavin, niacin, iodine and zinc necessary for maintenance:

> 1 tsp (5 ml) vegetable oil
> 2-3 oz (55-85 g) raw liver
> 100 mg zinc sulfate (20 mg elemental zinc)
> 1 drop tincture of iodine

These levels, however, are not considered therapeutic but are adequate for maintenance. Also they have little effect in controlling vitamin A- or zinc-responsive dermatoses.

Protein Deficiency

Proteins are needed as a source of amino acids, the building blocks of body proteins. The skin and hair require 25-30% of the animal's total daily protein intake for maintenance; therefore, a minimum of 12% of the caloric intake should be made up of protein. Since most commercial dog foods have more than adequate amounts of protein, protein deficiency is rare. It is seen only in animals fed a poor-quality diet or animals that are ill and unable to take adequate feedings. Clinical signs include a dry, brittle haircoat, scaling, patchy hair loss and perhaps crusting.

Treatment consists of providing a good-quality diet that contains adequate protein.

Fatty Acid Deficiency

Fats usually make up 5-20% of the dry matter of dog foods and may provide 25-50% of the daily caloric needs of the animal. Fats are a great source of fuel and supply 2.25 times more energy than either proteins or carbohydrates. They also provide essential fatty acids, increase the palatability of feeds, and provide a vehicle for absorption of fat-soluble vitamins. Though linoleic, linolenic and arachidonic acids are all considered essential fatty acids, linoleic acid is truly essential in that if it is adequately provided in the diet, the other 2 can be synthesized within the body. This is true only for dogs, since in cats arachidonic acid must also be supplied. Linoleic acid is the major unsaturated fatty acid in most vegetable oils and makes up 15-25% of poultry and pork fat. Essential fatty acids should constitute at least 1% of the diet, or 2% of the caloric intake. Since animals tend to regulate their food intake by energy needs, fats should not constitute more than 20% of the diet or the animal will not consume enough to meet maintenance requirements for other nutrients.

Poor-quality dog foods may be deficient in fatty acids. Dry foods especially are limited in the amount of fats that can be incorporated without causing rancidity. Antioxidants are normally added to foods to delay this process, but foods stored for long periods, especially at high temperatures, can lose their fatty acid content. Medical conditions that limit the body's ability to absorb or metabolize ingested fats can result in fatty acid deficiency.

Animals must normally be fed a fatty acid-deficient diet for many months before they begin to show signs. A dry, lusterless coat and prominent dandruff are often the first signs. Bacterial infections can further affect the skin and haircoat.

Therapy involves feeding good-quality food with adequate fat content, and supplementing the diet with a suitable fatty acid compound. This fatty acid supplement may be purchased commercially or formulated by adding to the diet equal parts of animal fats (*eg,* bacon drippings, chicken fat) and vegetable oils (*eg,* safflower, corn oil) to the animal's tolerance (until the stools become soft). Table 1 shows the fatty acid content of some animal and vegetable food materials. Caution should be exercised in animals with pancreatitis, gallbladder disease or malabsorption syndromes, in which increased dietary fat can have medical con-

Table 1. Fatty acid content of oils.

Oil	Linoleic Acid (%)
Corn	50-55
Safflower	70-80
Soybean	35-60
Linseed	15-25
Cod liver	—
Salmon	11.5
Herring	13
Pork lard	10-20

sequences. Excessively high levels of fatty acids can interfere with metabolism of vitamin E. Topical applications of essential fatty acids also result in some absorption directly through the skin. Antiseborrheic shampoos remove the scales and oiliness from the skin that often accompany the condition.

Zinc-Responsive Dermatosis

This condition is called zinc-responsive dermatosis and not zinc deficiency. Affected animals have a higher than normal requirement for zinc and their blood zinc levels are normal. Two syndromes have been recognized, one in rapidly growing puppies and one with a predisposition for sled dog breeds.

Zinc is a cofactor in over 100 metalloenzymes, and an essential cofactor of DNA and RNA polymerase. Some of the important functions of zinc in the body include stabilization of cell and lysosomal membranes, modulation of metalloenzyme function, regulation of neutrophil and macrophage function, interference with the complement system, and generation of specific molecules and cells of immunologic recognition. Zinc also affects ligand-receptor and receptor-target interactions, and functions as a mild mitogen for lymphocytes.

Some ingredients in dog foods and supplements, such as calcium, phytates, iron, tin and copper, decrease zinc absorption. This is another reason why general supplements that include a multitude of nutrients may actually do more harm than good. Anything that interferes with absorption of zinc, affects its longevity or function in the body, enhances its excretion or causes general body wasting and catabolism also reduces the body stores of zinc.

Some Siberian Huskies, Malamutes, Samoyeds and perhaps Great Danes and Doberman Pinschers may have a genetic defect that results in decreased ability to absorb zinc from the intestine. This may also then result in impaired metabolism of zinc.

The second syndrome involves dietary supplementation, especially with calcium and phytate-containing products in young, rapidly growing dogs. These dogs therefore suffer from a functional zinc imbalance.

Clinical Signs

The clinical presentation is usually one of tenacious crusts, redness and a variable degree of pruritus, the most affected areas including the face, footpads, elbows and hocks (Fig 31). It is quite likely that the condition formerly known as "dry pyoderma" was really zinc-responsive dermatosis. Young, rapidly growing dogs that have been oversupplemented (especially with calcium) may also have stunted growth, bone deformities and a poor appetite.

Diagnosis

Diagnosis of zinc-responsive dermatosis is based on history, clinical signs, biopsies for histopathologic examination and response to zinc supplementation. Biopsies normally reveal extensive parakeratotic hyperkeratosis, crusting and leukocytic exocytosis. Blood zinc levels are invariably normal and hair analysis is of questionable value.

Management

Treatment is relatively easy. Animals that have been oversupplemented respond to eliminating the supplementation and feeding a balanced diet. Animals with inherited defects probably require some form of zinc supplementation for life. The requirement for elemental zinc is 1.1 mg/kg/day for maintenance and double this amount during periods of growth or stress. Zinc sulfate is about 22% and zinc gluconate is about 13% elemental zinc. Most forms purchased in pharmacies list the content of elemental zinc on their label. Animals that absorb zinc poorly from the GI tract must be given zinc IV.

Additional Reading

1. Sanecki, RK *et al*: Extracutaneous histologic changes accompanying zinc deficiency in pups. *Am J Vet Res* 46:2120-2123, 1985.

2. Fadok, VA: Zinc responsive dermatosis in a Great Dane: A case report. *JAAHA* 18:409-414, 1982.

3. Van den Broek, A and Thoday, KL: Skin disease in dogs associated with zinc deficiency: A report of 5 cases. *J Small Anim Pract* 27:313-323, 1986.

4. Degryse, AD *et al*: Recurrent zinc-responsive dermatosis in a Siberian Husky. *J Small Anim Pract* 28:721-726, 1987.

5. Buffington, A: Nutrition and the skin. *Proc Kal Kan Sympos*, 1987. p 12.

Generic Dog Food Disease

Some years ago a condition that appeared to be caused by feeding generic dog foods was recognized. Since then, it has been confirmed that this entity does indeed exist, but it is uncertain what is in (or not in) the diet that causes the problem. Some generic dog foods may contain ingredients that cause a relative zinc imbalance.

Clinical Signs

Affected animals usually develop clinical signs 2-4 weeks after being given the generic diet as the sole food source. Animals are often healthy on physical examination but lethargic, depressed and covered by crusts (Fig 32). The predominant sites of involvement include the distal extremities, face, pressure points, mucocutaneous junctions and trunk. Pruritus is variable but enlarged lymph nodes are common.

Diagnosis

Diagnosis is by the history, clinical signs, biopsy for histopathologic evaluation of skin sections (orthokeratotic, parakeratotic and follicular hyperkeratosis, dyskeratosis, leukocytic exocytosis), and response to diet correction.

Management

Treatment involves dietary management only. Switching to a brand-name diet usually corrects the situation in 6-8 weeks. Ongoing dietary supplementation is unnecessary in these cases.

Additional Reading

1. Sousa, CA *et al*: Dermatosis associated with feeding generic dog food: 13 cases (1981-1982). *JAVMA* 192:676-680, 1988.

2. Huber, TL *et al*: Variations in digestibility of dry dog foods with identical label guaranteed analysis. *JAAHA* 22:571-575, 1986.

Vitamin A-Responsive Dermatosis

This is not a deficiency syndrome but rather a skin condition that responds to large doses of vitamin A supplementation. The principal breed affected is the Cocker Spaniel, but other breeds (*eg*, Labrador Retriever, Cairn Terrier) have also been affected.

Anything that interferes with absorption of vitamin A or enhances its excretion can result in a relative deficiency. Vitamin A has important roles in biosynthesis of mucopolysaccharides, labilization of lysosomal enzymes, inhibition of abnormal epithelial keratinization and proliferation, suppression of sebaceous-gland size and secretion, and modulation of various neutrophil and mononuclear cell functions and prostaglandin synthesis. Analogs of vitamin A, such as etretinate (Tegison: Roche) and isotretinoin (Accutane: Roche), have been used in a number of skin disorders in people, including psoriasis, ichthyosis and acne. The former product exerts more effect on keratinization disorders, and the latter on sebaceous-gland disorders.

Clinical Signs

The syndrome is characterized by dandruff, hair loss and marked crusting, especially on the back (Fig 33). The center of the problem is the hair follicle, from which the scaling and crusting (follicular keratosis) originates.

Diagnosis

Diagnosis is based on the history, clinical signs and biopsies for histopathologic evaluation. Biopsies reveal dyskeratosis (abnormal keratinization) and marked follicular hyperkeratosis. Blood vitamin A levels are invariably normal and hair analysis is of questionable value.

Management

Therapy includes megadose vitamin A administration on a daily basis (10,000-100,000 IU/day), usually for life. Though actual dosages have not been established, empiric use of 500-1,000

IU/kg body weight once daily is a good starting point. Twice-daily administration may be necessary initially to effect remission. Doses should then be tapered to an amount that maintains the patient with few or no lesions. Use of large doses of vitamin A should not be viewed lightly, since toxicities have been reported. Since vitamin A is stored in the liver, liver function evaluation should be an important component of any monitoring program.

Additional Reading

1. Scott, DW: Vitamin A-responsive dermatosis in the Cocker spaniel. *JAAHA* 22: 125-129, 1986.

2. Ihrke, PJ and Goldschmidt, MH: Vitamin A-responsive dermatosis in the dog. *JAVMA* 182:687-690, 1983.

Vitamin E and Skin Disease

Vitamin E is a fat-soluble vitamin that acts as a natural antioxidant and is a mild antagonist to formation of leukotrienes from arachidonic acid. Good natural sources include wheat germ, soybeans, vegetable oils, enriched flour, whole wheat, whole-grain cereals and eggs. Excessive supplementation with fatty acids can actually render vitamin E less available in the body. The stability of vitamin E varies considerably among the different forms available.

Clinical Signs

Dogs with experimentally induced vitamin E deficiency show a keratinization defect (seborrhea sicca), increased susceptibility to infection, erythroderma and visual defects resembling progressive retinal atrophy.

Management

In therapeutic levels (200-800 IU twice daily), vitamin E has been used in treatment of discoid and systemic lupus erythematosus, acanthosis nigricans, demodicosis, dermatomyositis and epidermolysis bullosa simplex. Though it has been recommended that vitamin E should not be given within 2 hours of mealtime, this contention could not be documented.

Additional Reading

1. Scott, DW and Sheffy, BE: Dermatosis in dogs caused by vitamin E deficiency. *Compan Anim Pract* 1(4):42-46, 1987.

Chapter 7

Dalmatian Bronzing Syndrome

Dalmatian bronzing syndrome is not a nutritional disease *per se*, but a condition that does respond to proper dietary management. In all likelihood it represents an inherited defect in metabolism of uric acid, accumulation of which can result in gout in people. Dalmatians, however, do not suffer from gout but can form urinary calculi, suffer from recurrent urinary tract infections, and may develop a "moth-eaten" coat that becomes secondarily infected and may even change color to a bronze hue (hence the name), especially along the back (Fig 34). The reason for this color change has not been determined.

The condition can easily be controlled by limiting the amount of protein (especially purines) in the diet and/or by treating with compounds that lower blood uric acid levels. Though such medications as allopurinol (Zyloprim), at 10 mg/kg TID then tapering, lower the blood uric acid levels and control the situation, when possible one should try to manage the condition by dietary means. A low-purine, low-protein diet (u/d: Hill's) can be purchased or formulated according to a diet recommended by Mark Morris Associates of Topeka, Kansas:

>   5 oz or 2 cups cooked rice
>   1 oz corn oil
>   2 large hard-cooked eggs
>   1 tsp salt
>   1 tsp calcium carbonate

This diet provides 12% protein calories, 38% fat calories and 50% carbohydrate calories.

A more complicated diet, recommended by the Dalmatian Research Foundation, is as follows:

Combine 2 1/2 cups rice, 5 cups water, 1/3 cup corn oil and 1 tbsp salt in a saucepan and mix thoroughly. Bring to a vigorous boil, stirring only occasionally, then reduce heat to low and cover. Simmer until the water has been completely absorbed, then set aside to cool.

Boil 10 oz of frozen chopped broccoli in 2 cups of water until tender, then combine with 3 1-lb cans (undrained) of greens (kale, dock, mustard-greens) and 3 1-lb cans (undrained) of carrots, peas, green beans or tomatoes in a large preserving kettle, mixing thoroughly. The mixture is then pureed into a second kettle blending sufficiently to make certain no lumps remain. The mixture should not be cooked, as this would reduce its vitamin content. Fill plastic 1-qt containers with the puree, cover and freeze.

Thaw the frozen puree as needed and add the cooled rice little by little, making certain the mixture is thoroughly blended. This mixture can then be fed at a rate of 1-2 cups of diet 3X/day for an adult, adding 1 heaping tbsp of cottage cheese to each feeding. Adding 1 brewers' yeast tablet twice daily and some fish oil helps supply B vitamins and vitamin A.

Additional Reading

1. Pukay, BP: Dalmatian bronzing syndrome. *MVP* 63:641-642, 1982.

Nutrients Affecting the Skin

Multi-Nutrient Supplements

Nutritional supplements for pets abound in the marketplace, yet few actually meet the requirements of a pet with a skin problem. Animals have a certain maintenance requirement for vitamins and minerals. During growth and times of stress, this requirement is essentially doubled. Therefore, if we appreciate that skin disease is a form of stress in nutritional terms, and a good balanced diet provides all of the maintenance requirements for animals, a dietary supplement should meet the stress requirements. For example, the maintenance requirement for zinc is about 1.1 mg/kg/day. Double this amount (*ie*, 2.2 mg/kg/day) is required during stress. In an animal stressed with skin disease but fed a good basic diet that provides zinc at 1.1 mg/kg/day, the animal would still benefit from a supplement of 1.1 mg/kg/day.

Despite the vast number of supplements on the market, it is still rare to see ones that meet the requirements for the important vitamins, minerals and fatty acids in skin disorders (vitamin A, zinc, vitamin E and linoleic acid). Most supplements were designed to generally augment the diet with a multitude of vitamins and minerals but not necessarily at stress levels and not specifically for skin disorders (Table 2).

Stress levels differ markedly from therapeutic levels. Though the maintenance level of vitamin E is 1.1 IU/kg/day, vitamin E is often given in doses of 200-800 IU twice daily in dogs with conditions that benefit from such therapy. Such is also the case with vitamin A and zinc. There is a limit to how much linoleic fatty

Table 2. Comparison of nutritional supplements based on content.

Product	Mfr/Distrib	Recommended Day, Dose for Maintenance per 9 kg (20 lb)	Nutrients in Daily Dose			
			Vit A (IU)	Vit E (IU)	Zinc (mg)	Linoleic Acid (mg)
BVMO Liquid	Schering	5 ml (1 tsp)	1667	—	—	—
BVMO Tablets	Schering	1 tablet	2000	—	—	30
Dermacare	Hagen	5 ml (1 tsp)	1163	2.1	—	2410
Derma Sheen	Vetrepharm	28 g (4 tbsp)	1680	9.8	28	454
Diaglo Liquid	Syntex	5 ml (1 tsp)	1000	10	10	2400
Diaglo Powder	Syntex	6.75 g (2 tsp)	783	3	.70	1846
EFA-Z Plus	Allerderm	7 ml (1/2 oz)	850	14	8.8	3400
EFA-Z Plus (New)	Allerderm	7 ml (1/2 oz)	850	14	14	3400
Geriatric Palatabs	Osborn	1/2 tablet	925	5	1	—
Geribits	Norden	1 tablet	1800	20	1	30
Linatone	Lambert Kay	5 ml (1 tsp)	1060	2.3	—	2410
Linatone Plus	Lambert Kay	5 ml (1 tsp)	1500	10	2.5	1900
Linoplex	Evsco	2 g (1 tsp)	529	1.3	—	1226
Mirracoat Liquid	Borden/MTC	3.33 ml (2/3 tsp)	366	3.3	—	977
Mirracoat Powder	Borden/MTC	6.25 g (2 tsp)	309	2.1	—	781
Nutrical	Evsco	12 g (3 tsp)	2117	12.7	—	—
Nutriderm	Norden	2.5 ml (1/4 tsp)	575	4.5	—	913
Nutrisol	Norden	2 ml	2000	10	4	150
Nutriform G	Vet-a-Mix	1 tablet	1100	22	11	—
Nutripet	Vetcom	12 g (3 tsp)	2117	12.7	—	—
Nutritabs	Upjohn	1 tablet	1100	2.5	2.5	—
Pet-F.A. Liquid	Beecham	5 ml (1 tsp)	1000	10	10	—
Pet-Tabs	Beecham	1 tablet	1000	2	1.5	30
Pet-Tabs Jr.	Beecham	2 tablets	1000	2	1.5	30
Pet-Tabs Plus	Beecham	1 tablet	1500	15	1.5	30
SA-37	Rogar/STB	1 g (1/3 tsp)	850	0.4	0.2	28
Unipet	Upjohn	1 tablet	1500	—	—	—
Unipet Senior	Upjohn	1 tablet	1500	10	1	—
Veterol X	UEC/Winthrop	5 ml (1 tsp)	—	1	—	1500
Visorbits	Norden	1 tablet	1250	2	—	20
Vitamin Palatabs	Osborn	1 tablet	1500	2	1.5	—
Vitatone	Fort Dodge	8 g (2 tsp)	1972	3.4	0.24	96
Vitpet	PVU	1 tablet	1500	—	—	—

acids may be given, because oversupplementation can result in diarrhea and decreased absorption of protein.

Additional Reading

1. Ackerman, L: Nutritional supplements for canine dermatoses. *Can Vet J* 28:29-32, 1987.

Omega 3 and Omega 6 Fatty Acids

Essential fatty acids are polyunsaturated fatty acids, of which 2 series have been described. The omega 3 (n3) series is derived from alpha-linolenic acid, while the omega 6 (n6) series is derived from cis-linoleic acid. Cis-linoleic acid and alpha-linolenic acid have no biologic activity of their own other than their capacity to provide energy from their oxidation. To function as essential fatty acids (EFA), they must be biochemically transformed in the body. A common enzyme, delta-6-desaturase, converts alpha-linolenic acid (with an elongation step) to eicosapentanoic acid, and cis-linoleic acid to gamma-linolenic acid. These products then have biologic activities as essential fatty acids and continue along different biochemical pathways.

The omega 3 fatty acids include eicosapentanoic acid (EPA), docosapentanoic acid (DPA) and docosahexanoic acid (DHA), their names denoting the position of the first double bond on the end of the carbon string. All are derivatives of linolenate and originate in phytoplankton and algae, which are consumed by larger marine life, such as fish. Some fish (*eg,* herring, mackerel, salmon) store these fatty acids in their muscles, while others (*eg,* cod) store them in their livers. Cod liver oil with 9-20% EPA and krill with 40% EPA are acceptable natural sources of the omega 3 fatty acids, but excessive supplementation of the diet with cod liver oil may result in vitamin D toxicity. Blubber from marine mammals also contains omega 3 fatty acids that may be suitable for supplementation as well.

Leukotrienes, formerly known as slow-reacting substance of anaphylaxis, are formed from metabolism of arachidonic acid. They modulate some signs associated with inflammation and hypersensitivity reactions. Eicosapentanoic acid is an analog of arachidonic acid and therefore competes for the enzymes that ultimately synthesize leukotrienes. This results in reduced migration of neutrophils and monocytes, and consequent suppression of the inflammatory response.

In people, omega 3 fatty acids decrease serum cholesterol and the risk of hypertension, atherosclerosis, stroke and heart disease. Some benefit may also be derived for gout, rheumatoid arthritis, psoriasis and asthma. In dogs, their principal use has been as a nonsteroidal alternative for symptomatic relief of allergies.

The omega 6 fatty acids include gamma linolenic acid. Evening primrose (*Oenothera biennis*) oil, which contains 9% gamma-linolenic acid, appears to be readily metabolized, and is the most common source of gamma-linolenic acid in dietary supplements. Other important sources of gamma-linolenic acid include black currant (*Ribes nigrum*) seed oil, fungal (*eg, Phycomycetes*) oil and borage (*Borago officinalis*) oil.

Defective enzyme function may be responsible for some clinical manifestations of atopic dermatitis in people (and dogs?). The positive effects of omega fatty acids are probably due to enyzme bypass, rather than correction of any immune defect.

Such products as Derm Caps (DVM), OFA-Plus (Nutri-Specialties), EFA-Z Plus (Allerderm) and EfaVet (Efamol) contain a combination of omega 3 and 6 fatty acids.

Additional Reading

1. Ackerman, L: Omega 3 fatty acids. *Bull Can Acad Vet Dermatol* 3:2, 1986.

2. Somer, E: The omega 3 fatty acids: A review. *Nutrition Rept* 4:42-48, 1986.

3. Ackerman, L: Fatty acid supplementation in the treatment of allergic inhalant dermatitis. *Vet Allergist* Fall: 4, 1987.

4. Radha, E et al: Krill as a dietary source of EFA and DHA in the prevention of cardiovascular disease. *Fed Proc* 45:353, 1986.

5. Hudson, BJF: Oilseeds as sources of essential fatty acids. *Hum Nutrit* 41:1-13, 1987.

Dimethylglycine

Dimethylglycine (N,N-dimethylglycine) was originally called vitamin B-15 or pangamic acid but is not actually a vitamin at all, but rather a tertiary amino acid. It is a naturally occurring "food factor" present in minute quantities in sunflower seeds, brewers' yeast, rice bran, wheat bran, whole grain cereals, oat grits, corn grits, pumpkin seeds, sesame seeds, wheat germ and liver.

DMG is considered a metabolic enhancer and in people has been used to improve function of the immune system, cardiovascular system and muscles. It appears to act as a key intermediary in the biologic pathway that supplies the body with methyl groups (transmethylation). Presumably it enhances oxygen utilization by tissue and complexes free radicals.

In people, DMG has been shown to affect humoral and cellular immunity. Potentiation of response of DMG-treated lymphocytes from normal individuals to phytohemagglutinin, con A and pokeweed mitogen have been observed *in vitro*.

DMG use has been advocated in people to maximize athletic performance and as a nonspecific stimulator of the immune response in patients with chronic viral infections or immune deficiency diseases. Its ability to enhance oxygen utilization has also prompted its use in coronary artery insufficiency, rheumatic heart disease, asthma, angina and atherosclerosis. It appears to be completely nontoxic when given orally. Veterinary applications remain largely unexplored. Though controlled studies have not been done, indications in animals might include chronic pyodermas, generalized demodicosis, animals on immunosuppressive therapies, and working animals. I have used DMG to a limited extent at 12.5-500 mg daily, depending upon the severity of the condition.

Additional Reading

1. Graber, CD *et al:* Immunomodulating properties of dimethylglycine in humans. *J Infect Dis* 143:101-105, 1981.

Germanium

Organic germanium (bis-beta-carboxyethyl germanium sesquioxide) is a mineral present in a number of plants, including garlic, aloe, comfrey, ginseng and waternut. Shelf fungus (Shiitake mushroom) and *Chlorella* represent additional sources. Germanium is present in whole grain but not in refined flours.

Germanium appears to be an oxygen catalyst, antioxidant, electrostimulant and immune enhancer. It may be regarded as an adaptogen, which is a nontoxic substance that helps the body adjust to stress. It also acts as a detoxifier by chelating mercury, cadmium and other metals.

Some studies in people have suggested that interferon is induced by oral administration of germanium and that germanium can modulate alterations in the immune response by restoring normal function of T-cells, B-lymphocytes, antibody-dependent cytotoxicity, natural killer cells' activities, activating macrophages and increasing the numbers of plasma cells.

Doses in animals range between 10 mg and 1 g daily, though no controlled studies have yet been performed in dogs. Indications for administration might include chronic cutaneous bacterial or fungal infections, demodicosis and burns.

Additional Reading

1. Kamen, B: *Germanium, A New Approach to Immunity.* Nutrition Encounter, Larkspur, CA, 1987. pp 1-38.

Bromelain

Bromelain was originally isolated as a proteolytic enzyme in pineapple. It is a glycopeptide, with at least 2 proteolytic fractions, acid phosphatase, a peroxidase and several protease inhibitors, and contains organically bound calcium and furulic acid. A bromelain plasminogen activator attached to the protease may also have pharmacologic action. Bromelain has proteolytic, fibrinolytic and antiinflammatory properties. There are several good reasons however to suspect that proteolytic activity is not the sole basis of bromelain's pharmacologic effect.

Bromelain is thought to act by altering cell membrane proteins and selectively inhibiting biosynthesis of proinflammatory prostaglandins. While nonsteroidal antiinflammatory agents inhibit the cyclooxygenase pathway and thus the biosynthesis of all prostaglandins, bromelain may act further down the arachidonic acid cascade at the thromboxane synthetase step. Therefore, bromelain may block synthesis of proinflammatory prostaglandins without interfering with production of antiinflammatory prostaglandins. Bromelain plasminogen activator may activate plasminogen to liberate plasmin, which in turn results in production of Hageman factor fragments, which in turn are potent activators of the kinin system.

Bromelain has been rarely used in veterinary medicine. It can be administered orally or used as a topical preparation. In dermatology, bromelain may be used as adjunctive therapy in pyodermas, cellulitis and burns. Other indications might include musculoskeletal injuries, trauma due to injuries or surgery, arthritis and digestive disorders. Controlled studies have been lacking in people and animals. I have used bromelain to a limited extent experimentally in doses of 50-400 mg daily, depending upon the severity of the condition.

Additional Reading

1. Taussig, SJ: The mechanism of the physiological action of bromelain. *Med Hypotheses* 6:99-104, 1980.

Chapter 8
Congenito-Hereditary Skin Disorders

Skin disorders in young dogs are always fascinating because the question often arises as to whether the condition may have been inherited from one or both of the parents. For heritable conditions, it may mean reevaluation of breeding selections, since animals with inherited disorders have irreversible defects that for the most part are not amenable to simple forms of therapy. It must be kept in mind that not all skin diseases seen in the young are inherited; some may occur as a fluke of nature. On the other hand, it behooves us to recognize inherited conditions so that their incidence may be lessened by conscientious breeding.

Some conditions that are inherited (*eg*, tendency to develop allergies, immunoincompetence, poor absorption or metabolism of essential nutrients) may not show up immediately in the newborn and may not manifest themselves until later in the animal's life. In the language of genetics, traits present at birth are referred to as congenital, while those that appear at some later date are called tardive. In addition, certain animals have purposely been bred to have abnormal skin, such as the hairless breeds (*eg*, Mexican Hairless, Abyssinian Dog, African Sand Dog, Chinese Crested Dog, Xoloitzcuintli, Turkish Naked Dog). Color mutant breeds include Blue Dobermans, Great Danes, Dachshunds, Whippets and Standard Poodles. Dogs with excessively folded skin include Shar Peis and Pugs.

Breed Predispositions to Skin Disorders

Many conditions have appeared to be especially prominent in some breeds. Sometimes a mode of inheritance is discernible but in many cases we must be satisfied with a genetically inadequate "breed predisposition" or "predilection." The following list has been constructed with this premise in mind. It reflects breed tendencies toward disorders rather than clear-cut genetic links, and in some instances reflects regional differences in the breed gene pool. These conditions are listed alphabetically, as are the breeds themselves, and do not reflect prevalence of those conditions for the breeds specified.

Breed	Condition
Afghan	Demodicosis
	Hypothyroidism
Airedale	Allergic inhalant dermatitis
	Growth hormone responsive dermatosis
	Melanoma
	Vascular nevi
Akita	Hypothyroidism
	Pemphigus foliaceus (?)
	Sebaceous adenitis (periappendageal dermatitis)
	Uveodermatologic syndrome (Vogt-Koyanagi-Harada-like syndrome)
Alaskan Malamute	Hypothyroidism
	Nasal solar dermatitis
	Zinc-responsive dermatosis
Basenji	Hypothyroidism
Basset Hound	Collagen nevi
	Idiopathic keratinization disorder (seborrhea)
	Interdigital pyoderma
	Sebaceous-gland tumors
Beagle	Allergic inhalant dermatitis
	Cutaneous asthenia
	Demodicosis
	Hemangiopericytoma
	Hepatoid-gland tumor
	Lipoma
	Lymphosarcoma
	Perianal-gland tumors
	Sebaceous-gland tumors
	Zinc-responsive dermatosis
Bearded Collie	Black hair follicular dysplasia
	Lupus erythematosus (?)
Belgian Tervuren	Vitiligo
Bernese Mountain Dog	Hemangiosarcoma
	Malignant histiocytosis
Borzoi	Primary lymphedema
Boston Terrier	Allergic inhalant dermatitis
	Demodicosis
	Fibroma
	Hyperadrenocorticism
	Mast-cell tumor
	Melanoma
	Sebaceous-gland tumors
	Tail fold pyoderma

Congenito-Hereditary Skin Disorders

Boxer	Acne
	Coccidioidomycosis
	Cutaneous asthenia
	Demodicosis
	Dermoid sinus
	Fibroma
	Hemangioma
	Hemangiosarcoma
	Hemangiopericytoma
	Histiocytoma
	Hyperadrenocorticism
	Hypothyroidism
	Interdigital pyoderma
	Lymphosarcoma
	Mast-cell tumor
	Melanoma
	Sertoli-cell tumor
	Squamous-cell carcinoma
	Sternal callus
Brittany Spaniel	Hypothyroidism
	Liposarcoma
Bull Terrier	Demodicosis
	Lethal acrodermatitis
	Mast-cell tumor
Bulldog	Acne
	Demodicosis
	Face fold pyoderma
	Hepatoid-gland tumor
	Hypothyroidism
	Interdigital pyoderma
	Mast-cell tumor
	Perianal-gland tumor
	Primary lymphedema
	Sterile pyogranuloma
	Tail fold pyoderma
Bull Mastiff	Acne
Cairn Terrier	Allergic inhalant dermatitis
	Vitamin A-responsive dermatosis
Chihuahua	Anal sacculitis
	Congenital alopecia
	Demodicosis
	Melanoma
	Sertoli-cell tumor
Chow Chow	Color mutant alopecia
	Demodicosis
	Follicular dysplasia
	Growth hormone-responsive dermatosis
	Hypothyroidism
	Melanoma
	Tyrosinase deficiency

Cocker Spaniel	Allergic inhalant dermatitis
	Anal sacculitis
	Basal-cell tumor
	Cutaneous T-cell-like lymphoma
	Demodicosis
	Fibrosarcoma
	Hemangiopericytoma
	Hepatoid-gland tumors
	Histiocytoma
	Hypothyroidism
	Hypotrichosis
	Keratinization disorders (seborrhea)
	Lip fold pyoderma
	Lipoma
	Lymphosarcoma
	Melanoma
	Nasodigital hyperkeratosis
	Papilloma
	Perianal-gland tumor
	Sebaceous-gland tumor
	Sweat-gland tumors
	Trichoepithelioma
	Vitamin A-responsive dermatosis
Collie	Adverse reactions to ivermectin
	Black hair follicular dysplasia
	Bullous pemphigoid
	Demodicosis
	Dermatomyositis
	Discoid lupus erythematosus
	Epidermolysis bullosa simplex
	Fibrous histiocytoma
	Gray Collie syndrome
	Intracutaneous cornifying epithelioma
	Juvenile panniculitis
	Nasal pyoderma
	Nasal solar dermatitis (?)
	Nodular panniculitis
	Pemphigus erythematosus
	Pemphigus foliaceus (?)
	Pyotraumatic dermatitis (hot spots)
	Sebaceous adenitis (periappendageal dermatitis)
	Systemic lupus erythematosus
Dachshund	Acanthosis nigricans
	Black hair follicular dysplasia
	Callus pyoderma
	Color mutant alopecia
	Cutaneous asthenia
	Cutaneous vasculitis
	Demodicosis
	Ear margin dermatosis

Congenito-Hereditary Skin Disorders

	Histiocytoma
	Hypothyroidism
	Hyperadrenocorticism
	Keratinization disorders (seborrhea)
	Interdigital pyoderma
	Juvenile cellulitis
	Juvenile panniculitis
	Linear IgA dermatosis
	Lipoma
	Liposarcoma
	Mast-cell tumor
	Pattern baldness
	Perianal tumors
	Pinnal alopecia
	Sebaceous-gland tumor
	Sterile pyogranuloma
Dalmatian	Allergic inhalant dermatitis
	Dalmatian bronzing syndrome
	Demodicosis
Doberman Pinscher	Acne
	Acral lick dermatitis
	Adverse reaction to sulfa drugs
	Bullous pemphigoid
	Callus
	Coccidioidomycosis
	Color mutant alopecia
	Demodicosis
	Flank sucking
	Focal mucinosis
	Hypopigmentation of lips
	Hypothyroidism
	Ichthyosis
	Interdigital pododermatitis
	Lipoma
	Systemic lupus erythematosus
	Vitiligo
	Zinc-responsive dermatosis
Fox Terrier	Fibroma
	Hemangiopericytoma
	Juvenile panniculitis
	Mast-cell tumor
	Nodular panniculitis
	Schwannoma
German Shepherd	Acral lick dermatitis
	Calcinosis circumscripta (tumoral calcinosis)
	Callus
	Collagen nevi
	Cutaneous asthenia
	Demodicosis
	Discoid lupus erythematosus
	Furunculosis

	Hemangioma
	Hemangiopericytoma
	Hemangiosarcoma
	Interdigital pyoderma
	Intracutaneous cornifying epithelioma
	Lymphosarcoma
	Nasal pyoderma
	Nasal solar dermatitis
	Nodular dermatofibrosis
	Perianal fistulae
	Perianal-gland tumor
	Pituitary dwarfism
	Primary lymphedema
	Pyotraumatic dermatitis
	Tyrosinemia
	Vitiligo
	Zinc-responsive dermatosis
Golden Retriever	Allergic inhalant dermatitis
	Collagen nevi
	Hypothyroidism
	Ichthyosis
	Juvenile cellulitis
	Lymphosarcoma
	Periappendageal dermatitis (sebaceous adenitis)
	Pyotraumatic dermatitis (hot spots)
	Uveodermatologic syndrome (Vogt-Koyanagi-Harada-like syndrome)
Great Dane	Acne
	Acral lick dermatitis
	Calcinosis circumscripta (tumoral calcinosis)
	Callus
	Color mutant alopecia
	Demodicosis
	Dermoid cyst
	Histiocytoma
	Hypothyroidism
	Interdigital pyoderma
	Primary lymphedema
	Sterile pyogranuloma
	Zinc-responsive dermatosis
Greyhound	Color mutant alopecia
	Cutaneous asthenia
Irish Setter	Acral lick dermatitis
	Allergic inhalant dermatitis
	Callus
	Color mutant alopecia
	Hypothyroidism
	Keratinization disorders (seborrhea)
	Melanoma
	Sebaceous adenitis (granulomatous)
	Uveodermatologic syndrome (Vogt-Koyanagi-Harada-like syndrome)
Irish Wolfhound	Hypothyroidism

Congenito-Hereditary Skin Disorders

Karelian Bear Dog	Pituitary dwarf
Keeshond	Growth hormone-responsive dermatosis
	Intracutaneous cornifying epithelioma
Kerry Blue Terrier	Dermoid sinus
	Papilloma
	Pilomatrixoma
	Sebaceous-gland tumor
	Spiculosis
	Vascular nevi
Labrador Retriever	Acral lick dermatitis
	Allergic inhalant dermatitis
	Contact allergy (?)
	Focal mucinosis
	Infantile pustular dermatosis (impetigo)
	Interdigital pododermatitis
	Lipoma
	Mast-cell tumor
	Periappendageal dermatitis (sebaceous adenitis)
	Primary lymphedema
	Pyotraumatic dermatitis (hot spots)
	Vascular nevi
	Vitamin A-responsive dermatosis
Lhasa Apso	Allergic inhalant dermatitis
Malamute	Eosinophilic granuloma
	Hypothyroidism
	Zinc-responsive dermatosis
Mexican Hairless	Congenital alopecia
Newfoundland	Callus
	Hypothyroidism
	Sterile pyogranuloma
Norwegian Elkhound	Intracutaneous cornifying epithelioma
	Sebaceous-gland tumor
	Squamous-cell carcinoma
Old English Sheepdog	Demodicosis
	Intracutaneous cornifying epithelioma
	Primary lymphedema
	Uveodermatologic syndrome (Vogt-Koyanagi-Harada-like syndrome)
Papillon	Black hair follicular dysplasia
Pekingese	Face fold pyoderma
	Squamous-cell carcinoma
Pointer	Acral mutilation syndrome
	Callus
	Demodicosis
	Juvenile cellulitis
	Nasal pyoderma
Pomeranian	Hyperadrenocorticism
	Growth hormone-responsive dermatosis
	Sertoli-cell tumor
Poodle	Allergic inhalant dermatitis
	Anal licking
	Anal sacculitis
	Basal-cell tumor

Chapter 8

	Color mutant alopecia
	Cutaneous T-cell-like lymphoma
	Growth hormone-responsive dermatosis
	Hyperadrenocorticism
	Hypothyroidism
	Hypotrichosis
	Ichthyosis
	Junctional epidermolysis bullosa
	Juvenile panniculitis
	Lipoma
	Nodular panniculitis
	Pilomatrixoma
	Primary lymphedema
	Periappendageal dermatitis (sebaceous adenitis)
	Sebaceous-gland nevi
	Sebaceous-gland tumor
	Sertoli-cell tumor
	Squamous-cell carcinoma
	Zinc-responsive dermatosis
Pug	Allergic inhalant dermatitis
	Demodicosis
	Face fold pyoderma
	Tail fold pyoderma
Rhodesian Ridgeback	Dermoid sinus
Rottweiler	Acne
	Hypothyroidism
	Interdigital pododermatitis
St. Bernard	Callus
	Cutaneous asthenia
	Lip fold pyoderma
	Pyotraumatic dermatitis (hot spots)
	Sterile pyogranuloma
Samoyed	Hepatoid-gland tumor
	Nasal solar dermatitis
	Perianal-gland tumor
	Sebaceous adenitis (granulomatous) (periappendageal dermatitis)
	Uveodermatologic syndrome (Vogt-Koyanagi-Harada-like syndrome)
	Zinc-responsive dermatosis
Schipperke	Black hair follicular dysplasia
Schnauzer	Allergic inhalant dermatitis
	Cutaneous asthenia
	Hypothyroidism
	Schnauzer comedo syndrome
	Sertoli-cell tumor
	Subcorneal pustular dermatosis
	Vitamin A-responsive dermatosis
Scottish Terrier	Allergic inhalant dermatitis
	Lymphosarcoma
	Melanoma

Congenito-Hereditary Skin Disorders

	Squamous-cell carcinoma
	Vascular nevi
Shar Pei	Allergic inhalant dermatitis
	Body fold pyoderma
	Demodicosis
	Face fold pyoderma
	Focal mucinosis
	Food allergy (?)
	Hypothyroidism
	Infantile pustular dermatitis (impetigo)
	Interdigital pododermatitis
	Keratinization disorders (seborrhea)
	Lip fold pyoderma
	Pemphigus foliaceus (?)
Shetland Sheepdog	Bullous pemphigoid (?)
	Dermatomyositis
	Discoid lupus erythematosus
	Epidermolysis bullosa simplex (?)
	Focal mucinosis
	Histiocytoma
	Nasal solar dermatitis
	Pemphigus erythematosus (?)
	Sertoli-cell tumor
	Systemic lupus erythematosus
Shih Tzu	Allergic inhalant dermatitis
	Dermoid sinus
Siberian Husky	Discoid lupus erythematosus
	Eosinophilic granuloma
	Sertoli-cell tumor
	Uveodermatologic syndrome (Vogt-Koyanagi-Harada-like syndrome)
	Zinc-responsive dermatosis
Springer Spaniel	Cutaneous asthenia
	Hemangiopericytoma
	Keratinization disorders (seborrhea)
	Lip fold pyoderma
	Melanoma
	Psoriasiform-lichenoid dermatitis
Staffordshire Terrier	Demodicosis
	Mast-cell tumor
Weimaraner	Lipoma
	Mast-cell tumor
Welsh Corgi	Cutaneous asthenia
	Nasal solar dermatitis
West Highland White Terrier	Allergic inhalant dermatitis
	Ichthyosis
	Keratinization disorders (seborrhea)
Whippet	Color mutant alopecia
	Hypotrichosis
Yorkshire Terrier	Allergic inhalant dermatitis
	Sertoli-cell tumor

Additional Reading

1. O'Neill, CS: Hereditary skin disease in the dog and cat. *Comp Cont Ed Pract Vet* 3:791-800, 1981.

2. Merton, DA: Selective breeding in the dog and cat. Part 1. Fundamentals of inheritance and planned breeding. *Comp Cont Ed Pract Vet* 4:251-258, 1982.

3. Merton, DA: Selective breeding in the dog and cat. Part 2. Known and suspected genetic diseases. *Comp Cont Ed Pract Vet* 4:332-356, 1982.

4. Clark, RD and Stainer, RD: *Medical & Genetic Aspects of Purebred Dogs.* Veterinary Medicine Publishing, Edwardsville, KS, 1983. p 576.

Color Mutant Alopecia

Color mutant alopecia describes the patchy poor haircoat that develops in affected animals. They are born with normal coats but later suffer from hair loss, dry skin and cutaneous bacterial infections (Fig 35). The condition often involves a maculopapular eruption with associated hair loss. If one looks closely, the skin disease is confined only to abnormally colored hairs.

The principal breeds involved include Blue Doberman Pinschers, Great Danes, Dachshunds, Whippets, Italian Greyhounds and Standard Poodles. Red Doberman Pinschers and Fawn Irish Setters may have milder forms of the disorder.

Diagnosis is based on clinical signs and biopsies for histopathologic examination. Most of these dogs are not hypothyroid and do not benefit from unwarranted supplementation of thyroxine. Similarly, zinc supplementation rarely improves the condition. Biopsies often reveal profound follicular hyperkeratosis and cystic dilatation of affected hair follicles. Perifolliculitis, hyperpigmentation of hair bulbs, and melanin-laden histiocytes about the hair bulb are other common findings.

Treatment is symptomatic and lifelong, since the abnormal hair follicles cannot be replaced. Antiseborrheic shampoos are normally prescribed to remove the prominent scale that forms on the skin surface. Therapy should be considered lifelong and affected animals should not be used for breeding.

Additional Reading

1. Briggs, OM and Botha, WS: Color mutant alopecia in a blue Italian Greyhound. *JAAHA* 22: 611-614, 1986.

Cutaneous Asthenia

Cutaneous asthenia (Ehlers-Danlos syndrome) represents a number of different biochemical disorders that result in skin fragility, overextensibility and possible laxity of the joints. These animals are the "rubber men" of the dog world. The changes are due to defects in creation of collagen, which is responsible for the strength and fibrous stabilization of the dermis. When the skin of affected dogs is pulled, it stretches excessively to the point where it can even tear. Affected breeds include the Beagle, Dachshund, Boxer, St. Bernard, German Shepherd, English Springer Spaniel, Greyhound, Schnauzer and mongrels. The genetic nature of the condition is complex, but there is much evidence to suggest a dominant trend.

The condition is usually easily diagnosed by clinical findings. A skin extensibility index, measured by a ratio of the maximum dorsal displacement of skin to total body length x 100, is inevitably >17%. A diagnosis may or may not be supported by biopsy results, since some forms of cutaneous asthenia show characteristic light microscopic changes, while others are only discernible by electron microscopy. Animals with defects in fibrillogenesis have abnormal segments of collagen fibers that can be identified by their failure to stain blue or green with trichrome stains.

There is no specific treatment for cutaneous asthenia because there is no method to overcome the inherited collagen defect. Large doses of vitamin C (vitamin C is a cofactor in collagen synthesis) and minimizing the potential for skin injury are the only steps that can be taken in management. These animals should definitely not be bred. Further, it is usually not safe for them to undergo surgery, even neutering.

Additional Reading

1. Minor, RR *et al*: Defects in collagen fibrillogenesis causing hyperextensible, fragile skin in dogs. *JAVMA* 182:142-148, 1983.

2. Prockop, DJ and Kivirikko, KI: Heritable diseases of collagen. *N Engl J Med* 311:376-386, 1984.

3. Freeman, LJ *et al*: Ehlers-Danlos syndrome in dogs and cats. *Sem Vet Med Surg* 2:221-227, 1987.

Dermatomyositis, Epidermolysis Bullosa Simplex

Dermatomyositis has been recently described in dogs. Cases earlier described as epidermolysis bullosa simplex may actually have been dermatomyositis. Since these conditions show such great clinical similarity, they will be discussed together. Junctional epidermolysis bullosa has recently been described in dogs but is an entity distinct from epidermolysis bullosa simplex.

Dermatomyositis is seen mostly in Collies, Shetland Sheepdogs and their crosses. Animals first begin to show signs at about 12 weeks of age. Lesions include scaling, ulcers and erosions most prevalent over the face, ears, elbows, hocks and other friction points (Fig 36). Hair may also be lost from the tip of the tail. In later stages, muscle wasting may also be seen, especially on the top of the head (temporalis muscles) and over the hindquarters. The condition is inherited as an autosomal dominant trait with variable expressivity. This means that if one parent is affected, most of the offspring will be affected. This is an important consideration, since parents may only be mildly affected themselves but should be closely scrutinized if they produce affected young.

Diagnosis

There is no blood test to identify carriers, and not enough data have been collected to permit pedigree analysis to select good breeding stock. Most cases are diagnosed on the basis of the history, clincial signs, electromyography and biopsy. Well-chosen biopsies often reveal interface dermatitis with hydropic degeneration of basal cells, subepidermal clefting and a mixed perivascular inflammatory infiltrate. Electromyographic abnormalities include fibrillation potentials, positive sharp waves and bizarre high-frequency discharges.

Treatment

Therapy is only symptomatic. Both vitamin E and corticosteroids have been used to relieve scaling and scarring. An antimalarial, hydroxychloroquine (Plaquinol), has been used to lessen the severity of cutaneous lesions in people, but I have tried it in too few cases (at 2-4 mg/kg BID) to recommend its routine use. Because of the potential risk of retinopathy with long-term use of antimalarials, periodic ophthalmologic examination is mandatory.

The disease usually determines its own path around the time of puberty, when some animals deteriorate further or recover spontaneously. Recovered animals should definitely not be bred, since offspring will undoubtedly be affected, at least to some extent.

Additional Reading

1. Hargis, AM *et al*: Familial canine dermatomyositis. *Am J Pathol* 120:323-325, 1985.

2. Hargis, AM *et al*: A skin disorder in three Shetland sheepdogs: Comparison with familial canine dermatomyositis of Collies. *Comp Cont Ed Pract Vet* 7:306-315, 1985.

3. Dunstan, RW *et al*: A mechanobullous disease (junctional epidermolysis bullosa) in a Toy Poodle. *Proc Ann Mtg Am Acad Vet Dermatol*, 1987. p 10.

Dermoid Sinus

Dermoid sinus refers to an abnormal congenital tract that connects the skin surface with the underlying spine (actually the supraspinous ligament or the dura mater) via a communicating tunnel. The tract is lined with skin; therefore, sebum, hair and debris eventually fill the channel and cause inflammation. Though the condition is most common in Rhodesian Ridgebacks, it has also been reported in the Boxer and Shih Tzu.

Diagnosis can usually be made on the basis of clinical signs and fistulography and can be confirmed by biopsy. Histopathologic evaluation reveals that the sinus is lined by a stratified squamous epithelium, complete with adnexa.

Complete excision is the only real cure, but individuals usually recover and appear completely normal. These animals should not be used for breeding.

Additional Reading

1. Hathcock, JT *et al*: Dermoid sinus in a Rhodesian Ridgeback. *Vet Med* 74:53-56, 1979.

2. Selcer, EA *et al*: Dermoid sinus in a Shih Tzu and a Boxer. *JAAHA* 20:634-636, 1984.

Disorders Of Pigmentation

Albinism

Albinism is extremely rare in dogs and is a hereditary lack of pigmentation supposedly transmitted as an autosomal recessive trait. Albinos have melanocytes but have a biochemical defect in that they lack the tyrosinase necessary to synthesize melanin.

Vitiligo

Vitiligo, describes a patchy loss of pigment that may be inherited or acquired. Thus, pigmentary loss may be due to such nongenetic factors as autoimmune disorders (*eg*, autoimmune vitiligo, lupus erythematosus, Vogt-Koyanagi-Harada-like syndrome), some cancers (*eg*, melanoma, cutaneous T-cell lymphoma) and postinflammatory change. A heritable form of vitiligo may be seen in Belgian Tervurens and Doberman Pinschers ("Dudley nose"), though the actual heritability has not been confirmed. A similar loss of pigment in Chow Chows is due to an inherited deficiency of tyrosinase, an enzyme important in pigment production.

Gray Collie Syndrome

Some Collie pups born with a silver-gray haircoat may be smaller and weaker than their normal littermates, and may have a light-colored nose. It appears to be transmitted as an autosomal recessive trait. By 8-12 weeks of age, they develop clinical signs that may include fever, diarrhea, conjunctivitis, arthralgia and a cyclic neutropenia at 11- to 14-day intervals. Neutropenia is followed by rebounding neutrophilia.

Diagnosis can be confirmed by sequential blood counts over a 14-day period. Therapy is invariably unsuccessful and most animals succumb during periods of neutropenia. Parents and littermates should not be used for breeding.

Lentigo

Lentigo (lentiginosis profusa) is a rare condition in which black macules are found on skin caused by focal increase in pigmentation. The Pug appears to be predisposed. The mode of inheritance may be autosomal dominant, though progeny studies have not yet been done. The animal's health status remains unaffected, but they become inadequate for show purposes. Transition to melanoma has not been reported in the dog. There is no practical therapy, though dermabrasion and electrodesiccation have been used in people.

Additional Reading

1. Guaguere, E and Alhaidari, Z, in Kirk, R: *Current Veterinary Therapy VIII.* Saunders, Philadelphia, 1989. p 628-632.

2. Mahaffey, MB *et al*: Focal loss of pigment in the Belgian Tervuren dog. *JAVMA* 173:390-396, 1970.

3. Briggs, OM: Lentiginosis profusa in the pug: Three case reports. *J Small Anim Pract* 26:675-680, 1985

Hair Follicle Defects

Congenital Hypotrichosis

Congenital hypotrichosis (alopecia) is a rare ectodermal defect reported in the Cocker Spaniel, Belgian Shepherd, Toy Poodle, Whippet, Bichon Frise, Basset Hound, Labrador Retriever and

Beagle. It is not known whether these animals were affected by the same or different genetic processes. Poodles and Basset Hounds may be predisposed, and males may be at increased risk.

Diagnosis is usually not a problem, as hair loss is readily apparent. Biopsies of affected areas usually demonstrate orthokeratotic hyperkeratosis, a normal epidermis and rudimentary hair follicles and adnexa. Therapeutic intervention is unsuccessful, as there are no normal follicles present from which to grow hair, and new follicles do not develop after birth.

Additional Reading

1. Chastain, CB and Swayne, DE: Congenital hypotrichosis in male Basset hound littermates. *JAVMA* 187:845-846, 1985.

2. Grieshaber, TL *et al:* Congenital alopecia in a bichon frise. *JAVMA* 188:1053-1054, 1986.

3. Kunkle, GA: Congenital hypotrichosis in two dogs. *JAVMA* 185:84-85, 1984.

Follicular Dysplasia

Follicular dysplasia is characterized by alterations in size, shape and orientation of hairs. Primary hairs are more commonly affected than secondary hairs. The condition is seen most commonly in animals <1 year of age, most frequently as a tardive trait.

Diagnosis is based on characteristic biopsies and normal hormonal assays. Biopsies often display follicles arrested in catagen, with involvement of predominantly primary follicles. Twisting and convolution of the glassy membrane are frequently noted. A breed-related dysplasia appears to occur in the Siberian Husky, in which guard hairs are shed and not replaced. The undercoat then takes on a rusty hue, and alopecia may result.

Black Hair Follicular Dysplasia

Black hair follicular dysplasia is seen in dogs with at least some black haircoat. Though the dogs are normal at birth, they later begin to lose only black hairs in certain areas. Nonblack hairs remain normal throughout. The condition has been reported in a number of breeds, including the Dachshund, Papillon, Bearded Collie, Schipperke and mongrels. Though the exact mode of inheritance has not been established, when 2 affected individuals are bred, most of the offspring are affected by 4 weeks of age.

Additional Reading

1. Gosselin, Y et al: Black hair follicular dysplasia in a dog. *Canine Pract* 9(2):8-15, 1982.
2. Stogdale, L et al: Congenital hypotrichosis in a dog. *JAAHA* 18:184-187, 1982.
3. Post, K et al: Hair follicle dysplasia in a Siberian husky. *JAAHA* 24:659-662, 1988.

Spiculosis

"Spiculosis" refers to a hair shaft disorder in Kerry Blue Terriers. In one report, affected dogs were 6-30 months old, and all 3 were male. Hairs on the face, trunk and extremities were brittle and thick, and had large "spicules." The spicules were so named because of spiny appearance on microscopic examination. These abnormal hairs may result from fusion of the primary and secondary hairshafts at the level of the hair bulb.

Additional Reading

1. Torres, SMF: Speculating on "spiculosis." *Proc Ann Mtg Am Acad Vet Dermatol*, 1988. p 25.

Ichthyosis

In ichthyosis, the surface of the skin is covered by a thick, tenacious scale. Various types of ichthyosis occur in people, the major groupings consisting of ichthyosis vulgaris, X-linked ichthyosis, lamellar ichthyosis and epidermolytic hyperkeratosis. Different forms of ichthyosis may be transmitted as autosomal dominant, sex-linked or autosomal recessive traits. It is uncertain as to which types the animal cases most resemble. The condition is rare but has been documented in West Highland White Terriers, Golden Retrievers, Doberman Pinschers, Standard Poodles and in a terrier mix. It is uncertain if all of these cases actually represent the same defect.

Diagnosis can usually be strongly suspected from clinical signs and histopathologic findings. Major histologic changes include marked orthokeratotic hyperkeratosis, dyskeratosis, hypergranulosis, and mitotic figures in the epidermis.

Treatment must be intense and results are usually disappointing. Strong antiseborrheic products, including sulfur and/or tar shampoos, are helpful, as are lactic acid and urea products available from drug stores. Some of the newer vitamin A derivatives, such as retinoids and especially etretinate, may have an important role in the management of patients with ichthyosis. Even intense treatment, however, will only mask the disorder. As with all hereditary defects, treatment is only palliative.

Additional Reading
1. Williams, ML and Elias, PM: Ichthyosis. *Arch Dermatol* 122:529-531, 1986.
2. Muller, GH: Ichthyosis in two dogs. *JAVMA* 169:1313-1316, 1976.

Lethal Acrodermatitis

Lethal acrodermatitis is a fatal disorder seen in Bull Terriers and inherited as an autosomal recessive trait. Thymic hypoplasia is likely a significant component of this disorder.

The syndrome is characterized by growth retardation, progressive acrodermatitis, pyoderma, paronychia, diarrhea, pneumonia, abnormal behavior and death by 16 months of age.

Affected pups have somewhat lighter pigmentation than unaffected littermates at birth; with time, this difference becomes progressively more evident. Eating is often difficult and most pups appear weaker than littermates. The feet become typically splayed and, by 6-10 weeks of age, dermatologic manifestations become evident. Clinical signs include mucocutaneous crusting dermatitis, hyperkeratotic footpads, interdigital pododermatitis, paronychia, facial erythroderma and generalized papulopustular dermatitis. Ocular changes include light and mottled pigmentation around the pupillary border of the iris and occasionally small zonular opacities in the lens.

Diagnosis is based on history, clinical signs, histopathologic examination and lymphocyte blastogenesis. Skin biopsies do not confirm the diagnosis, but typical changes include orthokeratotic and parakeratotic hyperkeratosis and a mixed perivascular inflammatory infiltrate. At necropsy, the thymus is absent or markedly hypoplastic.

The syndrome appears similar to lethal trait A46 in cattle and acrodermatitis enteropathica in people. Unlike those conditions, it is unresponsive to zinc supplementation. The underlying defect may involve multiple trace minerals, including zinc and copper. The metabolic defect appears to cause immune system dysfunction.

Additional Reading
1. Jezyk, PF *et al*: Lethal acrodermatitis in bull terriers. *JAVMA* 188:833-839, 1986.

Chapter 8

Acral Mutilation Syndrome

Acral mutilation syndrome is a bizarre condition reported in German Short Haired Pointer and English Pointer pups. It is probably inherited as an autosomal recessive trait. Because of a sensory neuropathy, affected individuals destroy their distal extremities by self-mutilation.

The condition first appears in animals 3-5 months of age as a loss of pain sensation in the toes. Chewing at the feet leads to mutilation. Paronychia, pododermatitis and swelling are commonly noted.

The condition is based on the history, clinical signs, electromyography and histopathologic examination. No denervation potentials are evident of electromyographic evaluation. Nerve changes are seen in tissue sections.

Additional Reading

1. Cummings, JF *et al:* Acral mutilation and nociceptive loss in English pointer dogs. *Acta Neuropathol* 53:119-122, 1981.

Chapter 9
Skin Tumors

Skin tumors are the most common neoplasms seen in dogs. Not all are harmful, and therefore a method of naming tumors has evolved to denote not only the original cell type of the cancer but also its biologic activity. Benign tumors are unlikely to have complications and are designated by the suffix -oma (*eg*, lipoma, a benign fatty tumor). Malignant tumors do much harm and may also metastasize. They are designated as to whether their origin is epithelial, by the suffix -carcinoma (*eg*, adenocarcinoma, a malignant glandular cancer) or nonepithelial, by the suffix -sarcoma (*eg*, liposarcoma, a malignant fatty tumor). The prognosis with skin tumors varies from good to poor, depending on the type of neoplasm involved.

Additional Reading

1. Conroy, JD: Canine skin tumors. *JAAHA* 19:91-114, 1983.

2. Bevier, DE and Goldschmidt, MH: Skin tumors in the dog. Part I. Epithelial tumors and tumorlike lesions. *Comp Cont Ed Pract Vet* 3:389-400, 1981.

3. Bevier, DE and Goldschmidt, MH: Skin tumors in the dog. Part II. Tumors of the soft (mesenchymal) tissues. *Comp Cont Ed Pract Vet* 3:506-516, 1981.

4. Goldschmidt, MH and Bevier, DE: Skin tumors in the dog. Part III. Lymphohistiocytic and melanocytic tumors. *Comp Cont Ed Pract Vet* 3:588-594, 1981.

5. Esplin, DG and Carr, SH: Skin tumors and other cutaneous masses. *MVP* 64:5-10, 1983.

6. Roszel, JF *et al*: Use of cytology for tumor diagnosis in private veterinary practice. *JAVMA* 173:1011-1014, 1978.

7. Meyer, DJ and Franks, P: Clinical cytology. Part 2. Cytologic characteristics of tumors. *MVP* 67:440-445, 1986.

8. Allen, SW and Prasse, KW: Cytologic diagnosis of neoplasia and perioperative implementation. *Comp Cont Ed Pract Vet* 8:72-80, 1986.

9. Barton, CL: Cytologic diagnosis of cutaneous neoplasia: an algorithmic approach. *Comp Cont Ed Pract Vet* 9:20-33, 1987.

10. Feldman, BF *et al*: Plasma fibronectin concentration associated with various types of canine neoplasia. *Am J Vet Res* 49:1017-1019, 1988.

Basal-Cell Tumor

Basal-cell tumors are common benign growths that may have some breed predisposition for Poodles and Cocker Spaniels. The tumors are found predominantly in middle-aged dogs (average is 9 years of age). Basal-cell tumors may develop on sun-damaged skin, though this has not been decidedly proven.

Clinical Signs

Most basal-cell tumors are solitary and usually arise on the head, neck and shoulders. They may be large or small lumps that are well encapsulated and move freely with the skin, not bound to underlying tissues.

Diagnosis

The tumors are usually easily diagnosed on histopathologic examination. A variety of patterns occur (solid, garland, medusoid, adenoid), though they all appear to have similar behavior. On cytologic examination, aspirates reveal clusters of small round cells with large oval nuclei and little cytoplasm.

Management

The tumors may be surgically removed or left without problem. Metastasis of basal-cell tumors has never been reported.

Basosquamous carcinoma is considered a different subset of basal-cell tumors and may even be a completely different entity. It has a much more aggressive behavior than basal-cell tumors and grows by infiltrating adjacent stroma. Metastasis to regional lymph nodes or lung may occur. Early excision is the treatment of choice, but local recurrence is a problem because the tumor is often poorly cirumscribed.

Additional Reading

1. Goldschmidt, MH: Basal- and squamous-cell neoplasms of dogs and cats. *Am J Dermatopathol* 6:199-206, 1984.

Cutaneous Cysts

Cutaneous cysts are derived from epidermal or pilosebaceous components and are diagnosed clinically many more times than they can be confirmed histologically.

Apocrine cysts result from retention of secretion from apocrine glands because of occlusion of the excretory duct. The most common cause is follicular hyperkeratosis, in which the hair follicle itself is blocked.

Dermoid cysts are usually congenital defects and most common in the Rhodesian Ridgeback, though they have been reported in other breeds. They are different from other keratinous cysts in that they have adnexa associated with the lining epithelium. Hair follicles containing hair project into the lumen of the cyst. Careful excision is curative.

Epidermal cysts are derived from the epidermis or the outer root sheath of hair follicles, and may occur in a dermal or subcutaneous location. They are most commonly found in the head, neck and sacral regions. Histologically, these cysts consist of well-differentiated stratified squamous epithelium lacking adnexa that undergoes gradual keratinization, with a granular cell layer. If the cyst ruptures, the keratin material results in a pronounced foreign body reaction in the dermis and/or subcutis. Excision is the treatment of choice for epidermal cysts.

Follicular cysts or pilar cysts, as they are sometimes known, may be further subclassified as trichilemmal or proliferating. Trichilemmal cysts are derived from the epithelium of the outer root sheath from the isthmus region of the follicle. The cysts are comprised of an epithelial lining that shows abrupt keratinization, without a granular layer. Sequelae may include rupture with associated foreign body reaction or calcification of keratin.

Proliferating follicular cysts are associated with epidermal hyperplasia and may contain secondary cysts. Basaloid cells and abrupt keratinization differentiate this cyst from intracutaneous cornifying epithelioma (keratoacanthoma).

Excision is curative for both types of follicular cysts.

Fibroma, Fibrosarcoma, Nodular Dermatofibrosis

Fibromas

Fibromas are uncommon benign tumors, seen more frequently in females and with a breed predisposition for Boxers, Boston Terriers and Fox Terriers.

Clinical Signs: Older animals are more commonly affected. The masses are firm to soft, usually solitary, noninvasive and non-metastatic. They are most commonly located on the limbs, flanks and perineum.

Diagnosis: Diagnosis is by finding a well-differentiated proliferation of fibrocytes and collagen in interlacing bundles on histopathologic examination. Cytologic examination is rarely helpful in diagnosing mesenchymal tumors.

Management: Excision is usually curative.

Fibrosarcomas

Fibrosarcomas are the malignant counterpart of fibromas. They are more common in females and may have a predilection for Cocker Spaniels. The average age of affected individuals is about 9 years.

Clinical Signs: The masses are often irregular in shape, poorly circumscribed and frequently ulcerated. Most fibrosarcomas are locally invasive and metastasize only in about 25% of cases. They are most commonly found on the limbs and trunk, and less often on the head, neck, oral cavity and mammary regions.

Diagnosis: Diagnosis is usually easily rendered on biopsy. Fibrosarcomas display poorly circumscribed proliferations of atypical, pleomorphic spindle-shaped cells. Mitoses are not infrequently found. Cytologic examination is less helpful for mesenchymal tumors than for other neoplasms.

Management: Incomplete excision may result in recurrence in about 30% of cases. Radiotherapy, hyperthermia, and even arterial cross-circulation have been proposed as alternative forms of therapy for fibrosarcoma.

Generalized Nodular Dermatofibrosis

Generalized nodular dermatofibrosis has been observed in German Shepherds with renal cystadenocarcinoma. Nodular dermatofibrosis is important because it is a cutaneous indication of internal malignancy.

Clinical Signs: This condition is characterized by collagenous papules and nodules, usually involving the head, trunk and back legs of adult dogs.

Diagnosis: The diagnosis is based on the history, appearance of the lesions, blood tests and biopsies. Histopathologic examination demonstrates nodules consisting of densely packed, mature-appearing fibrous connective tissue that infiltrates the dermis, panniculus and sometimes deeper structures. The clinical presentation varies, depending on the presence or absence of uremia, polyuria, polydipsia and metastasis.

Management: Treatment usually is not attempted unless the nodules interfere with movement, in which case excision should be attempted. Though some animals improve after the neoplastic kidney is resected, the prognosis must remain guarded.

Additional Reading

1. Brewer, Jr., WG and Turrel, JM: Radiotherapy and hyperthermia in the treatment of fibrosarcomas in the dog. *JAVMA* 181:146-150, 1982.

2. Hustead, DR *et al*: Fibrosarcoma: Therapy with arterial cross circulation. *Vet Med* 80:41-43, 1985.

3. Cosenza, SF and Seely, JC: Generalized nodular dermatofibrosis and renal cystadenocarcinomas in a German Shepherd dog. *JAVMA* 189:1587-1590, 1986.

4. Lium, B and Moe, L: Hereditary multifocal renal cystadenocarcinomas and nodular dermatofibrosis in the German Shepherd dog: macroscopic and histopathologic changes. *Vet Pathol* 22:447-455, 1985.

Hemangioma, Hemangiosarcoma

Hemangioma

Hemangiomas are uncommon benign tumors of blood vessels. The average age of affected individuals is about 8 years. Boxers may be at increased risk.

Clinical Signs: The masses are usually solitary, well-circumscribed and pigmented, and occur most commonly on the limbs, flank, neck and face.

Diagnosis: Diagnosis is on the basis of biopsy. Histologically, hemangiomas are typed as capillary or cavernous but both consist of proliferations of thin-walled vessels lined by typical endothelium; most of the vascular spaces contain erythrocytes.

Management: The tumors have a rich blood supply and may be treated by careful resection or conscientious neglect.

Hemangiosarcoma

The malignant form, the hemangiosarcoma, occurs more commonly in males. The average age of affected individuals is about

8 years. German Shepherds, Boxers and Bernese Mountain Dogs are predisposed.

Clinical Signs: Hemangiosarcoma can cause a wide variety of clinical signs, depending on the primary site and the degree of systemic metastatic involvement. They can arise from any blood vessel in the body, but primary tumors are most common in the right atrium and spleen in addition to cutaneous, subcutaneous and muscular locations. Internal tumor rupture can result in intermittent lethargy with pallor to acute collapse and shock.

Hemangiosarcoma is a poorly circumscribed neoplasm that causes marked inflammation of surrounding tissue. Most masses are a mixture of capillary and cavernous forms.

Diagnosis: On biopsy, the masses consist of sarcomatous endothelial cells with a high mitotic index and accompanying hemosiderin-laden macrophages. The growths are highly invasive and malignant. Metastasis occurs early because sarcomatous endothelium is easily shed into local blood vessels.

Management: Regardless of the form of therapy attempted, the prognosis is poor. Splenectomy may be warranted if this is a primary site of tumor involvement.

Additional Reading

1. Fees, DL and Withrow, SJ: Canine hemangiosarcoma. *Comp Cont Ed Pract Vet* 3:1047-1051, 1981.

2. Brown, NO: Hemangiosarcomas. *Vet Clin No Am* 15:569-576, 1985.

Hemangiopericytoma

Hemangiopericytomas are common benign tumors thought to originate from the tissue surrounding blood vessels. Boxers, German Shepherds, Cocker Spaniels, Springer Spaniels and Fox Terriers appear predisposed. Females are more commonly affected than males.

Clinical Signs

The tumors are usually firm and large, and occur most commonly on the limbs, but are occasionally found on the trunk, head, neck and mammary regions (Fig 37). The average age of affected individuals is about 9 years.

Diagnosis

Diagnosis is rendered on biopsy. Cytologic examination is not of much benefit (though a whorled or "fingerprint" pattern is suggestive). Histologically, the tumor displays proliferations of spindle-shaped cells arranged in sheets, and whorled perivascular patterns. Differentiating hemangiopericytoma from fibrosarcoma is not always easy.

Management

Resection is the the therapy of choice, but about one-fourth eventually recur following excision. Radiation therapy may be a useful adjunct when complete excision is impossible.

Additional Reading

1. Postorino, NC et al: Prognostic variables for canine hemangiopericytoma: 50 cases (1979-1984). JAAHA 24:501-509, 1988.

2. Fossum, TW et al: Treatment of hemangiopericytoma in a dog using surgical excision, radiation, and a thoracic pedicle skin graft. JAVMA 193:1440-1442, 1988.

Histiocytic Tumors

Histiocytoma

Histiocytomas are fairly common tumors often seen in young dogs, most <2 years of age. Histiocytomas are more prevalent in the Boxer, Cocker Spaniel, Great Dane, Shetland Sheepdog and Dachshund but may occur in any breed. The tumor may be induced by a virus, but this remains unsubstantiated.

Clinical Signs: Histiocytomas appear as a small, "red button" on the skin surface, usually on the head or ears (Fig 38).

Diagnosis: Diagnosis is based on clinical signs, cytologic examination and biopsy for histopathologic evaluation. Cytologically, histiocytomas are round-cell tumors, with a finely granular chromatin pattern and pale-blue cytoplasm with distinct margins. The tumor is comprised of poorly circumscribed collections of mononuclear cells, with associated accumulations of lymphocytes (more common peripherally) and zones of necrosis. On tissue sections, the tumor looks very aggressive, but in reality it usually spontaneously regresses without the need for medical or surgical intervention. Biopsies should be read by veterinary pathologists, since people do not get histiocytomas and human pathologists may read the biopsy as a malignant cutaneous histiocytoma, which warrants a poor prognosis.

Management: No treatment is necessary, as histiocytomas spontaneously regress. Only rarely do new tumors arise at the site of excision or at other sites.

Cutaneous Histiocytosis

Clinical Signs: Cutaneous histiocytosis involves dermal and pannicular infiltrates of histiocytic cells that appear as erythematous plaques and nodules that wax and wane, and appear in new sites, regardless of treatment.

Diagnosis: Diagnosis of histiocytosis is based on biopsies for histopathologic examination. The histiocytic nature of the infiltrating cells can be documented by using special staining techniques for detection of lysozyme activity.

Management: Therapy with corticosteroids and chemotherapy is only temporarily beneficial. Internal dissemination is not a feature of this condition. The histologic behavior and clinical presentation in many ways are more suggestive of an inflammatory process rather than a neoplastic process. Some pathologists believe this may represent a manifestation of leptospirosis, rather than a histiocytic disorder.

Malignant (Systemic) Histiocytosis

Malignant histiocytosis has recently been described in dogs. The Bernese Mountain Dog appears to be predisposed.

Clinical Signs: Malignant histiocytosis is characterized by a rapidly progressive and inevitably fatal course. Multiple cutaneous nodules are distributed on the body surface, but there may be a site predilection for the scrotum, nasal planum and eyelids. Clinical signs vary, but lethargy, anorexia, weight loss, lymphadenomegaly, anemia, hepatosplenomegaly, respiratory and CNS abnormalities predominate. The lungs were the primary site of tumor involvement in most cases.

Diagnosis: Diagnosis is based on biopsy. Histopathologic examination reveals atypical histiocytes, with frequent mitoses, invading the dermis and panniculus in a nodular to diffuse pattern.

Management: All forms of therapy have been ineffective. Immunomodulation remains an option worth attempting.

Fibrous Histiocytoma

Fibrous histiocytomas (nodular fasciitis) are uncommon. Research suggests that they may be granulomatous rather than neoplastic.

Clinical Signs: Fibrous histiocytomas occur in younger dogs (2-4 years average). Collies appear predisposed. The nodules and plaques are most commonly seen on the face, especially the lips and sclera, but occasionally on the feet. Ophthalmologists usually refer to the condition as nodular (granulomatous) episcleritis.

Diagnosis: Diagnosis is based on typical histopathologic findings of fibroblasts and histiocytes in a swirling stroma. A lymphocytic-plasmacytic infiltrate is usually evident peripherally.

Management: Oral or sublesional corticosteroids are the treatment of choice. In unresponsive or refractory cases, azathioprine is a logical alternative.

Malignant Fibrous Histiocytoma (Giant-Cell Tumor)

Malignant fibrous histiocytoma is a rare malignancy believed to be of histiocytic origin.

Clinical Signs: The tumors are nodular and locally invasive to deeper tissues but are apparently slow to metastasize. There may be a site predilection for the limbs and neck.

Diagnosis: Histologically, malignant fibrous histiocytoma is characterized by an infiltrative collection of pleomorphic histiocytes, fibroblasts and multinucleated giant cells with mitotic figures not infrequently seen.

Management: The therapy of choice is radical excision.

Additional Reading

1. Calderwood Mays, LMB and Bergeron, JA: Cutaneous histiocytosis in dogs. *JAVMA* 188: 377-381, 1986.

2. Tully, RC: Cutaneous histiocytosis vs. leptospirosis. *JAVMA* 188:1142-1143, 1986.

3. Rosin, A *et al*: Malignant histiocytosis in Bernese mountain dogs. *JAVMA* 188:1041-1045, 1986.

4. Bender, WM and Muller, GH: Multiple, resolving, cutaneous histiocytoma in a dog. *JAVMA* 194:535-537, 1989.

Intracutaneous Cornifying Epithelioma

Intracutaneous cornifying epithelioma (also known as keratoacanthoma) usually develops in younger dogs (<5 years). Males are more often affected than females.

Clinical Signs

In most breeds, the tumor is solitary and often has a pore on the top. In such breeds as the Norwegian Elkhound, Old English Sheepdog and Keeshond, the lesions may be generalized and range in number from a few growths to several hundred.

Diagnosis

Diagnosis is by biopsy. Histologically, the tumor consists of a keratin-filled cavity lined by stratified squamous epithelium and including nests of keratinocytes that sporadically form horn cysts.

Management

Treatment for the solitary lesions is resection. Intracutaneous cornifying epitheliomas neither recur following excision nor metastasize. For the generalized form, observation without therapy may be a realistic alternative. Some of the newer vitamin A derivatives, such as etretinate (Tegison), have successfully been used to treat generalized keratoacanthomas in people. I have had some limited success with similar treatments in dogs, though the product is currently not licensed for this use.

Additional Reading

1. Stannard, AA and Pulley, LT: Intracutaneous cornifying epithelioma (keratoacanthoma) in the dog: A retrospective study of 25 cases. *JAVMA* 167:385-388, 1975.

Keratoses

Keratoses are accumulations of keratin. They may be seborrheic, actinic, lichenoid or proliferative (cutaneous "horns").

Seborrheic keratoses are nodular to plaque-like growths that often are hyperpigmented and have a greasy texture. On biopsy they show extreme orthokeratotic hyperkeratosis and papillomatous epidermal hyperplasia.

Actinic keratoses are caused by excessive exposure of skin to ultraviolet light. They form on lightly haired or lightly pigmented skin, which receives a comparatively large amount of ultraviolet irradiation from sunlight. Biopsy shows dysplastic epidermal cells and hyperkeratosis. Actinic keratosis may be a premalignant lesion that can develop into squamous-cell carcinoma.

Proliferative keratoses (cutaneous horns) form from accumulations of compact lamellated orthokeratotic hyperkeratosis that may overlay tumors, virus-induced lesions or other keratoses.

Lichenoid keratoses are generally solitary lesions confined to the ears and infrequently result in clinical problems. They appear as grouped plaques and often have a scaly surface. Biopsy shows irregular epidermal hyperplasia and interface dermatitis with a lichenoid band of mononuclear inflammatory cells.

Lipoma

Lipomas are common benign tumors arising from subcutaneous fat. They are most common in older dogs (8 years average). Some predilection exists for obese females and Cocker Spaniels, Dachshunds, Weimaraners, Labrador Retrievers and Terriers.

Clinical Signs

They are usually fair-sized, soft to flabby and well circumscribed, and most commonly located around the neck, chest, abdomen and limbs. Most lipomas are innocuous, but large tumors may undergo necrosis and calcification.

Diagnosis

Further diagnostic testing is usually not warranted but confirmation can easily be rendered by biopsy. Histologically the tumors are composed of proliferations of adipocytes with pyknotic nuclei.

Management

Most lipomas can be neglected, but some that compromise the function of other organ systems or are a nuisance to the animal may be surgically removed. Putting the dog on a diet beforehand not only lessens the risk of surgery, but also helps delineate the tumor. An alternative to surgery is injecting 10% calcium chloride into the lipoma in a volume estimated to be half of that of the lipoma itself. Skin overlying injected tumors may slough.

Liposarcoma

Liposarcomas are rare tumors that are less well circumscribed than lipomas. They are rapid-growing and invasive neoplasms that do not arise from preexisting lipomas.

Diagnosis

Histologically, liposarcomas can be classified as well differentiated, round-cell, myxoid and pleomorphic. The frequency of mitosis is variable, though bizarre features may become apparent. Metastasis is uncommon.

Management

Treatment for liposarcoma may involve complete surgical excision and chemotherapy, if warranted.

Infiltrative Lipomatosis

Infiltrative lipomas can interfere with movement because the proliferative fat cells inflitrate or replace muscle or collagen. Complete resection is difficult and recurrence is common, though metastasis has not been reported.

Additional Reading

1. Albers, GW and Theilen, GH: Calcium chloride for treatment of subcutaneous lipomas in dogs. *JAVMA* 186:492-494, 1985.

2. Strafuss, AC *et al*: Lipomas in dogs. *JAAHA* 9:555-561, 1973.

3. Ackerman, LJ and Silver, JN: Abdominal liposarcoma in a dog. *MVP* 65:468-469, 1984.

4. Kramek, BA *et al*: Infiltrative lipoma in three dogs. *JAVMA* 186:81-82, 1985.

5. Romatowski, J: Canine liposarcomatosis. *MVP* 66:707-709, 1985.

Lymphosarcoma

Cutaneous lymphosarcoma is a malignant disorder of lymphocytes. As outlined in the introductory section on the immune system, the 2 varieties of lymphocytes, B-cells and T-cells, each may be involved in a cancerous process.

B-Cell Lymphosarcoma

B-cell lymphosarcoma is more common in elderly dogs, with males 3 times more frequently affected than females.

Clinical Signs: Affected animals may have strictly cutaneous lesions, such as nodules, plaques or a maculopapular rash, or may have systemic involvement, including leukemia and/or liver, spleen and lymph node enlargement.

Diagnosis: Diagnosis is by cytologic examination (including blood smears) and biopsies for histopathologic examination. A complete blood count is indicated, as are a biochemical profile and serum protein electrophoresis to help detect internal disease. Strictly cutaneous B-cell lymphosarcoma is quite rare.

Histologically, lymphoid proliferation is noted within the dermis and subcutis but usually not in the most superficial dermis. In time, neoplastic cells invade the epidermis and cause necrosis, ulceration, and exudation. Metastasis may affect the lymph nodes or lungs.

Management: Treatment of B-cell lymphosarcoma is usually attempted with corticosteroids and combination chemotherapy using several anticancer drugs (*eg,* cyclophosphamide, azathioprine, vincristine, L-asparaginase, doxorubicin, chlorambucil). L-asparaginase (Elspar: MSD), given at 400 IU/kg daily IM, IP, SC or IV, is very effective for induction of chemotherapy and rapidly decreases lymph node size. Because the product is quite antigenic, pretreatment with antihistamines is recommended to help prevent anaphylaxis. Combination therapy with cyclophosphamide (Cytoxan), vincristine (Oncovin: Lilly) and prednisone is commonly used in treatment of lymphosarcoma as follows:

Cyclophosphamide: 2.2 mg/kg PO 3-4 days per week.

Vincristine: 0.025 mg/kg or 0.5 mg/m^2 weekly for 3 weeks, then every 3 weeks.

Prednisone: 2.2 mg/kg daily for 1 week, then 1.1 mg/kg daily.

Doxorubicin: This is used as a final option and is particularly indicated in dogs with thymic or multicentric lymphosarcoma. It is given IV at 30 mg/m^2 every 3 weeks for a maximum of 5-8 cycles.

T-Cell-Like Lymphoma

T-cell-like lymphoma (mycosis fungoides) is a slightly less malignant process in which lesions evolve from a red scaly exfoliative rash (erythroderma) through a plaque stage to large cutaneous nodules (Fig 39). This evolution of lesions is quite protracted and may occur over months to years. Cocker Spaniels and Poodles appear overrepresented.

Diagnosis: Cutaneous T-cell-like lymphoma is best diagnosed by histopathologic examination, but early cases may be very difficult if not impossible to confirm. In people, it is not unusual to do serial biopsies over some time until characteristic changes are seen and a diagnosis is rendered. These characteristic changes include a strong affinity for invading the epidermis (epidermotropism), abnormal convoluted lymphocytes in the dermis (MF cells), and collections of these neoplastic cells in clusters within the epidermis (Pautrier's microabscesses).

Management: Treatment of T-cell lymphomas can be undertaken with the realization that, for the most part, by the time a diagnosis is made, the tumor has already spread. In affected people, it is assumed that the neoplasm originates from an individual clone of neoplastic cells, and therefore >1 lesion implies hematologic spread. At this time, I am not certain whether any form of therapy increases survival time, though it does frequently improve the animal's condition.

T-cell lymphoma has a very protracted course. Treatment with corticosteroids or topical mechlorethamine (nitrogen mustard) may be of some benefit. Topical nitrogen mustard as an anhydrous ointment may be prepared as follows: Add 1.0 ml of absolute or isopropyl alcohol to a 10-mg vial of mechlorethamine. Filter off the sodium choride precipitate. Blend the remaining mechlorethamine solution with 100 mg of an absorbent ointment base to yield a 10-mg/dl product. Apply daily at first (wearing gloves), then less often.

Combination chemotherapy may be beneficial for T-cell lymphomas, as it is for B-cell lymphomas. An additional form of therapy involves daily intradermal injections of placental lysate (A-510: Scott Biologicals). This may offer an alternative to traditional chemotherapy, but more research is needed to document its efficacy.

Woringer-Kolopp Disease

Pagetoid reticulosis, or Woringer-Kolopp disease, is a rare disorder with some features similar to T-cell lymphoma.

Clinical Signs: Affected animals have exfoliative and plaque-like lesions that may have a site predilection for the oral cavity and footpads (too few cases have been reported to be specific).

Diagnosis: Diagnosis relies totally on histologic interpretation. Skin sections show intraepidermal accumulation of large pale-staining cells that resemble Paget cells, hence the descriptive term pagetoid.

Management: For now, treatment options should include those discussed for T-cell lymphoma.

Additional Reading

1. Ackerman, L: Cutaneous T cell-like lymphoma in the dog. *Comp Cont Ed Pract Vet* 6:37-42, 1984.

2. McKeever, PJ: Canine cutaneous lymphoma. *JAVMA* 180:531-536, 1982.

3. MacEwen, EG *et al*: Cyclic combination chemotherapy of canine lymphosarcoma. *JAVMA* 178:1178-1181, 1981.

4. Harris, CK and Macy, DW: Diagnosis and treatment of lymphosarcoma in dogs. Part 1. *MVP* 66:244-247, 1985.

5. Harris, CK and Macy, DW: Diagnosis and treatment of lymphosarcoma in dogs. Part 2. *MVP* 66:313-316, 1985.

6. Bender, WM: Nontraditional treatment of mycosis fungoides in a dog. *JAVMA* 185:900-901, 1984.

7. Ladiges, WC *et al*: Phenotypic characterization of canine lymphoma using monoclonal antibodies and a microlymphocytotoxicity assay. *Am J Vet Res* 49:870-872, 1988.

8. Postorino, NC *et al:* Single agent therapy with adriamycin for canine lymphosarcoma. *JAAHA* 25:221-225, 1989.

Mammary Tumors

Mammary tumors may not be entirely a dermatologic concern but are included here because of the prevalence and obvious cutaneous involvement. Dogs have a higher incidence of mammary neoplasia than do women (3X the incidence of breast cancer in women) or any other domestic animal. Though mammary tumors are obviously a heterogenous population, some trends are apparent. Estrogen and progesterone receptors have been identified in canine mammary tumors, but their role in prognosis has not been characterized. Increased levels of growth hormone have been noted in the pituitary gland of dogs with mammary tumors but the role of growth hormone in etiopathogenesis has not been characterized either. About 60% of all mammary tumors are in the fourth and fifth mammary glands, which are thought to be the most hormonally active.

Bitches ovariohysterectomized before their first heat have <1% of the risk of developing mammary cancer than intact bitches. The risk becomes equal when bitches are allowed to have >4 heats before neutering. Therefore, neutering at the time of tumor evaluation or removal will not affect the survival time of affected bitches.

Clinical Signs

Mammary gland tumors may be nodular and unattached to underlying tissues or more infiltrative masses invading both the skin and deep structures. Differential diagnoses for mammary nodules include septic mastitis, fibrotic nodules, fibrocystic disease (a form of mammary dysplasia), galactoceles, skin tumor and inguinal hernia. About half of mammary tumors are benign and half malignant. Half of all mammary tumors are multicentric. Metastasis is common and may occur by direct extension or via the blood or lymphatics. Lymphatic metastasis is usually associated with the inguinal (glands 4, 5) and axillary (glands 1, 2) nodes, though other lymph nodes may be involved. Other common metastatic sites include the lungs, skin, liver, kidney, heart, bone and brain.

Diagnosis

Diagnosis is based on cytologic examination and biopsies for histopathologic examination. Cytologic examination is not always valuable for a number of reasons: mammary tumors are not composed of a solid mass of tumor cells; carcinoma cells have a varied appearance; mammary fluid may not contain cells if the duct draining the tumor is occluded; a trained cytopathologist is needed for interpretation; and clusters of neoplastic cells can be confused with clusters of epithelial cells that are often seen with benign mammary neoplasms or subsequent to pregnancy and pseudocyesis.

Histologically, the more common tumors include papillomas, complex adenomas, fibroadenomas and mixed mammary tumors, which are benign and tubular, and papillary adenocarcinomas, solid carcinomas, spindle-cell carcinomas, carcinosarcomas (malignant mixed tumor) and anaplastic carcinomas, which are malignant. Some benign mammary tumors are thought to become malignant with time. All lesions should be excised, as different tumor types may exist in different glands. Draining lymph nodes should also be examined to aid in clinical staging and prognosis.

Management

Therapy of mammary neoplasia for animals in good health and <12 years of age warrants radical resection after careful evaluation. This evaluation should include survey thoracic radiographs, complete blood counts and a biochemical profile. Radiation therapy may be of value in preventing local recurrence in the absence of metastases. Very little information is available on use of chemotherapy and immunotherapy in canine mammary tumors and even less on antiestrogen hormonal manipulation.

Additional Reading

1. Brodey, RS et al: Canine mammary gland neoplasms. JAAHA 19: 61-90, 1983.
2. Ferguson, HR: Canine mammary gland tumors. Vet Clin No Am 15:501-511, 1985.
3. Mann, FA: Canine mammary gland neoplasia. Canine Pract 11(6):22-26, 1984.

Mast-Cell Tumor

Mast-cell tumors are relatively common in dogs. The average age of affected individuals is 8 years. They are most prevalent in Boxers, Boston Terriers, English Bulldogs, Bull Terriers, Fox Terriers, Staffordshire Terriers, Labrador Retrievers, Dachshunds and Weimaraners. No sex predilection has been reported.

Clinical Signs

The clinical appearance is highly variable. They usually are more common on the trunk, anogenital region and limbs (Fig 40). In addition to the skin lesions, GI bleeding and lack of blood clotting may also be noted. These tumors may be either benign or malignant in their behavior. Thus, all mast-cell tumors should be treated as being potentially malignant; those affecting the anogenital area and digits usually are.

Systemic mastocytosis is uncommon and usually a sequel to cutaneous mast-cell tumor. Regional dissemination, edema, ulceration, lymph node enlargement and abscessation are seen in most cases. Such systemic signs as anorexia, vomiting and diarrhea are seen in about half of affected dogs. The lymph nodes, spleen and liver are most commonly involved.

Diagnosis

Diagnosis is by the history, clinical examination, cytologic examination and biopsy. Cytologic examination is an important but underused tool for a rapid diagnosis. Mast-cell tumors exfoliate readily. Representative cells are easily identified on fine-needle aspirates and stain exceptionally well with such products as Diff-Quik. Mast cells are round cells with nuclei often obscured by cytoplasmic granules. Eosinophils are often admixed with the neoplastic cells. Mast-cell tumors can not be graded by cytologic evaluation; therefore, tumors diagnosed by cytologic examination should still be submitted for histopathologic examination.

Histologically, mast-cell tumors consist of sheets of round cells with round or oval nuclei and several nucleoli. Metachromatic cytoplasmic granules are better stained with toluidine blue or Giemsa but are usually discernible with hematoxylin-eosin. A variable number of eosinophils is also commonly associated with mast-cell tumors. Other less common features include foci of collagen necrosis, perivascular hyalinization, and focal accumulations of lymphocytes and plasma cells. The degree of differentiation of the neoplastic cells is of some prognostic significance, since poorly differentiated mast-cell tumors are more aggressive and associated with shorter survival time than well-differentiated tumors.

Biopsy specimens of mast-cell tumors are often graded by the pathologist to help form a prognosis. Grade-I tumors are anaplastic, immature and poorly differentiated, and carry a mean survival time of about 18 weeks following diagnosis. Grade-II tumors are intermediate in their differentiation, with a mean survival time of about 28 weeks. Grade-III tumors are well differentiated and offer a mean survival time of about 52 weeks.

Additional diagnostic tests include lymph node aspirates, buffy coat smears (centrifuge a microhematocrit tube of blood, break it at the level of the buffy coat, express the buffy coat onto a microscope slide and evaluate for circulating mast cells), bone marrow biopsy, occult blood tests on stool (for GI bleeding) and radiography (for tumor metastasis).

Management

Treatment may be accomplished by a number of mechanisms. Solitary tumors are best excised, while multiple tumors usually require some form of chemotherapy. Cryosurgery has been useful, especially for multiple small skin tumors. A wide margin of normal tissue must be frozen to lessen the chance of recurrence. Corticosteroids are often given PO (prednisone) or injected into the tumors (triamcinolone). Cimetidine (Tagamet), an H2-specific antihistamine, is often given at 4 mg/kg QID if there is evidence of GI bleeding.

Where available, radiation therapy, in 10 equal treatments of 400 rads each for 3 days per week, is used for lesions not amenable to complete excision. Radiation therapy is an effective treatment of mast-cell tumor in dogs. Surgical debulking of the tumors is normally done before irradiation. As a final alternative, intralesional injections of preparations of *Propionibacterium acnes* (ImmunoRegulin: Immunovet) or mycobacteria (Regressin or Stimune) may result in some tumor regression after 3-4 months.

Additional Reading

1. Tams, TR and Macy, DW: Canine mast-cell tumors. *Comp Cont Ed Pract Vet* 3:869-878, 1981.

2. Pukay, BP: Disseminated mastocytosis in a dog. *Can Vet J* 25:351-352, 1984.

3. Patnaik, AK *et al*: Canine cutaneous mast cell tumor: Morphologic grading and survival time in 83 dogs. *Vet Pathol* 21:469-474, 1984.

4. O'Keefe, DA *et al*: Systemic mastocytosis in 16 dogs. *J Vet Int Med* 1:75-80, 1987.

5. Tinsley, PE and Taylor, DO: Immunotherapy for multicentric malignant mastocytoma in a dog. *MVP* 68:225-228, 1987.

6. Turrel, JM *et al*: Prognostic factors for radiation treatment of mast cell tumor in 85 dogs. *JAVMA* 193:936-940, 1988.

Melanoma

Melanomas are tumors of the pigment-producing melanocytes. They may be benign or malignant. Scottish Terriers, Boston Terriers, Airedale Terriers, Cocker Spaniels, Boxers, Irish Setters, Chow Chows, Chihuahuas and Springer Spaniels have a higher incidence of melanomas than other breeds. Males appear to be affected more often than females. The tumors arise most commonly around the mouth, genitalia and mammary glands.

As a general rule, those arising on skin are more likely to be benign than those originating on mucous membranes.

Clinical Signs

Benign melanomas are usually small, dark mole-like nodules in the skin, while malignant melanomas are usually larger and frequently ulcerated.

Diagnosis

Diagnosis is by histopathologic examination, but there is not always a clear-cut distinction between benign and malignant variants. Benign melanomas are normally subdivided into those with junctional activity and benign cellular or fibrous dermal melanomas. Malignant melanomas are classified according to cell type as epithelioid, spindle cell, mixed and pleomorphic. Transformation of preexisting benign melanomas to malignant melanomas is apparently uncommon, though in one report, 40% of tumors thought to be benign on histopathologic evaluation showed metastasis.

Management

The therapy of choice for any melanoma is radical excision, regardless of histopathologic interpretation. No correlation exists between prognosis and microscopic appearance of the tumor, mitotic index, degree of pigmentation, timing of surgery, tumor volume or type of surgery.

Additional Reading

1. Reed, RJ: A classification of melanocytic dysplasias and malignant melanomas. *Am J Dermatopathol* 6:195-206, 1984.
2. Harvey, HJ *et al*: Prognostic criteria for dogs with oral melanoma. *JAVMA* 178:580-582, 1981.

Myxoma, Myxosarcoma

Myxoma

Myxomas are rare neoplasms that arise from fibroblasts altered to produce mucin in the intercellular matrix. They are similar to fibromas but the end product is mucin rather than collagen.

Clinical Signs: Myxomas are often unencapsulated soft infiltrative growths. There is no breed or sex predilection but the tumors typically occur in older dogs. Myxomas may occur more commonly on the limbs, back and groin.

Diagnosis: Diagnosis is by biopsies for histopathology.

Management: The treatment of choice is wide excision. Recurrence is not uncommon because of the infiltrative nature of the tumor.

Myxosarcoma

Clinical Signs: Myxosarcoma is the malignant counterpart of myxoma and is similarly soft, infiltrative and unencapsulated. Metastasis, though uncommon, may occur; the lungs are usually the first site affected.

Diagnosis: Diagnosis is by biopsy but it is not always easy to distinguish between the benign and malignant varieties.

Management: Therapies considered for myxosarcomas should be the same as for fibrosarcomas and include wide excision and irradiation.

Nasal Tumors

Nasal tumors are not strictly a dermatologic concern but are included here for completeness. There does not appear to be any breed or sex predilection but nasal tumors are usually seen in older dogs, with an average of 8-10 years of age. The tumors are malignant in 80% of cases and most are carcinomas, such as adenocarcinomas and squamous-cell carcinomas. Mesenchymal tumors, such as chondrosarcomas, fibrosarcomas, osteosarcomas and the lymphosarcomas and transmissible venereal tumors may also invade this area. Tumors in the nasal passages are usually primary and do not usually result from metastasis, nor do they frequently metastasize. Most benign nasal tumors are fibromas and papillomas.

Clinical Signs

Clinical signs include nasal discharge, sneezing, facial deformity, and dyspnea. Systemic signs of disease are not common though bacterial infection is a frequent sequel.

Diagnosis

Diagnosis is by radiography, rhinoscopy and biopsy.

Early nasal tumors may be difficult to recognize radiographically because of the similarities of presentation between neoplasia and some inflammatory processes. The radiographic view that provides the most information is the open-mouth ventrodorsal, which allows visualization of the entire turbinate region. The radiographic appearance of nasal tumors is variable and diagnosis cannot be based on radiography alone.

Rhinoscopy can be diagnostic if the tumors are in a rostral position and not completely obscured by nasal discharges. An otoscope speculum can be used for this purpose and is also useful for detecting foreign objects.

Aspiration biopsy may be performed with a large-bore (7 mm) plastic tube, such as the protective covering of an IV catheter. The length of the tube should not exceed the distance from the external nares to the medial canthus of the eye. It may be entered into the nostril until it contacts the tumor (located by radiography), connected to a 12-ml syringe, and negative pressure applied to obtain the biopsy. Negative pressure is maintained as the tube is withdrawn from the nasal passage. The tissue can then be blotted gently with gauze before being preserved in 10% buffered formalin. Extreme caution must be used to ensure that hemorrhage is controlled, that aspiration is not a problem, and that the tube does not approach the cribriform plate (brain biopsies rarely improve the prognosis). Punch biopsies can also be achieved with a Tru-Cut disposable biopsy needle (Travenol). Practitioners should thoroughly review the references listed below before attempting any of these procedures. Surgical exposure of the nasal passages may be necessary to confirm a diagnosis when other attempts fail.

Management

Treatment of nasal tumors may involve surgery and radiation therapy. Surgery does little to prolong the animal's life (median survival time is 6-9 months) but may make the animal more comfortable. Radiotherapy with preirradiation surgical cytoreduction appears to offer the best prognosis (12-15 months). A grave prognosis must be given for all nasal malignancies.

Additional Reading

1. Legendre, AM *et al:* Canine nasal and paranasal sinus tumors. *JAAHA* 19:115-123, 1983.

2. Beck, ER and Withrow, SJ: Tumors of the canine nasal cavity. *Vet Clin No Am* 15:521-533, 1985.

3. Laing, EJ and Binnington, AG: Surgical therapy of canine nasal tumors: A retrospective study (1982-1986). *Can Vet J* 29:809-813, 1988.

4. Adams, WM *et al*: Radiotherapy of malignant nasal tumors in 67 dogs. *JAVMA* 191:311-315, 1987.

Nevi

A nevus (cutaneous hamartoma) is a well-demarcated developmental skin defect. The predominant component of a nevus determines its classification (sebaceous nevus, collagen nevus, epidermal nevus, etc).

Sebaceous nevi begin at birth as alopecic plaques that develop into proliferative hyperplastic yellow-orange plaques around puberty. On biopsy they are indistinguishable from sebaceous-gland hyperplasia, but clinically this distinction is obvious. Treatment involves excision or lifelong topical antiseborrheic therapy.

Collagenous nevi appear as asymptomatic nodules, usually on the limbs. Usually dogs of various breeds >3 years of age are affected; German Shepherds seem predisposed. The surface of the nevus is often dimpled and resembles an orange peel (peau d'orange). Biopsies show collagenous hyperplasia, which must be differentiated from fibroma. The course is often progressive, and therapy is often impractical if the lesions cannot be excised.

Epidermal nevi are often present at birth or develop shortly thereafter. They appear as linear bands of hyperkeratotic plaques. On tissue section, epidermal nevi may be indistinguishable from papillomas, seborrheic keratosis and ichthyosis, but they are easily distinguished clinically. Treatment involves extensive excision or lifelong topical antiseborrheic therapy.

Vascular nevi (angiomatous hamartomas) often appear as plaques and nodules consisting of a proliferation of blood vessels. They must be differentiated from hemangiomas and other vascularized neoplastic and inflammatory lesions.

Melanocytic nevi are maculopapular to papulonodular pigmented lesions seen most commonly on the trunk. Malignant transformation has not been reported. Biopsies reveal benign, hyperplastic melanocytes in superficial dermal nests or even within the epidermis.

Organoid nevi occur as single or multiple papules, plaques or vegetative structures occurring more commonly on the face, head or limbs. Biopsies reveal proliferation of the follicular appendages and adnexa.

Additional Reading

1. Scott, DW *et al*: Nevi in the dog. *JAAHA* 20:505-512, 1984.

2. Roudebush, P and MacDonald, JM: Mucocutaneous angiomatous hamartoma in a dog. *JAAHA* 20:168-170, 1984.

Oral Tumors

Oral neoplasms, unless they involve the mucocutaneous junction, are out of the realm of dermatology but will be briefly discussed here because they represent an overlap area of the specialties dermatology, dentistry, internal medicine and oncology. More complete descriptions are available in texts of these other areas.

Oral tumors arise most commonly in adult dogs (average age 8-10 years). Males may be affected more often than females.

Clinical Signs

The oral cavity may be involved in both benign and malignant neoplastic processes. Of malignant oral neoplasms, melanoma, squamous-cell carcinoma and fibrosarcoma are by far the most common. Less common malignancies include adenocarcinoma, odontogenic tumor, hemangiosarcoma and invading tumors from contiguous tissues (*eg*, osteosarcoma, chondrosarcoma, mast-cell tumor, nasal tumors). The most common benign tumors of the oral cavity include epulis, ameloblastoma and papillomatosis.

Melanomas may involve the gingiva, buccal or labial mucosa, hard and soft palate, and tongue. They are locally invasive and highly metastatic via veins and lymphatics and commonly spread to the lungs. The neoplasm itself may be pigmented (melanotic) or nonpigmented (amelanotic).

Squamous-cell carcinoma most commonly occurs in the tonsillar crypts and gingiva, and the sites are important prognostic indicators. Gingival squamous-cell carcinoma appears as a nodular mass, with frequent involvement of bone. They metastasize to the regional lymph nodes <10% of the time. Tonsillar squamous-cell carcinomas show early metastasis to regional lymph nodes in >95% of cases; most also show distant metastasis.

Fibrosarcomas occur most often along the maxillary gingiva and occasionally on the hard palate. They appear as large nodular masses that are often secondarily infected with bacteria.

Epulides are the most common class of benign oral neoplasms that arise from the periodontal ligament. Fibromatous epulis contains periodontal ligament stroma, while ossifying epulis contains osteoid matrix within this stroma. Acanthomatous epulis contains sheets of epithelial cells associated with the underlying stroma. Acanthomatous epulis, with its epithelial component, may invade regional tissues.

Odontogenic tumors frequently have enamel inclusions, dental pulp stroma or organized dental structures present; these features are never seen in epulides. These rare odontogenic tumors arise from the dental laminar epithelium and include ameloblastomas, keratinizing ameloblastoma, ameloblastic fibroodontoma, compound odontoma and complex odontoma. They appear as soft-tissue tumors of the gingiva.

Diagnosis

Diagnostic testing should include survey radiography of the oral cavity and thorax, excisional or incisional biopsies of tumor and enlarged lymph nodes, and determination of hematologic and blood chemistry values.

Management

Treatment of oral neoplasms depends on tumor type, aggressiveness and patient suitability. Epulides are most commonly treated with excision or cryosurgery, with or without irradiation/hyperthermia. Local recurrence is common if treatment is not aggressive. Most odontogenic tumors require radical surgical intervention, such as mandibulectomy or partial maxillectomy. Wide excision is the most effective form of therapy for malignant melanoma; partial maxillectomy may be warranted.

Tonsillar squamous-cell carcinoma, because of its rapid rate of metastasis, is unlikely to respond to treatment. Nontonsillar squamous-cell carcinoma may respond to wide excision, electrocautery or cryotherapy. Fibrosarcomas are poorly responsive to irradiation, chemotherapy and immunotherapy, but wide excision and possibly mandibulectomy or partial maxillectomy may be effective.

Additional Reading

1. Harvey, HJ: Oral tumors. *Vet Clin No Am* 15:493-500, 1985.

2. Richardson, RC *et al:* Oral neoplasms in the dog: A diagnostic and therapeutic dilemma. *Comp Cont Ed Pract Vet* 5:441-446, 1983.

3. Werner, Jr., REF: Canine oral neoplasia: A review of 19 cases. *JAAHA* 17:67-69, 1981.

Papilloma, Papillomatosis

Papilloma

Clinical Signs: Papillomas (warts) are common skin tumors that usually occur as small, solitary lobulated masses on the head, feet and genitalia of middle-aged to older dogs. These tumors are not related to the papovavirus-induced papillomatosis, described below.

Diagnosis: The lesion consists of hyperplastic dermal extensions or digitations with associated epidermal hyperplasia and orthokeratotic hyperkeratosis. Hyperplastic epidermis should not invade the dermis, as is seen with squamous-cell carcinoma.

Management: A good prognosis may be given whether the mass is excised or left in place.

Papillomatosis

Clinical Signs: Viral papillomatosis is a different disorder from cutaneous squamous papilloma. It is caused by a papovavirus and results in oral proliferative lesions in young dogs.

Diagnosis: Diagnosis rests on clinical presentation and histopathologic findings. Biopsies show proliferative epidermal changes with viral inclusions.

Management: Treatment is usually unnecessary, as most cases spontaneously regress, but a "wart vaccine" can be formulated if necessary.

Perianal (Hepatoid-Gland) Tumors

Hepatoid-gland tumors are derived from modified sebaceous glands, usually located around the anus but occasionally found on the genitalia, tailhead, caudal back and hind limbs.

Hepatoid-Gland Adenoma

Clinical Signs: Hepatoid-gland adenomas are quite common and occur with greater frequency in males than in females. Cocker Spaniels, English Bulldogs, Samoyeds and Beagles appear to be at increased risk. They are seen most frequently in animals ≥ 8 years.

Diagnosis: Diagnostic testing may include fine-needle aspirates and biopsies for histopathologic examination. Cytologic examination reveals clustered epithelial cells that resemble hepatic parenchymal cells. The masses consist of lobular patterns of large eosinophilic polygonal cells, with prominent vascularization.

Management: Since the growth of these tumors is influenced by the male sex hormone testosterone, castration or injecting the tumor with 10-20 mg of diethylstilbestrol (DES) on 3 separate occasions usually shrinks the tumor to a size that it is amenable to complete surgical removal. The tumor may recur in about a third of cases, especially if castration was not performed. Resection must be carefully performed to avoid damage to perineal nerves and fibrosis around the anal sphincter.

Hepatoid-Gland Adenocarcinoma

Clinical Signs: Hepatoid-gland adenocarcinomas tend to grow more rapidly, ulcerate and metastasize widely. They occur in older pets; there is no sex predilection.

Diagnosis: Diagnosis is by cytologic and histopathologic evaluation. On cytologic examination, the "hepatoid" epithelial cells show more nuclear variability and atypical forms. Histologically, there is less well circumscribed growth with mitotic figures and nuclear atypia ("bird's eye" cells). Invasion of lymphatics by neoplastic cells is an important feature.

Management: Carcinomas warrant a poor prognosis. Treatment requires complete excision, which is often difficult because of the invasive natue of these cancers. Radiation therapy may be warranted if internal metastasis has not yet occurred.

Additional Reading

1. Umphlet, RC and Bertoy, R: Tumors of the perianal gland: A case report and review. *Compan Anim Pract* 2(3):30-32, 1988.

Periocular Tumors

Tumors of the eye and conjunctivae are best covered in a text of ophthalmology. The following discussion is limited to neoplasms commonly involving the eyelids.

Clinical Signs

Palpebral tumors are generally seen in older animals (average 9-10 years). There may be some breed predisposition for Beagles, Siberian Huskies and English Setters. Most eyelid tumors (75%) are benign, but some may be troublesome because of their location. The most common benign tumors include sebaceous tarsal-gland adenomas, benign melanomas, papillomas and acrochordons. Malignancies involving the eyelids include malignant melanoma, adenocarcinoma, basosquamous carcinoma, mast-cell tumor, squamous-cell carcinoma, malignant histiocytosis, fibrous histiocytoma and hemangiosarcoma.

Diagnosis

Diagnosis is by biopsy or cytologic examination.

Management

Eyelid tumors are best managed by blepharoplasty or cryosurgery.

Additional Reading

1. Roberts, SM *et al:* Prevalence and treatment of palpebral neoplasms in the dog: 200 cases (1975-1983). *JAVMA* 189:1355-1359, 1986.

2. Krehbiel, JD and Langham, RF: Eyelid neoplasms of dogs. *Am J Vet Res* 36:115-119, 1975.

Pilomatrixoma

Clinical Signs

Pilomatrixomas are thought to be derived from the pilar portion of the hair matrix. They are usually single firm masses on the shoulders, back, flanks or legs. Kerry Blue Terriers and

Poodles appear to have a higher incidence than other breeds. They may appear similar to trichoepitheliomas and other skin tumors.

Diagnosis

Diagnosis is confirmed by histopathologic examination of tissue sections, in which a connective tissue capsule surrounds a zone of basophilic cells (hair matrix cells of the hair bulb?). At the center of the nodule are degenerated "shadow" cells that often show focal calcification. The transition from basophilic cells to shadow cells is abrupt.

Management

Like trichoepitheliomas, pilomatrixomas rarely recur or metastasize, though malignant variants have been reported.

Plasmacytoma

Cutaneous plasmacytomas are tumors of plasma-cell origin that may arise as primary tumors or may represent metastasis of primary osseous multiple myeloma. This tumor may be mistaken for a number of different neoplasms histologically.

Clinical Signs

There appears to be no breed or sex predilection for cutaneous plasmacytomas; the average age of occurrence is 10 years. It is perhaps advantageous to separate plasmacytomas into cutaneous and mucocutaneous variants, as the prognosis appears to differ. Cutaneous plasmacytomas are dome-shaped nodules that may become ulcerated. They are most frequently seen on the lips, trunk, digits and ears. Mucocutaneous plasmacytomas are most frequently seen in the oral cavity and rectum.

Diagnosis

Diagnosis is based on histopathologic examination of tissue sections which contain compact cords and nests of neoplastic round cells, and show cellular atypia and frequently multiple nuclei. Toward the periphery of the mass, cells gradually and progressively decrease in size and acquire more obvious plasmacytoid features. Most cells have cytoplasmic staining with methyl green pyronine and show immunoreactivity with vimentin markers. Some tumors have detectable immunoglobulin, especially IgG and occasionally IgA.

Management

Cutaneous plasmacytomas generally display benign behavior, though recurrence is occasionally reported. In contrast, mucocutaneous tumors of the oral cavity and rectum are more often invasive and offer a poor prognosis.

Sebaceous-Gland Tumors

Benign Sebaceous-Gland Tumor

Clinical Signs: Tumors of the sebaceous glands are common in dogs and are mostly seen in animals >9 years of age. They are most frequently reported in Cocker Spaniels, Poodles, Beagles, Dachshunds and Boston Terriers, with a slight predilection for females. Benign sebaceous adenomas and benign sebaceous adenomatous hyperplasia are far more common than malignant adenocarcinomas. Most benign sebaceous growths are misdiagnosed as warts but have the same good prognosis. They normally appear as small, lobulated, sometimes greasy nodules not connected with any underlying structures and are most prevalent on the abdomen, thorax, hindlimbs, head, neck, shoulders, eyelids, forelimbs and ears.

Diagnosis: Cytologically, benign sebaceous-gland tumors appear as clusters of large epithelial cells containing lipid droplets. On tissue sections, the tumors appear as discrete clusters of sebaceous glandular epithelium.

Management: Resection is curative or lesions may be left intact without problems.

Sebaceous-Gland Carcinoma

Clinical Signs: Sebaceous-gland carcinomas are much rarer than their benign counterparts; Cocker Spaniels may be at increased risk. The average age of affected individuals is 9 years. Most tumors are located on the head, thorax, abdomen and forelimbs. These tumors have a rapid rate of growth and frequently ulcerate, but do not usually metastasize.

Diagnosis: Diagnosis is by histopathologic examination, which reveals that nuclei of the epithelial cells are of variable size and contain large nucleoli. Cords of neoplastic cells infiltrate the dermis and subcutis distinguishing these tumors from the benign processes.

Management: Treatment should involve complete excision, but local recurrence is possible if the tumor was incompletely removed.

Additional Reading

1. Strafuss, AC: Sebaceous gland adenomas in dogs. *JAVMA* 169:640-642, 1976.

Squamous-Cell Carcinomas

Squamous-cell carcinomas are the most malignant epithelial tumors of canine skin. Some of these occur secondary to chronic sun exposure.

Clinical Signs

There may be some increased incidence in the Scottish Terrier, Pekingese, Boxer, Poodle and Norwegian Elkhound. Involvement of the toes is thought to be the most malignant form. The tumors are most commonly located on the limbs, trunk, head and neck. The clinical appearance is highly variable. They may appear as a proliferative, cauliflower-type growth, or as an ulcerative process covered by crusts. Most squamous-cell carcinomas are locally invasive but some, like those affecting the toes, are quick to metastasize to the lymph nodes and lungs.

Diagnosis

Diagnosis is usually by histopathologic examination. The process is comprised of cords and masses of keratinocytes that infiltrate the dermis and subcutis. The more differentiated tumors display squamous "pearls" or horn cysts, while those more poorly differentiated show cellular and nuclear atypia.

Management

When the area is completely excised, the prognosis is good. For digital squamous-cell carcinomas and those showing aggressive features on histopathologic evaluation, the prognosis becomes more guarded. Therapy with platinum compounds (*eg,* cisplatin), hyperthermia, cryosurgery, electrosurgery and radiation therapy may also be used with variable success.

Additional Reading

1. Strafuss, AC *et al:* Squamous cell carcinoma in dogs. *JAVMA* 425-428, 1976.

2. Barrie, KP *et al:* Eyelid squamous cell carcinoma in four dogs. *JAAHA* 18:123-127, 1982.

3. Madewell, BR *et al:* Multiple subungual squamous cell carcinomas in five dogs. *JAVMA* 180:731-734, 1982.

4. Himsel, CA *et al*: Cisplatin chemotherapy for metastatic squamous cell carcinoma in 2 dogs. *JAVMA* 189:1575-1578, 1986.

Sweat-Gland Tumors

Sweat-gland tumors of the apocrine or eccrine sweat glands are uncommon in dogs. Most sweat-gland tumors are derived from apocrine glands.

Apocrine-Gland Adenoma

Clinical Signs: Apocrine-gland adenomas may be subdivided into papillary syringoadenomas, cystadenomas or mixed tumors, according to a classification from the World Health Organization. Apocrine adenomas predominantly occur in dogs >8 years of age and are more common in males. Cocker Spaniels may have an increased incidence. They are most frequently reported on the head and neck.

Diagnosis: Diagnosis is confirmed by histopathologic evaluation, which reveals multiple acinar or cystic structures lined by a single layer of cuboidal to columnar epithelial cells, thrown into papillary extensions. Mixed tumors are characterized by proliferation of both glandular and myoepithelial cells. It is often difficult or impossible to differentiate among hyperplastic, dysplastic or neoplastic processes on the basis of cytologic findings.

Management: Excision is usually curative.

Apocrine-Gland Adenocarcinoma

Clinical Signs: Apocrine adenocarcinomas are often clinically indistinguishable from adenomas and mixed tumors, and have a predilection for the back, flanks and feet.

Diagnosis: Apocrine adenocarcinomas may be subclassified as papillary, tubular, solid or signet-ring carcinomas. The poorly differentiated epithelial cells arranged in these patterns often have observable lymphatic vessel invasion. There is often nuclear and cellular pleomorphism. Apparently, metastasis is most common with the solid carcinomas.

Management: Excision is the treatment of choice for apocrine adenocarcinomas, but local recurrence is not uncommon. Site irradiation should be contemplated if there is doubt as to whether the tumor was completely removed. Metastases may occur via the lymphatics to local lymph nodes and the lungs.

Eccrine adenomas are very rare and limited to the footpads. These tumors can be classified as papillary syringoadenomas if they are derived from ducts or spiradenomas if from the secretory portion of the eccrine sweat glands.

Clear-cell hidradenocarcinomas are very infrequently reported in dogs. Though the actual cell type is being disputed, it is presumed to be of eccrine sweat gland origin. Too few cases have been reported to make generalizations.

Additional Reading

1. Conroy, JD and Breen, PT: Apocrine sweat gland carcinoma with lymphatic invasion in a dog. *Vet Med* 67:297-298, 1972.

2. Jabara, AG and Finnie, JW: Four cases of clear-cell hidradenocarcinomas in the dog. *J Comp Pathol* 88:525-532, 1978.

Transmissible Venereal Tumors

Transmissible venereal tumor (TVT) was the first transplantable and transmissible tumor to be recorded. The tumor is not composed of host cells transformed to cancerous cells but acts more like a tissue graft. The tumor even has a different number of chromosomes (often around 59) than do normal dog cells (78). It is transmitted from dog to dog by sexual contact and direct contact associated with social behavior, and is thus seen most commonly on the genitalia and face.

Clinical Signs

The tumors are often large cauliflower-like growths seen most commonly on the genitalia or face. Metastasis is possible but not frequent and likely reflects traumatic inoculation of neoplastic tissue. Tumors within the nasal cavity may result in nose bleeds (epistaxis) and sneezing.

Diagnosis

Diagnosis is confirmed by histopathologic and cytologic examination. Vacuoles are often observed within the cytoplasm of cells on cytologic preparations. Mitotic figures are common. Histologically, TVT must be differentiated from cutaneous lymphosarcoma, histiocytoma and poorly differentiated mast-cell tumor.

Management

Spontaneous regression has not been reported, so therapeutic intervention is required. Unlike many forms of neoplasia, a total cure is possible with TVT. Where feasible, the tumor should be completely excised. For localized areas not amenable to surgery, irradiating the lesions at 1500 rads divided weekly for 1-3 weeks is often effective. For systemic or metastatic disease, treatment should be commenced with either doxorubicin HCl (Adriamycin) IV at 30 mg/m² every 3 weeks or vincristine sulfate at 0.5 mg/m² weekly until complete remission is achieved. This often requires about 6 weeks of therapy.

Additional Reading

1. Richardson, RC: Canine transmissible venereal tumor. *Comp Cont Ed Pract Vet* 3:951-956, 1982.

2. Calvert, CA *et al:* Vincristine for treatment of transmissible venereal tumor in the dog. *JAVMA* 181:163-164, 1982.

3. Dass, LL *et al*: Malignant transmissible venereal tumor. *Canine Pract* 13(3):15-18, 1986.

Trichoepithelioma

Clinical Signs

Trichoepitheliomas are derived from the hair matrix and occur predominantly in adult dogs. There is no breed or sex predilection. They appear as round masses, usually on the back. They are freely movable and unattached to underlying tissues. The skin overlying the mass may be hairless and ulcerated due to trauma.

Diagnosis

Diagnosis is by histopathologic evaluation, which shows dermal and/or subcutaneous proliferation of basaloid and squamous cells in solid or branching patterns, with abrupt keratinization of keratin cysts.

Management

The lesions are usually slow growing and benign in behavior, and rarely metastasize or recur when removed.

Additional Reading

1. Norris, AM and Withrow, SJ: A review of cancer chemotherapy for pet animals. *Can Vet J* 25:153-157, 1984.

2. Rosenthal, RC: Principles of chemotherapy. *Comp Cont Ed Pract Vet* 3:358-362, 1981.

3. Henderson, RA *et al:* Surgical management of cancer. *MVP* 65:615-621, 1984.

4. Zacarian, SA: Cryosurgery of cutaneous carcinomas. *J Am Acad Dermatol* 9:947-956, 1983.

5. Core, DM: Hyperthermia and cancer. *Comp Cont Ed Pract Vet* 4:719-722, 1982.

6. Grier, RL *et al:* Hyperthermic treatment of superficial tumors in cats and dogs. *JAVMA* 177:227-233, 1980.

7. Bowles, CA *et al:* Experience with *Staphylococcus aureus* and Protein A in the treatment of canine malignancies. *J Biol Resp Modif* 3:260-265, 1984.

Chapter 10
Miscellaneous Skin Disorders

Acanthosis Nigricans

Clinical Signs

Acanthosis nigricans is an uncommon condition that may occur as a primary or secondary disease. The primary condition is seen almost exclusively in Dachshunds, suggesting that it is an inherited problem. Most affected dogs are quite young when they first begin showing signs. The condition normally begins with increased pigmentation in the axillary areas (Fig 41) and then may spread to the groin area and then the entire undersurface of the body may become involved. Hair loss, thickening of the skin, bacterial infections and a greasy texture to the skin develop over time. Secondary acanthosis nigricans is identical but occurs in traumatized areas, such as those chewed, irritated or chafed on frictional surfaces (*eg*, axillae, groin, folds of skin).

Diagnosis

Acanthosis nigricans is diagnosed by the history, clinical signs and biopsies for histopathologic examination.

Management

Treatment of primary acanthosis nigricans is symptomatic. Antiseborrheic shampoos remove much of the skin's greasiness and odor, but are unlikely to lighten the pigmentary changes. The condition often improves markedly with continued use of corticosteroids, melatonin or vitamin E. Antiinflammatory doses of corticosteroids usually must be continued indefinitely.

Melatonin is a pineal gland extract that supposedly counteracts MSH. A dose of 2 mg is given every other day for 4 treatments, then bimonthly, monthly or as needed. Absolute ethanol (2-3 ml) and 90% DMSO (2-3 ml) are used to dissolve 100 mg of melatonin. Then the solution is diluted with distilled water to a volume of 75-100 ml. Melatonin can be acquired from Rickards Research Foundation, 18001 Euclid Ave, Cleveland, OH 44112.

Large doses of vitamin E (200 IU BID) are considered a very safe and effective form of therapy for acanthosis nigricans, with improvement being observed about 30 days after commencement of therapy. Secondary acanthosis nigricans can only be cleared when the underlying cause is identified and treated.

Additional Reading

1. Scott, DW and Walton, DK: Clinical evaluation of oral Vitamin E for the treatment of primary canine acanthosis nigricans. *JAAHA* 21:345-350, 1986.

2. Anderson, RK: Canine acanthosis nigricans. *Comp Cont Ed Pract Vet* 1:466-471, 1979.

Acral Lick Dermatitis

Clinical Signs

Acral lick dermatitis or lick granuloma is a common condition in which the dog traumatizes a body part, usually the legs, for no apparent reason. Before this diagnosis is rendered, however, organic causes of the problem must be ruled out before the condition is explained away as due to neurotic behavior. Doberman Pinschers, Great Danes, German Shepherds, Labrador Retrievers and Irish Setters are most commonly affected. Dogs with acral lick dermatitis may have mild sensory polyneuropathy.

Affected dogs begin licking at a site, removing the hair, causing inflammation and finally removing layers of the skin, sometimes down to the bone (Fig 42). The area becomes raw and weeping, and the chronic trauma itself becomes irritating, further stimulating the dog to lick and chew.

Diagnosis

Diagnosis cannot be confirmed by clinical signs alone. Bacterial and fungal cultures, cytologic examination and biopsies must be performed to rule out organic causes.

Management

With true acral lick dermatitis, treatment must be directed at both the psychological impairment and the skin disorder. The first step, of course, is to remove any underlying psychological problem. Boredom and stress are often important features of the condition. If the cause cannot be determined, mood-altering drugs, such as tranquilizers, female sex hormones (*eg,* medroxyprogesterone acetate at 20 mg/kg IM or SC once or repeated in 4-6 months) or narcotic antagonists (naltrexone at 2.2 mg/kg SID or BID) can be used until the skin lesion is cleared up. Pimozide (Orap: McNeil), a drug used to treat people with delusions of parasitosis, may have some applications here.

Elizabethan collars or modified buckets occasionally must be placed over the dog's head to deny access to the lesion. Then the skin can be treated by a number of methods to relieve inflammation. Corticosteroids injected into the lesion or applied topically with a penetrating agent, such as DMSO, offer the most successful options. The most common form of therapy is to add 3 ml of flunixin meglumine (Banamine: Schering) to a container of fluocinolone and DMSO (Synotic: Syntex), and apply it to the affected area daily. An alternative is to inject 5 mg of orgotein (Palosein) intralesionally and repeat treatment in 1 week. Many other approaches, including narcotic antagonists (*eg,* naltrexone at 2.2 mg/kg SID-BID), injecting cobra antivenin, amitryptilline (2.2 mg/kg BID), pentazocine (2.2 mg/kg BID), radiation therapy, cryosurgery and excisional surgery, have been tried with limited success. Undoubtedly, this is one of the most difficult conditions in veterinary dermatology to completely resolve.

Additional Reading

1. Scott, DW and Walton, DK: Clinical evaluation of a topical treatment for canine acral lick dermatitis. *JAAHA* 20:565-570, 1984.

2. van Nes, JJ: Electrophysiological evidence of sensory nerve dysfunction in 10 dogs with acral lick dermatitis. *JAAHA* 22:157-160, 1986.

3. White, SD: Treatment of acral lick dermatitis with the endorphin blocker naltrexone. *Proc Ann Mtg Am Acad Dermatol,* 1988. p 37.

4. Dodman, NH *et al*: Use of narcotic antagonists to modify stereotypic self-licking, self-chewing, and scratching behavior in dogs. *JAVMA* 193:815-819, 1988.

Alopecia

Alopecia is a loss of hair due to either an absolute decrease in the number of hairs, or hairs that are normal in number but shorter than normal. The disorder may be further subclassified as scarring or nonscarring, and congenital or acquired. Alopecia is not a dignosis but a description. A diagnostic key for alopecias can be found in the Introduction.

Congenito-hereditary alopecias and disorders of hair follicles are discussed in Chapter 8. Similarly, alopecia may result from parasitic infections (especially demodicosis and *Pelodera* dermatitis), fungal infections (especially dermatophytosis), immune-mediated disorders (alopecia areata, lupus erythematosus, scleroderma), endocrinopathies (hypothyroidism, hyperadrenocorticism, growth hormone-responsive dermatosis, sex hormone-related dermatoses), neoplastic disorders (T-cell-like lymphoma, Sertoli-cell tumor) and others (periappendageal dermatitis, epidermal dysplasia, toxicities, adverse reactions to such drugs as methotrexate and cyclophosphamide, keratinization defects, etc), covered in the appropriate chapters. Alopecia may also occur secondary to self-trauma (licking, chewing).

Telogen effluvium (defluxion) refers to hair loss following stressful periods, such as severe illness, fever, shock, pregnancy or surgery. The hairs are forced into a resting stage, and hair loss may be profound before a new wave of hair growth commences 4-8 weeks after the insult.

Pattern baldness is a regional hair loss that may be associated with aging or testosterone levels, or may be breed predisposed. The pinnae and dorsum are usually affected the most. There is usually no underlying ailment requiring treatment.

Periodic alopecia tends to wax and wane over time. It has been seen in a number of breeds, including Poodles, Dachshunds and Airedales. Airedales may show significant hyperpigmentation in alopecic regions. No underlying cause has been determined.

Management

Alopecias should be treated on the basis of their underlying problem. Specific treatments are discussed throughout this book in association with the specific problem. Idiopathic alopecias reflect an inability to arrive at a correct diagnosis and are best treated with conscientious neglect. An alternative in pattern alopecias, if the owner insists on treatment, is minoxidil (Rogaine: Upjohn), a potent vasodilator effective in treatment of severe hypertension in people. Hypertrichosis occurs in 70-80% of people taking the drug systemically (Loniten: Upjohn) and the product was reformulated by the company to be used topically in treatment of male pattern baldness and alopecia areata. The drug is not licensed for use in dogs, and because of the potent vasodilator effect, cardiac monitoring is important for canine cases.

Anal Sac Disorders

The anal sacs, often mistakenly referred to as anal glands, act as reservoirs for the secretions of the anal sac glands. Anal sac secretions are periodically released through 2 ducts on either side of the rectum. Normal anal sac fluid is brown and slightly granular, and has a distinctly disagreeable odor (an understatement). Presumably the odor and fluid are associated with social recognition and territorial marking among dogs.

Anal sac fluid is normally emptied with each bowel movement, but a number of conditions can impede its release, causing discomfort as the sacs are expanded by their contents. Predispositions to anal sac disease include thick secretions of large quantity, an abnormally small duct system, anal irritation, changes in muscle tone or fecal form, and following diarrhea or estrus. Diarrhea appears to be the most common predisposing cause of anal sac impaction. It is assumed that the lack of a formed stool prevents the normal emptying of the sacs by the exertion of pressure on the sac during defecation. This may lead to increased bacterial fermentation or occlusion of the duct with flocculent secretory material. The specific relationship of estrus and anal sac disease is not known.

Conditioned hyperirritability or autosensitization dermatitis is a phenomenon in which dermatitis on one area of the body results in a more generalized hyperirritability of the skin even in distant areas. The specific mechanisms involved are not known but it is believed that anal sac problems can be related to acute moist dermatitis, chronic or recurrent pyoderma, otitis externa, pododermatitis, periorbital dermatitis, anal ulcers and perianal fistulae. Perhaps the infected anal sacs act as a subclinical source or reservoir for chronic pyoderma.

Clinical Signs

It is not uncommon to see dogs with anal sac problems "scoot" on their backsides or chew at the anal area. Anal sacs should be periodically checked and their contents expressed, if necessary.

The anal sacs, due to their anatomy and location, are prone to a number of disorders, including impaction, infection, abscessation and neoplasia.

Diagnosis

Diagnostic testing might involve palpation, cytologic examination, and bacterial culture and sensitivity tests. Bacteria cultured most frequently from diseased anal sacs are *Streptococcus faecalis, Clostridium welchii, E coli, Proteus* spp, micrococci, *Staphylococcus* spp and diphtheroids. Normal resident flora include micrococci, *E coli, Streptococcus faecalis* and *Staphylococcus* spp.

Microscopic examination of anal sac secretions can yield valuable diagnostic information. Diseased anal sacs contain a large number of leukocytes and numerous intracellular and extracellular bacteria. Biopsy of the anal sac is usually only warranted if neoplasia is suspected.

Management

Some problems can be treated by expressing the sacs regularly and some by flushing with antiseptics and antibiotics. With recurrent problems, oral antibiotics should also be added to the regimen. Some problems refractory to medical management require anal sac resection. Anal sacculectomy is indicated in cases of recurrent anal sacculitis, impaction or abscessation, or in association with neoplasia, perianal fistulae, or a verified concomitant dermatosis (autosensitization dermatitis). Other complicating clinical signs include anal itching, recurring bacterial infections, interdigital inflammation, recurrent ear problems, anal ulcers and draining tracts (perianal fistulae — see Chapter 2). Carcinoma of the anal sac glands offers a poor prognosis and is variably associated with hypercalcemia and hypophosphatemia. Metastasis may occur to the iliac and sacral lymph nodes, causing obstruction of the pelvic inlet.

Additional Reading

1. Anderson, RK: Anal sac disease and its related dermatoses. *Comp Cont Ed Pract Vet* 6:829-837, 1984.

2. Nesbitt, GH: Anal sacculitis. *Vet Reports* 1:5, 1988.

3. Nesbitt, GH: Diseases of the anal sacs: A review. *Vet Focus* 1(1):16-18, 1989.

Cutaneous Vasculitis

Clinical Signs

Cutaneous vasculitis is not a specific entity but rather a collection of disorders in which the underlying problem includes destructive and inflammatory changes in the blood vessels. Most vasculitic syndromes are associated with immune complex deposition in the blood vessel walls. The location of the blood vessels affected and the severity of the damage are important determinants of how the skin lesions are manifested. While vasculitic lesions may occur anywhere in the body, they are most frequent on the dependent parts of the body, feet and ears (Fig 43). The most common lesion visualized and felt is an elevated bruise, so-called "palpable purpura." A red, pigmented (petechiae, purpura) or an erosive-ulcerative process is inevitable at some stage of the disease. In later stages, when the blood vessels have been thoroughly compromised, the tissue may die, leaving a depressed area. It should be kept in mind that the same process may be going on internally, where lesions are hidden from view.

Cutaneous vasculitis may occur secondary to a number of processes, including infections (bacterial, mycoplasmal, rickettsial, viral, fungal), drug reactions, eruptions due to foods and food additives, immune-mediated disorders (systemic lupus erythematosus, scleroderma, dermatomyositis, rheumatoid arthritis, polyarteritis), exposure to cold, trauma, reactions to injections (vaccinations), chronic diseases (diabetes mellitus, chronic respiratory disease, neoplasia), arthropod bites or for no apparent reason.

Diagnosis

Diagnosis is based on history and clinical findings, and is confirmed on tissue sections, with or without immunopathologic evaluation. Specific tests may be warranted, depending on the clinical signs (*eg*, ANA, rheumatoid factor, hypoallergenic food trial, bacterial or fungal culture of skin or blood, titers).

Management

Treatment should be directed at the underlying cause if it is known. If no cause has been determined, therapy is often initiated with antiinflammatory or immunosuppressive doses of corticosteroids. Dapsone, a product marketed to treat leprosy in people, has been used successfully in dogs. Bone marrow and liver function must be monitored on a regular basis.

Additional Reading

1. Wilcock, BP and Yager, JA: Focal cutaneous vasculitis and alopecia at sites of rabies vaccination in dogs. *JAVMA* 188:1174-1177, 1986.

2. Randall, MG and Hurvitz, AI: Immune-mediated vasculitis in five dogs. *JAVMA* 183:207-211, 1983.

3. Ekenstam, E and Callen, JP: Cutaneous leukocytoclastic vasculitis *Arch Dermatol* 120:484-489, 1984.

4. Crawford, MA and Foil, CS: Vasculitis: Clinical syndromes in small animals. *Comp Cont Ed Pract Vet* 11:400-415, 1989.

Dermatitis Herpetiformis

In people, dermatitis herpetiformis is a chronic, extremely pruritic dermatitis in which groups of papules, vesicles and urticaria-like plaques are located primarily on the extensor surfaces of the extremities, buttocks, sacrum, shoulders, neck and scalp. Affected patients have an associated gluten-sensitivity enteropathy, circulating gluten antigenemia, significant elevation of IgA circulating immune complexes and irregular granular deposits of IgA in the papillary dermis.

The pathogenesis is unknown but immune complexes of gluten and antigluten may be trapped in skin by reticulin-bound antireticulin antibodies, which cross-react with gluten. The IgA deposited in skin originates from plasma cells in the lamina propria of the intestine. Patients generally respond well to a gluten-free diet or therapy with dapsone, sulfapyridine or colchicine.

Clinical Signs

Dermatitis herpetiformis has only rarely been suspected in dogs. Suspects have shown a papulocrustous, pruritic eruption involving principally the trunk, head, ears and feet.

Diagnosis

The early papules are characterized microscopically by collections of neutrophils and a varying number of eosinophils at the tips of the edematous dermal papillae, which eventually form subepidermal bullae and clefts.

These findings closely approximate those reported in people, but no canine case has ever been substantiated by positive direct immunofluorescence or detection of IgA circulating immune complexes. To properly confirm a diagnosis, an animal should have appropriate clinical signs, characteristic histopathologic lesions, a positive direct immunofluorescence test for IgA in granular deposits in the dermal papillae, and a favorable response to dapsone.

Management

The preferred treatment for confirmed diagnosis of dermatitis herpetiformis is dapsone. Patients should be carefully monitored via blood counts, and liver function profiles.

Additional Reading
1. Ackerman, L: Dermatitis herpetiformis-Does it exist? *JAVMA* 185:633-635, 1984.
2. Thiers, BH: Dermatitis herpetiformis. *J Am Acad Dermatol* 5:114-117, 1981.

Ear Problems

Otitis Externa

Otitis externa is common in dogs. Contributing factors include a long, relatively narrow ear canal, pendulous ears in some breeds, hair growth within the ear canal, and a number of skin diseases, including bacterial, fungal and yeast infections, parasitic infestations, allergies, autoimmune diseases, nutritional disorders, keratinization disorders, environmental causes, neoplasia and foreign body reactions which affect this region.

Clinical Signs: When the problem is noted within the external ear canal, bacterial, fungal, parasitic and foreign body causes are usually first evaluated. When the pinna is inflamed, one must suspect that the ear problem is merely an extension of an internal problem. It is important to make this distinction, since an ear problem secondary to an internal or generalized problem will never completely resolve if treatment involves only applying medication to the ear canal.

Hair loss confined to the pinnae without concurrent inflammation may be seen with a number of conditions, including pinnal alopecia (seen most commonly in Dachshunds, Chihuahuas and Whippets), periodic alopecia (seen in Poodles) and congenito-hereditary disorders. Hormonal disorders (hypothyroidism, ovarian imbalance type II), dermatophytosis, demodicosis and alopecia areata may or may not be associated with inflammatory reactions. The pinnae may also be involved in a number of systemic disorders, including allergic inhalant dermatitis, food allergy, ear-margin dermatosis, cutaneous vasculitis, pemphigus erythematosus and foliaceus, systemic and discoid lupus erythematosus, dermatomyositis, lichenoid dermatoses and keratinization disorders.

Diagnosis: It is not usually difficult to diagnose otitis externa. Head shaking is a common feature, as is a painful reaction when the ear is touched. Head shaking may be so pronounced that small blood vessels are damaged and a hematoma forms in the pinna. Persistent infections or irritations within the ear canal result in a red and very thickened ear canal lining, further narrowing the opening. This makes the problem worse. Exudates in the ear canal may produce a foul smell. They recur quickly even after they have been thoroughly removed by cleaning.

Successful management of the condition requires knowledge of the underlying cause. The most important diagnostic test is a thorough examination of the ear canal, to the level of the eardrum. This usually requires heavy sedation or general anesthesia, as such examination is very painful with severe ear canal inflammation. Undiagnosed rupture of the eardrum is one of the most common reasons for treatment failure.

The ear must be thoroughly irrigated to remove debris and waxy deposits. This not only aids in diagnosis but also allows medication to penetrate to the real site of the problem. Also, some antibacterials, especially gentamicin, may be inactivated by pus. Before irrigation, swabs can be used to obtain specimens for microscopic evaluation for mites, for cytologic examination, or for bacterial and/or fungal culture as necessary.

The color of the exudate may be a diagnostic clue. Mites often produce a black discharge. Gram-positive bacteria are often associated with a brown exudate. Gram-negative infections are often associated with a yellow exudate. Cytologic evaluation is the single most helpful diagnostic test in ear problems. A smear can be stained (*eg,* Gram stain or Diff-Quik) and yeasts, bacteria, inflammatory cells and wax easily visualized. Whether organisms are intracellular or extracellular is of great importance.

Culture and sensitivity tests of ear exudates are less productive, since opportunistic bacteria are invariably present and drug sensitivities are only applicable when blood levels of antibiotics are anticipated. Since most otic products are instilled directly into the ear canal and not used systemically, sensitivities can often be predicted for the organisms recovered. Also, despite sensitivities reported following culture, the antibiotics are being applied directly in much higher concentrations than could ever be attained in the blood, such that organisms apparently resistant to certain antibiotics may actually be sensitive when they contact the product directly. Staphylococci, alpha- and nonhemolytic streptococci, *Micrococcus* spp, *Corynebacterium*, *Malassezia pachydermatis* and occasionally coliforms are commonly recovered from ear canals of normal dogs. Organisms that attain significance in the inflamed ear include *Staphylococcus intermedius*, beta-hemolytic streptococci, *Pseudomonas*, *Proteus*, coliforms and occasionally yeasts.

Management: Treatment can begin while the animal is still sedated or anesthetized. Hairs can be plucked, debris removed by flushing and antiseptics (chlorhexidine and povidone-iodine) or wax-dissolving substances (propylene glycol, dioctyl sodium sulfosuccinate or aluminum acetate) can be instilled deeply into the ear canal.

Debris must be removed by flushing, not with swabs. A swab can pack the material deeply into the ear canal. Flushing removes the material from bottom to top. A swab or cotton ball can then be used to remove excess liquid, or suction can be gently applied to the canal. Treatment can then begin for the specific problem.

Mildly inflamed ears for which no apparent infectious cause can be determined may suggest an allergic cause. In the meantime, mild corticosteroid or combination antibiotic-corticosteroid topical preparations may relieve some inflammation (Tables 1-7). Ears with heavy bacterial colonization usually benefit from desiccating the ear canals. Vinegar and water in a 1:1 or 1:2 ratio produce dramatic bacterial and yeast kill, are relatively easy to use and inexpensive, and offer few disadvantages.

Long-term use of potent antibiotics within the ear canal can lead to drug resistance and may also cause allergic drug reactions and overgrowth of yeasts and resistant bacteria. Eliminating the underlying cause or treating with safe products, such as vinegar and water, antiseptics or drying agents, greatly reduces the incidence of these adverse effects, making long-term treatment safer. It is now more common to give antibiotics systemically for a week or so in the treatment of otitis externa than in the past,

Table 1. Anticipated patterns of antibacterial response in ear infections.

Organism	Characteristics	Frequently Sensitive	Frequently Resistant
Beta-hemolytic Streptococci	Gram-positive coccus beta hemolytic, catalase negative	Ampicillin, amoxicillin, penicillin B, bacitracin, erythromycin, novobiocin	Aminoglycosides, tetracyline, polymixin B
Coliforms	Gram-negative rods, lactose fermenting	Cephalosporins, gentamicin, polymixin B, trimethoprim-sulfa, chloramphenicol	Penicillins, tetracycline, lincomycin, erythromycin, bacitracin, novobiocin
Malassezia pachydermatis	Bottle-shaped budding yeast	Miconazole, ketoconazole, clotrimazole, thiabendazole nystatin, acetic acid	Antibacterials, griseofulvin
Proteus	Gram-negative rod, catalase positive, oxidase positive	Cephalosporins, gentamicin	Penicillins, lincomycin, erythromycin, bacitracin, novobiocin
Pseudomonas aeruginosa	Gram-negative rod, oxidase positive, catalase positive	Polymixin B, carbenicillin, amikacin, ticarcillin, cephalosporins	Penicillins, cephalosporins, neomycin, tetracycline
Staphylococcus intermedius	Gram-positive coccus, coagulase positive, catalase positive, hemolytic	Potentiated penicillins, amoxicillin-clavulanate, lincomycin, erythromycin, cephalosporins, trimethoprim-sulfa, chloramphenicol, aminoglycosides	Ampicillin, amoxicillin, tetracycline, polymixin B

Table 2. Antibacterial otic preparations.

Ingredients	Examples	Manufacturer
Chloramphenicol	Chloralean Drops Pentamycetin Otic	MTC Pentagone
Polymixin B sulfate, neomycin sulfate, gramicidin	V-Sporin Solution	Wellcome
Polymixin B, gramicidin	Polysporin	Wellcome
Polymixin B, gramicidin lidocaine	Lidosporin	Wellcome

Table 3. Corticosteroid otic preparations.

Ingredients	Examples	Manufacturer
Fluocinolone acetonide	Synalar Solution	Syntex
Fluocinolone acetonide, DMSO	Synotic	Syntex
Hydrocortisone, acetic acid, colloidal sulfur	ClearX	DVM
Hydrocortisone, salicylic acid, precipitated sulfur	Stearotic Lotion, Cerex	Upjohn

Table 4. Antibacterial corticosteroid otic preparations.

Ingredients	Examples	Manufacturer
Chloramphenicol, prednisolone, tetracaine, squalene	Liquichlor	Evsco
Gentamicin sulfate, betamethasone valerate	Gentocin Otic	Schering
Neomycin sulfate, hydrocortisone acetate	Neo-Cortef Drops	Upjohn
Neomycin sulfate, hydrocortisone acetate	Neo-Cortef Ointment	Upjohn
Neomycin sulfate, isoflupredone acetate	Neo-Predef	Upjohn
Neomycin sulfate, methylprednisolone acetate	Neo-Medrol	Upjohn
Neomycin sulfate, prednisolone acetate	Neo-Delta-Cortef	Upjohn
Neomycin sulfate, polymixin B, hydrocortisone acetate	Cortisporin Otic	Wellcome
Polymixin B, neomycin sulfate, hydrocortisone	V-Sporin HC Otic	Wellcome

when treatment was limited to topical therapy. Apparently, systemic therapy is less likely to interfere with the normal flora of the ear canal. Systemic therapy with antibiotics is crucial with eardrum rupture and otitis media.

Yeast infections within the ear are almost always secondary to some other underlying process. The most common yeast, *Malassezia pachydermatis* (formerly *Pityrosporum canis*) is a normal inhabitant of the ear canal and only overgrows if there is debris to feed on. The yeast acts as a parasite and rarely damages the skin

Table 5. Antibacterial-antifungal-corticosteroid otic preparations.

Ingredients	Examples	Manufacturer
Neomycin sulfate, thiabendazole, dexamethasone	Tresaderm	MSD Agvet
Neomycin sulfate, thiostrepton, nystatin, triamcinolone acetonide	Panolog	Solvay
Neomycin sulfate, bacitracin, nystatin, triamcinolone, lidocaine	Oribiotic	MTC
Nitrofurathiazide, griseofulvin, undecylenic acid, tetracaine dexamethasone	Fulvidex Otic Solution	Schering

Table 6. Antiparasitic otic preparations.

Ingredients	Examples	Manufacturer
Pyrethrins 0.15%	Flea-Off Ear Mite Lotion	Adams/Norden
Carbaryl, neomycin, tetracaine, mineral oil, sulfacetamide	Mitox Liquid	Norden
Pyrethrins, squalene	Cerumite	Evsco
Thiabendazole, dexamethasone, neomycin sulfate	Tresaderm Oticare-M	MSD Agvet Ar Labs

Table 7. Miscellaneous ear preparations.

Ingredients	Examples	Manufacturer
Acetic acid 2.5%	Vinegar and water	—
Alcohol and boric acid	Panodry	Solvay
Aloe vera gel, dioctyl NA sulfosuccinate, propylene glycol, sulfur, urea	Liquid Ear desiccant	Adams
Aluminum acetate	Buro-Sol Otic Domeboro Otic	TCD Miles
Carbamide (urea) peroxide	Cer-Otic Murine Panoprep	Syntex Abbott Solvay
Dioctyl calcium sulfosuccinate	Surfak	Hoechst
Dioctyl sodium sulfosuccinate, aloe vera gel, glycerine	Panotic	Adams
Docusate sodium	Ear-Groom Cerusol EPI-Otic ClearX	Lambert Kay Burns Biotec Allerderm DVM
Hydrocortisone, salicylic acid, precipitated sulfur	Cerex	Upjohn
Propylene glycol	—	—
Resorcinol bismuth subgallate, bismuth subnitrate, zinc oxide, calamine, juniper	Pellitol	Pitman-Moore
Squalene	Cerumene	Evsco

lining the ear canal. Yeast infections are easy to diagnose and easy to treat with a variety of products, including clotrimazole, miconazole, povidone-iodine, chlorhexidine and even vinegar and water. Yeast infections recur as long as there is material for the yeast to feed on. Since the yeast is a normal inhabitant of the skin surface and normally is harmless, it is senseless to try to eliminate it to remedy an ear problem. *Candida* yeasts may damage the lining of the ear canal and usually indicate a faltering immune system. This yeast may be killed by a variety of products, such as nystatin.

Parasites, such as mites and ticks, are usually controlled by common antiparasitic products (pyrethrins, rotenone, thiabendazole) specially formulated for otic use (*eg,* Cerumite: Evsco, Canex:Pitman-Moore, Tresaderm:MSD Agvet, OtiCare M:ARC).

As a final option, ear problems due to chronic lack of ventilation can be surgically corrected by resecting the lateral aspect of the vertical ear canal, giving the ear canal better exposure (Zepp or Lacroix procedure). About 50% of patients subjected to this surgery benefit significantly. Chronically inflamed and scarred ears or ones in which the horizontal ear canal has been markedly narrowed show the least favorable results.

Aural Hematomas

Aural hematomas are a consequence of a variety of ear problems in which trauma plays at least some role. The usual management involves surgical drainage to retain a cosmetically acceptable pinna, though it has recently been proposed that large doses of corticosteroids may offer similar benefits and that there might be an immune-mediated component. An ANA test should probably be a component of the diagnostic workup.

Additional Reading

1. Griffin, CE: Otitis externa. *Comp Cont Ed Pract Vet* 3:741-749, 1981.

2. Harvey, CE: Ear canal disease in the dog: Medical and surgical management. *JAVMA* 177:136-139, 1980.

3. Rausch, FD and Skinner, GW: Incidence and treatment of budding yeasts in canine otitis externa. *MVP* 59:914-915, 1978.

4. Dubielzig, RR *et al:* Pathogenesis of canine aural hematomas. *JAVMA* 185:873-875, 1984.

5. Kuwahara, J: Canine and feline aural hematomas: Results of treatment with corticosteroids. *JAAHA* 22:641-647, 1986.

6. Griffin, C, in: *The Complete Manual Of Ear Care.* Veterinary Learning Systems, Lawrenceville, NJ, 1986. pp 21-36 and 612-618.

7. McKeever, PJ and Richardson, HW: Otitis externa Part 3: Ear cleaning and medical treatment. *Compan Anim Pract* 2(6):24-30, 1988.

Eosinophilic Granuloma

Clinical Signs

Canine eosinophilic granuloma appears to be an immune-mediated disorder, most commonly affecting Siberian Huskies, males and dogs <3 years of age. The masses are most commonly found within the mouth but are occasionally seen on the underside and flanks. Affected dogs are healthy and the lumps are neither painful nor itchy.

Diagnosis

Diagnosis is based on the classic changes seen on tissue sections including collagenolysis and granuloma formation with eosinophils, lymphocytes and histiocytes. Histologically the condition resembles linear granuloma in the cat, collagenolytic granuloma in the horse and Well's syndrome in people.

Management

Most dogs are treated with antiinflammatory to immunosuppressive doses of corticosteroids successfully. Some lesions undergo spontaneous regression. Though the syndrome is poorly understood, it is considered quite responsive to therapy.

Additional Reading

1. Turnwald, GH *et al:* Cutaneous eosinophilic granuloma in a Labrador retriever. *JAVMA* 179:799-801, 1981.

2. Madewell, BR *et al:* Oral eosinophilic granuloma in Siberian husky dogs. *JAVMA* 177:701-703, 1980.

Erythema Multiforme

Erythema multiforme is an uncommon self-limiting syndrome of distinctive skin lesions, with or without concurrent lesions in the oral cavity or other mucous membranes. The disease is presumably immune-mediated. In people, most cases are secondary to recurrent *Herpes simplex* or mycoplasmal infection and drug reactions. The name, which literally means "redness of the skin appearing in a multitude of forms," is a very apt description (Fig 44).

Clinical Signs

The eruption is usually symmetric and often involves the limbs. Manifestations include spots (macules), bumps (papules), hives (urticarial plaques) and blisters (vesicles or bullae). Lesions often spread centrifugally, leaving a central clear area, commonly referred to as a "target" or "iris" lesion.

Diagnosis

Biopsies taken for histopathologic evaluation often reveal individual keratinocyte necrosis and hydropic degeneration of basal cells. These findings support a diagnosis but on their own are nonconfirmatory.

Management

In people, the prognosis is good, and the condition subsides without treatment in about 3 weeks. If the underlying problem has not been identified or corrected (*eg, Herpes simplex* infection), recurrence of the lesions at some future date is a good possibility. Most cases in dogs have been secondary to staphylococcal folliculitis or reactions to drugs.

Additional Reading

1. Scott, DW *et al*: Erythema multiforme in the dog. *JAAHA* 19:453-459, 1983.

2. Huff, JC *et al*: Erythema multiforme: A critical review of characteristics, diagnostic criteria, and causes. *J Am Acad Dermatol* 8:763-775, 1983.

Focal Mucinosis

Clinical Signs

Focal mucinosis is a rare disorder characterized grossly by bumps or lumps (papules, plaques or nodules) and microscopically by accumulation of mucin and proliferation of fibroblasts. The condition is asymptomatic and affected animals are in no medical distress. There are no apparent site predilections. Breeds at increased risk include the Shar Pei and Doberman Pinscher. Shetland Sheepdogs and Labrador Retrievers have also been affected. Females may also be at increased risk.

Diagnosis

The diagnosis is based on the characteristic biopsy findings.

Focal mucinosis is probably not a true entity but likely reflects a number of conditions that cause collection of mucin (usually hyaluronic acid) in the dermis. In the Shar Pei, this may be an inherited defect. In fact, some degree of mucinosis in this breed is probably normal and accounts to some extent for the characteristic folding of the skin. In other dogs, especially those with more generalized lesions, such differential diagnoses as hypothyroidism, inherited mucopolysaccharidoses, immune-mediated diseases (especially lupus erythematosus), dermatomyositis, scleroderma and eosinophilic granuloma should be considered.

Management

Any therapies undertaken should be directed at the underlying cause.

Additional Reading

1. Dillberger, JE and Altman, NH: Focal mucinosis in dogs: Seven cases and review of cutaneous mucinoses of man and animals. *Vet Pathol* 23:132-139, 1986.

2. Rosenkrantz, WB *et al*: Idiopathic cutaneous mucinosis in a dog. *Compan Anim Pract* 1(3):39-42, 1987.

Footpad Diseases

Diseases of the footpads are often referred to as hyperkeratotic footpads, since the pads tend to become thickened, cracked and scaly when diseased. Footpad diseases have various causes. In the past, many cases were undoubtedly due to infection with distemper virus (hard pad disease). Since the advent of modern vaccination programs, distemper is now rare; however, some vaccinated animals may demonstrate signs normally attibutable to distemper.

With today's sophisticated methods of diagnosis, many different conditions have been implicated in footpad disorders, including parasitism (hookworms, *Pelodera*), bacterial infections, fungal infections (dermatophytes, yeasts, intermediate and deep fungi), contact allergy, autoimmune diseases (lupus erythematosus, pemphigus foliaceus), nutritional skin diseases (zinc-responsive dermatosis, generic dog food disease), congenito-hereditary diseases (lethal acrodermatitis, tyrosinemia), neoplasms (squamous-cell carcinoma), foreign body penetration, contact irritation, acral mutilation syndrome and nasodigital hyperkeratosis.

Acral Mutilation Syndrome

Acral mutilation syndrome is a bizarre inherited condition most commonly seen in Pointer pups. Nerve dysfunction causes the pups to chew their feet to the point of mutilation. Treatment is only palliative. Since the nerve defect is inherited, the parents should not be used for further breeding. Acral mutilation syndrome is covered more completely in Chapter 8.

Lethal Acrodermatitis

Lethal acrodermatitis is a syndrome in Bull Terriers, characterized by growth retardation, progressive acrodermatitis, chronic pyoderma and paronychia, diarrhea, pneumonia, abnormal behavior and death by 16 months of age.

The syndrome appears to be transmitted as an autosomal recessive trait and resembles lethal trait A46 in cattle and acrodermatitis enteropathica in people. Unlike those conditions, it is unresponsive to zinc supplementation. The underlying defect may involve multiple trace minerals, including zinc and copper. The metabolic defect appears to cause immune system dysfunction. The condition is covered in more detail in Chapter 8.

Tyrosinemia

Tyrosinemia was recently observed in a German Shepherd. This condition mimics tyrosinemia II or Richner-Hanhart syndrome in people. The disorder is transmitted as an autosomal recessive trait in people, but this has not been confirmed in dogs. Erosions and ulcerations of the footpads and nose, and ophthalmic lesions were noted.

The diagnosis is based on elevated serum and urine levels of tyrosine. Skin biopsies stained with Millon's stain may reveal orange-stained dermal granules. Treatment is supportive and includes a low-phenylalanine, low-tyrosine diet.

Nasodigital Hyperkeratosis

Nasodigital hyperkeratosis is a strange entity in which excessive layers of the shingle-like stratum corneum accumulate on the nose and/or footpads. The cause is unknown. The condition is diagnosed by excluding the other causes of hyperkeratotic lesions listed above. Treatment is attempted by shaving away the excess dead tissue and applying hydrating ointments to increase shedding of the accumulated material.

Additional Reading

1. Anderson, RK: Canine pododermatitis. *Comp Cont Ed Pract Vet* 2:361-371, 1980.

2. Jezyk, RF *et al*: Lethal acrodermatitis in Bull Terriers. *JAVMA* 188:833-839, 1986.

3. Kunkle, GA *et al*: Tyrosinemia in a dog. *JAAHA* 20:615-620, 1984.

4. Machino, H *et al*: Successful dietary control of tyrosinemia II. *J Am Acad Dermatol* 9:533-539, 1983.

Juvenile Cellulitis

Clinical Signs

Juvenile cellulitis or puppy strangles is an immune-mediated disease in which the face and head are swollen, inflamed, nodular and indurated (Fig 45). Dachshunds, Golden Retrievers and Pointers are most commonly affected.

Diagnosis

Biopsies reveal underlying cellulitis. Bacterial cultures may reveal organisms, though they do not appear to be of primary significance.

Management

Treatment with a bactericidal antibacterial and immunosuppressive doses of corticosteroids is required for about 2 weeks. The condition usually responds completely, with little chance of recurrence.

Keratinization Disorders

Keratinization disorders (seborrhea, erythroderma, exfoliative dermatitis) refer to a broad classification of clinical entities ranging from simple dandruff to severe, red, crusting and scaly skin. The normal process of epidermal renewal involves the orderly turnover of epidermal cells, progressing from the basal cell layer to the shingle-like stratum corneum in about 21-23 days. In keratinization disorders, there is an increased turnover rate. The entire epidermis may be replaced in as little as 2-4 days, leaving scale on the skin surface.

The term seborrhea is a poor one, since it literally means "flow of sebum" and most keratinization disorders have little or nothing to do with sebum production. Much better descriptive terms for the condition include "disorders of keratinization," which implies some problem with epidermal cell turnover, "erythroderma," which means scaly skin that may be reddened or have some inflammatory component, or "exfoliative dermatitis," which means increased production and shedding of scale from the skin surface. Unfortunately, this scaling reaction is not specific for any one condition. Dozens of different disorders with different causes and different treatments have been lumped together under the heading "seborrhea" in the past. Hopefully, most conditions now are better diagnosed and specific therapy rendered.

Some animals undoubtedly are born with a defect in their keratinization process. These congenital conditions can be considered primary, but they are rare. Most disorders are secondary to an underlying disorder. Pups born with ichthyosis (Chapter 8) have tenacious scale adherent to the skin surface caused by a primary inherited defect of keratinization. By far, most keratinization disorders occur secondary to underlying problems. Thus, it is always best to identify a specific cause to which a specific treatment can be applied.

Some common conditions that can result in keratinization disorders are included in Table 8.

Table 8. Some conditions that may cause keratinization disorders.

Allergies	Inhalant, food, drug, contact
Immune-mediated	Pemphigus foliaceus, pemphigus erythematosus, systemic and discoid lupus erythematosus
Endocrine	Hypothyroidism, hyperadrenocorticism, growth hormone-responsive dermatosis
Fungi	Dermatophytosis (ringworm)
Miscellaneous	Bacterial hypersensitivity, seborrheic dermatitis, acanthosis nigricans, metabolic disorders, toxicities, granulomatous sebaceous adenitis, psoriasiform-lichenoid dermatitis, epidermal dysplasia
Neoplastic	Cutaneous T-cell lymphoma
Nutritional	Fatty acid deficiency, zinc-responsive dermatosis, vitamin A-responsive dermatosis
Parasites	*Cheyletiella, Sarcoptes*

Clinical Signs

Scaling, crusting, greasiness and hair loss are the primary clinical signs of keratinization disorders. Secondarily, variable degrees of inflammation, scratching, self-trauma and bacterial dermatitis are evidenced in some cases. The normal bacterial flora of 100-200 organisms per cubic centimeter of skin may be increased to over 16,000 per cubic centimeter in keratinization disorders. The most common offending bacterium is *Staphylococcus intermedius*. The combination of bacteria and abnormal surface debris may create a foul odor on the animal.

Diagnosis

Diagnosis is based on clinical examination, history, skin scrapings, bacterial and fungal cultures, blood tests and biopsies for histopathologic examination, with or without immunopathologic assay. Other tests may be performed as warranted. A nonspecific diagnosis of keratinization disorder (seborrhea) should only be made after all other possible underlying causes have been excluded.

Management

Treatment is very successful when the underlying provoking factors have been identified and corrected. Thus, hypothyroidism can be corrected by thyroid replacement therapy, nutritional problems by dietary supplementation, infections by antibiotic therapy, etc. For disorders in which the underlying condition has not been identified, treatment must be vigorous and intensive, though in most cases the animal's overall health status is not terribly compromised. Frequent bathing and topical treatment of the skin, as well as perhaps dietary supplementation, may make the condition more tolerable. This usually means bathing from twice weekly to once every few weeks with an antiseborrheic shampoo.

Ingredients considered antiseborrheic include sulfur, salicylic acid, tar, selenium sulfide and benzoyl peroxide (Appendix 2). One should always use tar shampoos with some caution, since they may irritate the skin and can result in contact dermatitis in the person doing the bathing. *Always wear gloves when using tar shampoos.* Benzoyl peroxide can dry the skin and can bleach many fabrics. Therefore, it should not be used in dogs with overly dry skin unless the bath is followed by an emollient rinse or spray. Benzoyl peroxides are particularly helpful in cases of follicular hyperkeratosis, such as seen with Schnauzer comedo syndrome and vitamin A-responsive dermatosis. To maximize the effect of all antiseborrheic shampoos, they should be left on the animal's skin (not just the haircoat) for 5-15 minutes after thorough lathering, or as recommended by the manufacturer. Proper rinsing is essential, and animals should be preferably air-dried or towel-dried rather than blown dry.

Seborrheic pets often benefit from a good basic diet. Supplementing that diet with polyunsaturated oils (corn, safflower, peanut) and saturated fats (pork, beef, chicken) on a regular basis may help alleviate some of the scaling associated with the condition. Alternatively, there are many useful commercial supplements on the market. In people, some keratinization disorders of metabolic origin have responded to retinoids, derivatives of vitamin A, especially etretinate (Tegison). I have been conducting some trials with this compound and have had some limited success, despite the expense and potential toxicity of the product.

Additional Reading

1. Austin, VH: A clinical approach to abnormal keratinization diseases of the dog. *Comp Cont Ed Pract Vet* 5:890-897, 1983.

2. Anderson, RK: Exfoliative dermatitis in the dog. *Comp Cont Ed Pract Vet* 3:885-890, 1981.

3. Halliwell, REW: Seborrhea in the dog. *Comp Cont Ed Pract Vet* 1:227-236, 1979.

4. Dicken, CH: Retinoids: A review. *J Am Acad Dermatol* 11:541-552, 1984.

5. Fadok, VA: Treatment of canine idiopathic seborrhea with isotretinoin. *Am J Vet Res* 47: 1730, 1986.

6. Scott, DW: Granulomatous sebaceous adenitis in dogs. *JAAHA* 22:631-634, 1986.

7. Baker, BB and Maibach, HI: Epidermal cell renewal in seborrheic skin of dogs. *Am J Vet Res* 48:716-718, 1987.

Lichenoid Dermatoses

"Lichenoid" has very different meanings when used to describe clinical or histopathologic findings. Clinically, lichenoid refers to a dense grouping of papules or plaques. Skin sections may show collections of inflammatory cells at the dermal-epidermal junction, with hydropic degeneration of basal cells, Civatte bodies and pigmentary incontinence.

Histologically, lichenoid refers to interface dermatitis, in which an inflammatory infiltrate obscures the dermal-epidermal junction. Lichenoid tissue reactions have been associated with lupus erythematosus, pemphigus, pemphigoid, erythema multiforme, cutaneous T-cell-like lymphoma, uveodermatologic syndrome (Vogt-Koyanagi-Harada-like syndrome), toxic epidermal necrolysis, contact dermatitis, cheyletiellosis, lichenoid keratosis, lichenoid psoriasiform dermatitis and idiopathic lichenoid dermatitis.

Clinical lichenoid dermatoses are uncommon in dogs and include idiopathic lichenoid dermatosis, lichenoid keratosis and lichenoid-psoriasiform dermatitis of Springer Spaniels.

Lichenoid-Psoriasiform Dermatitis of Springer Spaniels

This condition should perhaps be included in the chapter on congenito-hereditary dermatoses. However, since no data are available to suggest any mode of inheritance, I have included it here in the miscellaneous category. The name connotes a pathologic description (psoriasiform dermatitis with a lichenoid tissue reaction) in a specific breed. To date, no other breeds have been affected. This suggests that inheritance has a role in the etiology.

The dermatitis usually is manifested as bumps or wart-like or cauliflower-like projections of the pinnae and ventral abdomen. Occasionally the lesions are generalized (Fig 46). Affected dogs are often <3 years of age. The condition is more of a cosmetic defect than a health concern.

Treatment with corticosteroids, antibiotics or vitamin A does not alter the course of the disease, which waxes and wanes. Topical use of vitamin A derivatives may offer some benefit, but treatment should not be overdone, since the condition does not affect the health of these otherwise normal dogs.

Additional Reading

1. Ackerman, L: Lichenoid-psoriasiform dermatosis in a Springer Spaniel. *MVP* 69:32-33, 1988.

2. Mason, KV *et al*: Characterization of lichenoid-psoriasiform dermatosis of Springer Spaniels. *JAVMA* 189:897-901, 1986.

3. Gross, TL *et al*: Psoriasiform lichenoid dermatitis in the Springer Spaniel. *Vet Pathol* 23:76-78, 1986.

4. Scott, DW: Lichenoid reactions in the skin of dogs: clinicopathologic correlations. *JAAHA* 20:305-317, 1984.

Metabolic Dermatosis

A number of medical conditions have been associated with ill-defined dermatoses over the past few years. These have been referred to by such terms as diabetic dermatopathy, hepatic dermatopathy, glucagonoma syndrome and necrolytic migratory erythema. Diabetes mellitus, hepatobiliary disease, renal disease, neoplasia and defects of bile acid and uric acid metabolism have all been implicated.

Clinical Signs

An ulcerative dermatosis has recently been observed in dogs with diabetes mellitus and liver disease. The condition has some similarities to necrolytic migratory erythema or glucagonoma syndrome in people, a paraneoplastic condition most often associated with glucagon-secreting pancreatic tumors. Few affected dogs also had a documented pancreatic tumor. I have also seen the condition associated with transitional-cell carcinoma, cholangiohepatitis and Fanconi syndrome. The pathogenesis is unknown but perhaps metabolic disorders, such as diabetes mellitus and liver disease, result in lowering of certain factors such as amino acids, tryptophan or niacin, or increase in glucagon levels, which is normally degraded by the liver.

The condition is characterized by an erythematous, ulcerative, crusting dermatitis or exfoliative dermatosis, with a predilection for the face, external genitalia, feet and footpads. Polyuria and polydipsia may be observed if diabetes mellitus is the underlying cause.

Diagnosis

Diagnosis is based on the history, physical examination, blood chemistry profile (including glucose, lipase, amylase, uric acid, bile acids), survey radiographs, ultrasonography and skin biopsies. Skin sections typically show intra- and extracellular edema in the superficial epidermis, focal epidermal necrosis, parakeratotic hyperkeratosis and irregular epidermal hyperplasia. Serum glucagon levels may indicate pancreatic neoplasia.

Management

Treatment usually is supportive, in addition to treating the underlying cause. Pancreatic neoplasia warrants surgery.

Additional Reading

1. Walton, DH et al: Ulcerative dermatosis associated with diabetes mellitus in the dog: a report of 4 cases. JAAHA 12:79-88, 1986.

2. Rosychuk, RA: Endocrine, metabolic, internal, and neoplastic causes of pruritus in the dog and cat. Vet Clin No Am 18:1101-1110, 1988.

3. Vandersteen, PR and Scheithauer, BW: Glucagonoma syndrome: a clinicopathologic, immunochemical and ultrastructural study. *J Am Acad Dermatol* 12:1032-1039, 1985.

Nail and Nailbed Diseases

Diseases of the nails (more correctly termed claws) and nail beds (ungual folds) are uncommon in dogs but may be seen with bacterial infections (paronychia), fungal infections (onychomycosis), yeast infections (*Candida* paronychia), autoimmune disorders (lupus erythematosus), inherited defects, nutritional imbalances, cardiopulmonary disease and parasitism (demodicosis). Bacterial paronychia is not uncommon but the underlying cause may be difficult to discern. Immune-mediated causes for involvement of the ungual folds include systemic lupus erythematosus, vasculitis, pemphigus vulgaris, bullous pemphigoid, erythema multiforme and drug eruption. The bacterial component can often be managed by appropriate antibiotic therapy and antiseptic flushes with chlorhexidine or iodides. If no underlying cause can be determined, long-term antibiotic therapy may be warranted or, alternatively, surgical removal of the affected nails. Samples for culture should be obtained from biopsy specimens.

Candida paronychia can often be diagnosed on the basis of cytologic smears, in which Gram staining reveals oval yeast bodies and pseudohyphae. Treatment with nystatin or ketoconazole, and antiseptic flushes are palliative.

Onychomycosis may occur with dermatophytosis, sporotrichosis and blastomycosis. The diagnosis is based on cultures, cytologic examination and biopsies for histopathologic examination. Treatment is often unrewarding but ketoconazole is the drug of choice, together with antiseptic flushes.

Onychorrhexis describes brittle nails, most commonly caused by chronic low-grade infection. Other causes can be genetic, nutritional or senile. If the underlying problem can be identified, treatment should be specific and accompanied by filing of the nails rather than trimming.

Onychomadesis is sloughing of the horny claw caused by clefting within the keratinizing layers of the claw. Causes include a multitude of immune-mediated disorders (lupus erythematosus, pemphigus, pemphigoid), vascular compromise, trauma and infection. In addition to a thorough physical examination, a minimum data base should include a CBC, biochemical profile, urinalysis and antinuclear antibody test. Cardiovascular assessment may also be warranted.

Treatment is aimed at correcting the underlying problem and treating symptomatically with soothing baths. As a last resort, the affected nails can be resected. Nutritional supplementation with zinc, methionine or gelatin (Knox gelatin in food at 1 packet/15 lb body weight daily) may help some affected dogs.

Additional Reading

1. White, SD: How I treat nail diseases. *Proc Seminar DVM, Inc*, 1987.
2. Foil, CS: Disorders of the feet and claws. *Proc 11th Ann Kal Kan Symp*, 1987. pp 23-32.

Nasal Dermatitis

Nasal dermatitis describes a number of very different conditions that may affect the skin of the nose. It was formerly referred to as "Collie nose," which is inappropriate since any breed may be affected. It is now known that many different diseases may be manifested as nasal dermatitis; therefore, correct treatment depends on definitive diagnosis of the underlying cause.

In the past it was thought that animals with so-called Collie nose were prone to damage from the sun's rays (photodermatitis); therefore, their noses were tattooed with black ink to offer some protection. It is now known that few if any of these dogs had primary photodermatitis, though many conditions can be worsened by exposure to ultraviolet light.

Conditions that have been implicated in nasal dermatitis include: external parasitism (especially demodectic mange); bacterial infections (nasal pyoderma, dermatophilosis); fungal infections (dermatophytosis, intermediate and deep mycoses); allergies (inhalant, food, contact); autoimmune skin diseases (pemphigus foliaceus, pemphigus erythematosus, bullous pemphigoid, systemic and discoid lupus erythematosus, Vogt-Koyanagi-Harada-like syndrome); nutritional skin diseases (vitamin A-responsive dermatosis, zinc-responsive dermatosis, generic dog food disease); neoplasms (cutaneous T-cell lymphoma, squamous-cell carcinoma); hereditary diseases (dermatomyositis, epidermolysis bullosa simplex, tyrosinemia); trauma; drug eruption; and perhaps photodermatitis. Most Collies with suspected Collie nose probably had discoid lupus erythematosus or pemphigus erythematosus, to which this breed appears to be particularly prone.

Diagnostic testing should include skin scrapings, bacterial and fungal cultures, and preferably biopsies for histopathologic and perhaps immunopathologic examination. Other tests may be performed as warranted. Treatment must be directed at the specific cause.

Additional Reading

1. Miller Jr, WH: Canine facial dermatoses. *Comp Cont Ed Pract Vet* 1:640-650, 1979.

2. Kaufman, GM and Blakemore, JC: Facial dermatitis in a dog. *Comp Cont Ed Pract Vet* 6:109-112, 1984.

Nodular Panniculitis

Nodular panniculitis is an inflammatory reaction in the subcutaneous fat, with several known and possibly many more unknown causes. Progression of degenerative changes in the adipose tissue is directly related to the degree of compromise of the tissue's vasculature. Interference with the arterial supply results in diffuse degeneration of the fat lobules (lobular panniculitis). Venous disorders result in alterations of the fibrous septae and the peripheral portions of the fat lobules (septal panniculitis).

Lesions can be localized or generalized, and vary in size up to several centimeters (Fig 47). Sometimes painful, they often become evident as deep subcutaneous nodules occurring singly or in groups. The nodules can subsequently ulcerate and drain, and resultant scarring can be pronounced.

Because nodular panniculitis is not an entity but rather a descriptive term, in each case it is necessary to further define the condition to establish a suitable therapeutic regimen. The condition can be subdivided into the following 5 categories: benign (or juvenile) panniculitis, connective tissue panniculitis, pancreatic panniculitis, immune-mediated panniculitis and chronic relapsing panniculitis.

Benign Panniculitis

Benign or juvenile panniculitis involves dogs <6 months of age, though older animals can display similar syndromes. The most commonly affected breeds are Dachshunds, Toy Poodles, Collies and Wirehaired Fox Terriers. Clinically, benign panniculitis appears as crops of subcutaneous nodules principally localized on the neck, trunk and proximal extremities. The nodules can rupture and discharge an oily, purulent material or regress spontaneously, leaving depressed, atrophic scars. The characteristic histologic lesion is a circumscribed area of panniculitis primarly containing neutrophils centrally and macrophages peripherally. Juvenile panniculitis responds rapidly and completely to antiinflammatory or immunosuppressive doses of corticosteroids for 1-2 weeks, with minimal chance of relapse. Additional therapy, such as water soaks with aluminum acetate or antiseptics (*eg,* chlorhexidine, benzoyl peroxide) can help cleanse and dry up draining lesions.

Connective Tissue Panniculitis

Connective tissue diseases, such as lupus erythematosus, dermatomyositis and scleroderma, can involve the subcutaneous fat as part of the overall inflammatory condition of the blood vessels and connective tissues. A variant of lupus erythematosus, called lupus profundus has been recognized in the dog. The resultant subcutaneous nodules tend to ulcerate and are histologically characterized by both lobular and septal panniculitis. The inflammatory infiltrate is principally mononuclear and plasmacytic, with evident focal areas of leukocytoclastic vasculitis. Treatment must be geared to the underlying condition and may be undertaken with many different forms of medication, though immunosuppressive doses of corticosteroids or other forms of chemotherapy are sometimes warranted.

Pancreatic Panniculitis

Pancreatic panniculitis is a misleading name because the underlying event appears to be digestion of subcutaneous fat by pancreatic enzymes, not necessarily as a sequel to pancreatic disease. Manifestations of pancreatitis and pancreatic cancer can be overt or inapparent; pancreatic disease may not even be present. Pancreatic panniculitis consists of enlarging papules and nodules that rupture and leave deep subcutaneous ulcers primarily distributed on the skin of the neck and the trunk. Histologically, it appears as foci of subcutaneous fat necrosis. Ghost-like anucleated cells with thick, shadowy walls are present in affected areas and surrounded by an inflammatory cellular infiltrate primarily composed of neutrophils and lymphocytes. Secondary hemorrhage and dystrophic calcification can appear in areas of necrosis. Successful therapy must be directed at the internal as well as the dermatologic disorder. It is also crucial to differentiate between inflammatory and neoplastic underlying processes.

Immune-Mediated Panniculitis

Erythema nodosum, a condition of undetermined origin, often appears to be an hypersensitivity reaction to an infectious agent or medication (including vaccination). In addition to the presence of subcutaneous nodules, the syndrome is associated with fever, depression and arthralgia. Signs usually abate spontaneously after 3-6 weeks. The histologic hallmark of erythema nodosum is septal panniculitis characterized by a predominantly lymphocytic cellular infiltration. Treatment with analgesics can hasten recovery.

Chronic Relapsing Panniculitis

Chronic relapsing panniculitis is a general term describing cases of panniculitis that elude specific diagnosis or recur following cessation of therapy. These cases might represent the yet undescribed canine versions of a number of human conditions, or they may be the test-negative cases of the conditions already discussed. Some of these cases are autoimmune in nature and thus would be expected to respond to immunosuppressive therapy. Treatment must be individualized, and dogs receiving long-term therapy may not be able to be weaned onto alternate-day therapy. Other affected dogs entirely fail to respond. These reflect inadequate diagnosis and/or inappropriate treatment of the underlying condition.

Other Causes of Subcutaneous Nodules

Subcutaneous nodules are a nonspecific sign of panniculitis and can occur in a variety of other conditions, including bacterial infections, fungal infections, skin tumors, cutaneous cysts, foreign body penetration, trauma and reaction to injections. For this reason, a systematic diagnostic approach must be used, incorporating some or all of the following steps: a complete history; thorough physical examination; impression smear cytologic examination or fine-needle aspiration; bacterial and fungal cultures; pancreatic enzyme evaluation; antinuclear antibody test; and biopsies for histopathologic examination, with or without immunopathologic assay.

Additional Reading

1. Ackerman, LJ: Canine nodular panniculitis. *Comp Cont Ed Pract Vet* 6:818-824, 1984.

2. Shanley, KJ: Panniculitis in the dog: A report of five cases. *JAAHA* 21:545-550, 1985.

3. Scott, DW and Anderson, WI: Panniculitis in dogs and cats: A retrospective analysis of 78 cases. *JAAHA* 24:551-559, 1988.

Pododermatitis

Pododermatitis is a descriptive term denoting inflammation of the feet and interdigital spaces. One or more feet may be involved. See Table 9 for a variety of causes of pododermatitis.

Furunculosis is probably the most common cause of interdigital pododermatitis. It is seen most frequently in English Bulldogs, Great Danes, Boxers, Doberman Pinschers, Rottweilers, Shar Peis, Dachshunds and Labrador Retrievers. Pododermatitis results from folliculitis and furunculosis, then consequent foreign body granulomatous reaction to displaced keratin. Dogs with chronic relapsing pododermatitis should be evaluated for possible allergy (inhalant, food), hypothyroidism, dermatophytosis and immunoincompetence. A major distinction must be made between microbial or parasitic causes and immune-mediated processes since the method of treatment is so dissimilar.

Pododermatitis is often a frustrating disorder to treat, especially if the underlying cause is unknown. A minimum data base must include skin scrapings, cytologic examination and microbial cultures. Histopathologic examination of biopsies is often necessary.

Table 9. Causes of pododermatitis.

Allergic	Contact, inhalant, food, drug eruption
Bacterial	Folliculitis/furunculosis, bacterial granuloma, actinomycotic mycetoma
Fungal	Dermatophytosis (ringworm), *Candida*, eumycotic mycetoma
Miscellaneous	Trauma, foreign body reaction, psychogenic, immunodeficiency, sterile pyogranuloma
Neoplastic	Squamous-cell carcinoma, melanoma, mast-cell tumor, cysts
Parasitic	Demodicosis, *Pelodera*, hookworm, ticks

Treatment is aimed at the underlying cause. Most forms are amenable to therapy, but chronic deep interdigital pyoderma and immunodeficiencies often warrant a poor prognosis. In addition to antibiotics, surgical debridement often hastens recovery.

Periappendageal Dermatitis

Periappendageal dermatitis (sebaceous adenitis) is a description rather than a diagnosis and implies an inflammatory reaction centered on the follicular appendages. The term is superior to granulomatous sebaceous adenitis since the dermatitis is not always granulomatous and the sebaceous glands are not always involved. Sebaceous adenitis is a collection of disorders most often observed in Standard Poodles, though Samoyeds, Irish Setters and Collies have also been affected. These disorders are grouped collectively because of our current limited knowledge of their etiology.

Granulomatous sebaceous adenitis appears to be familial in Standard Poodles, but a mode of inheritance has not yet been elucidated. Destruction of the sebaceous glands by a pyogranulomatous infiltrate appears to lead to scaling and hair loss. Fibrosis eventually leads to areas devoid of sebaceous glands.

Clinical Signs

Most dogs are initially affected at 1-5 years of age. Symmetric nonpruritic scaling and hair loss begin on the dorsal midline and progress. Secondary bacterial infection is common and may cause pruritus.

Another type of periappendageal dermatitis is a nodular to plaque-like dermatitis of the head and face. This condition is seen most commonly in Golden and Yellow Labrador Retrievers. The clinical appearance and histopathologic characteristics are very different from the granulomatous type of adenitis.

Diagnosis

The diagnosis is based on the history, clinical signs and histopathologic examination of biopsies, which show orthokeratotic hyerperkeratosis (scale) and periappendageal inflammation. In the early stages, a granulomatous to pyogranulomatous to lymphoplasmacytoid inflammatory reaction is centered around the follicle and adnexa. Later, follicular and adnexal structures are absent and there is some perifollicular fibrosis.

Management

Treatment is only palliative, in that sebaceous glands do not regenerate. Early treatment with corticosteroids may halt progession of the disease. Later, frequent antiseborrheic shampooing and application of emollients may be beneficial. Treatment with isotretinoin (Accutane: Roche) at 1 mg/kg daily may also be beneficial but animals must be carefully monitored for adverse effects. This product is not licensed for use in dogs.

Additional Reading

1. Rosser, EJ et al: Sebaceous adenitis with hyperkeratosis in the Standard Poodle: a discussion of 10 cases. JAAHA 23:341-345, 1987.

2. Scott, DW: Granulomatous sebaceous adenitis in dogs. JAAHA 22:631-634, 1986.

3. Carpenter, JL et al: Idiopathic periadnexal multinodular granulomatous dermatitis in 22 dogs. Vet Pathol 24:5-10, 1987.

Sterile Eosinophilic Pustulosis

Clinical Signs

Sterile eosinophilic pustulosis is a rare pustular disease with no apparent age, breed or sex predilection. Primary skin lesions include papules and pustules and pruritus is moderate to severe. Scaling, crusting, hair loss and hyperpigmentation are common sequelae.

Diagnosis

Diagnosis is by biopsy and ruling out other potential causes of follicular and nonfollicular pustules. Skin scrapings, bacterial culture, fungal culture, intradermal allergy testing and direct immunofluorescence are invariably negative.

Biopsies reveal intraepidermal pustules and often associated folliculitis or furunculosis. Eosinophils are the predominating cell type involved.

Management

Treatment consists of antiinflammatory dosages of corticosteroids (prednisone at 0.5-2.0 mg/kg) daily or on alternate days, long-term. Relapses are common when therapy is discontinued.

Additional Reading

1. Scott, DW: Sterile eosinophilic pustulosis in dog and man: Comparative aspects. *J Am Acad Dermatol* 16:1022-1026, 1987.

2. Scott, DW: Sterile eosinophilic pustulosis in the dog. *JAAHA* 20:585-589, 1984.

Sterile Pyogranuloma

Sterile pyogranuloma is an uncommon nonbacterial cause of foot disorders (pododermatitis) in dogs. Great Danes, St. Bernards, Newfoundlands, Dachshunds and English Bulldogs appear to be predisposed.

Clinical Signs

The condition appears as firm red nodular lesions between the toes, indistinguishable from those of any of the other types of pododermatitis.

Diagnosis

The diagnosis is based on bacterial culture and sensitivity tests (negative or only contaminant growth) and histopathologic examination of biopsies.

Management

Therapy consists of either resection or treatment with antiinflammatory doses of corticosteroids, suggesting that the underlying problem is immune-mediated.

Subcorneal Pustular Dermatosis

Subcorneal pustular dermatosis is a rare, presumably immune-mediated skin disease. Though there is no apparent age or sex predilection, Miniature Schnauzers appear to be predisposed.

Clinical Signs

The condition appears as a generalized pustular dermatitis, most concentrated over the trunk and head (Fig 48). Since the pustules are extremely short-lived, only a rash or keratinization disorder (seborrhea) may be noted. The disease often waxes and wanes despite therapy with antibiotics and corticosteroids. The overall health of the animal is not compromised.

Diagnosis

The diagnosis is based on the clinical presentation, biopsies for histopathologic examination and direct immunofluorescence studies, and response to therapy. Though biopsies from affected dogs have not been positive with direct immunofluorescence, this may represent a limitation of the testing procedure.

Management

Therapy is often undertaken with dapsone at 1 mg/kg TID, then tapering the dosage, or with sulfasalazine (Azulfidine or Salazopyrin) at 10-20 mg/kg TID. Dogs must be monitored during treatment, since these drugs may cause side effects (keratoconjunctivitis sicca, hemorrhagic diathesis, liver toxicity).

Additional Reading

1. McKeever, PJ and Dahl, MV: A disease in dogs resembling human subcorneal pustular dermatosis. *JAVMA* 170:704-707, 1977.

Toxic Epidermal Necrolysis

Clinical Signs

Toxic epidermal necrolysis is a life-threatening disease involving the mucosal and skin surfaces. In affected people, drugs and other chemicals usually initiate the condition, though infections may also be responsible. The disease is characterized by cutaneous pain, erythema and ulceration. A positive Nikolsky sign may also be evident. This consists of separation of the dermis and epidermis when the skin is stretched. It is commonly present in dogs with pemphigus but may also be present with toxic epidermal necrolysis.

Diagnosis

The diagnosis is based on the history, clinical appearance and characteristic histopathologic findings on biopsies.

Management

Treatment is aimed at eliminating the underlying chemical or microbial cause, with supportive care (corticosteroids, IV fluids) as needed.

Additional Reading

1. Daniel, GB and Patterson, JS: Toxic epidermal necrolysis: a case report. *JAAHA* 21:631-635, 1985.

2. Merot, Y and Saurat, JH: Clues to pathogenesis of toxic epidermal necrolysis. *Intl J Dermatol* 24:165-168, 1985.

Tumoral Calcinosis

Tumoral calcinosis or calcinosis circumscripta is a condition involving dystrophic calcification not associated with systemic disorders of calcium metabolism or renal disease. A plausible pathomechanism is not known, but further studies of affected animals are needed to elucidate calcium, phosphorus, parathormone and vitamin D abnormalities or genetic factors that might contribute to the problem.

Clinical Signs

The condition occurs predominantly in young, large-breed dogs and the German Shepherd appears to be predisposed. Clinically, lesions consist of one or more well circumscribed, nonpainful, subcutaneous, nodular swellings that may ulcerate and even discharge a white pasty material. Most lesions occur in the periarticular regions of the distal extremities but may occur in the cervical region, footpads and even the oral cavity.

Diagnosis

Diagnosis may be suspected on the basis of clinical signs and radiography but can only be confirmed by biopsy. Histopathologic examination usually reveals nodular to diffuse dermatitis and panniculitis, in which occurs dystrophic mineralization. Metabolic profiles, including calcium, phosphorus, their fractional urinary clearances and parathormone, might be helpful, though trends have not yet been established. It is also important to distinguish this condition from dystrophic mineralization due to hyperadrenocorticism, collagenolytic granuloma and calcifying tumors. In addition, calcinosis cutis has been associated with percutaneous absorption of calcium salts into dermal tissue.

Management

Treatment involves complete excision. This will likely remain the only mode of treatment until a plausible pathomechanism is proposed.

Chapter 10

Additional Reading

1. Roudebush, P *et al:* Canine tumoral calcinosis. *Comp Cont Ed Pract Vet* 10:1162-1164, 1988.

2. Legendre, AM and Dade, AW: Calcinosis circumscripta in a dog. *JAVMA* 164:1192-1194, 1974.

3. Paradis, M and Scott, DW: Calcinosis cutis secondary to percutaneous penetration of calcium carbonate in a Dalmatian. *Can Vet J* 30:57-59, 1989.

4. Scott, DW and Buerger, RG: Idiopathic calcinosis circumscripta in the dog: A retrospective analysis of 130 cases. *JAAHA* 24:651-658, 1988.

Appendix 1
Systemic Therapy

Antiparasitics

Pyrethrins

Pyrethrins are natural insecticides derived from certain species of chrysanthemums. They are a rapid-acting, so-called "quick-kill" insecticide with very little toxicity to mammals. Their effects are often potentiated by synergists, such as piperonyl butoxide and n-octyl bicycloheptene dicarboxamide, which are not themselves insecticides but enhance the killing ability of the pyrethrins for fleas and ticks.

Though they are relatively safe, pyrethrins are degraded rapidly in the environment, especially in sunlight, and therefore give very little residual effect. This disadvantage has been somewhat overcome by microencapsulation of the product (*eg,* Sectrol: 3M), which allows for slow release of the pyrethrins. This not only increases the residual effect of the insecticide but also further reduces its toxicity. In microencapsulated form, however, small beads of insecticide persist in the environment. Vacuuming must be temporarily halted after application or the insecticide will be removed and will have no residual effect. Synthetic pyrethrins or pyrethroids (*eg,* resmethrin, allethrin, d-trans allethrin, fenvalerate, d-phenothrin, tetramethrin) often have stronger insecticidal ability and a slightly more residual action than the natural pyrethrins.

Carbamates

Carbamates are derivatives of carbamic acid and kill moderately quickly, as compared to pyrethrins. They have good residual effect. Some important carbamates include carbaryl, bendiocarb and propoxur. Toxicity varies considerably among products. Compounds are also available to treat the outdoor environment, since the products are not rapidly broken down by sunlight (*eg,* Sevin: Carson). Carbamates are toxic by virtue of their ability to block the enzyme acetylcholinesterase, which is important in nerve impulse transmission. This feature is shared with organophosphate insecticides. Signs of carbamate toxicity in an animal (pinpoint pupils, vomiting, diarrhea, seizures) should be treated as an emergency. Carbamate products generally are safe if used exactly as recommended by the manufacturer.

Organophosphates

Organophosphates originated as nerve gas in World War II and are considered to be one of the most toxic insecticides to mammals. Their residual activity varies with the chemical structure from slight to very persistent. Important organophosphates include chlorfenvinphos, chlorpyrifos (dursban), cythioate, diazinon, dichlorvos, dioxathion, fenthion, malathion, propetamphos, temephos, tetrachorvinphos and phosmet.

Commercially available organophosphates may be given PO, such as cythionate (Proban:Haver) at 3.3 mg/kg every 3 days. Others are dabbed on the skin, such as fenthion (Prospot: Haver), sprayed into the environment, such as dursban (Duratrol: 3M) or diazinon (Diazotrol: Rogar/STB), used as a topical dip, such as phosmet (Paramite: Vet-Kem), or allowed to vaporize in a room, such as dichlorvos (Vapona: Shell). Some organophosphates are microencapsulated (Duratrol: 3M) to help decrease toxicity while increasing residual action.

Malathion is an organophosphate with fairly low toxicity but also only fair residual activity.

Like the carbamates, organophosphates block the enzyme acetylcholinesterase and can result in toxicities if not carefully handled.

Sometimes products intended for large animal use, such as fenthion (Spotton: Haver), trichlorfon (Neguvon: Haver) or fenchlorphosronnel (Ectoral), are used for troublesome parasitisms in dogs. It must be appreciated, however, that they are not licensed for this use and are to be administered with caution in all instances. Fenthion (Spotton) is commonly used for treatment of flea-bite hypersensitivity in dogs despite its lack of licensure and the fact that an approved small animal formulation of fenthion is available (Prospot: Haver) though not as effective. Fenthion 20% is applied at a rate of 1 ml/10 kg body weight directly to the skin on the dorsal midline every 2-4 weeks as necessary. Fenthion significantly depresses serum cholinesterases but reactivation is substantial by 2 weeks. Persons applying the product should wear gloves. Veterinarians must caution owners about contact with their organophosphate-coated pet, advise them not to be in a confined poorly ventilated space (*eg,* car with windows rolled up) with their pet, and notify them that the product is not licensed for use in this manner. I routinely have owners sign a release form whenever using unlicensed products.

Chlorinated Hydrocarbons

Chlorinated hydrocarbons represented the first attempt at synthetic pesticides. Because of their extremely residual nature in the environment and their carcinogenicity, they have all but disappeared commercially. They are especially toxic to cats. Some chlorinated hydrocarbons still marketed include lindane and methoxychlor.

Insect Growth Regulators

Insect growth regulators are not insecticides but rather hormone-like compounds that prevent flea larvae from developing into adults. Methoprene (Precor: Zoecon) appears to be safest for indoor use but is of no benefit when applied to animals or outdoors because it is rapidly inactivated by sunlight. Indoors, however, it is very residual and persists for 75-90 days. Because it is not an insecticide, there are few concerns about toxicity. The drawback is that since the product is not an insecticide, it does not kill adult fleas but only prevents adults from developing from eggs and larvae already in the environment. Because of this, new products (*eg,* Siphotrol Plus: Vet-Kem) combine the residual effect of methoprene with the adult flea-killing ability of such insecticides as pyrethrins. A new topical methoprene (Ovitrol: Vet-Kem) is claimed to inhibit hatching of flea eggs even after the eggs fall off the pet into the environment.

Natural Insecticides

Natural products have been used in flea control. Rotenone, derived from the derris root, is a safe and fairly effective product used not only for flea control but also for control of ticks and some species of mites and lice. It is uncommonly used in commercial preparations today, since more potent (and more toxic) chemical insecticides have become available.

Lime sulfur is marketed as a fungus-killing orchard spray, and is a safe and effective treatment for some forms of mange. It is used as a 2.5% solution.

A product derived from citrus pulp, d-limonene, has been marketed for flea control. Though one would expect it to be remarkably safe, it has been implicated in some cat deaths.

Brewers' yeast and garlic have been regarded by breeders for years to be good flea deterrents, but clinical trials have shown no such merit. An Avon product, Skin-So-Soft, in a diluted form (5%) was found by researchers at the University of Florida to offer some flea repellent activity.

Ivermectin

Ivermectin, a derivative of a soil organism, is effective in treatment of many internal and external parasites. It paralyzes nematodes and arthropods by its stimulatory effect on the neurotransmitter gamma-aminobutyric acid (GABA). Unfortunately, it has little effect on fleas or demodectic mange mites but is quite effective against *Cheyletiella*, *Sarcoptes* and *Otodectes* (ear) mites, usually at 0.2 mg/kg PO or SC.

Currently ivermectin is not licensed for use in dogs (in forms other than a heartworm preventive) and cats, and any use in these species is at the risk of both the veterinarian and pet owner. It has, however, been found to be quite safe except in the Collie (and perhaps Shetland Sheepdog?) and their crosses, in which it appears to be profoundly or even fatally toxic. Dosages of 0.05 mg/kg and less are unlikely to be toxic for these breeds but still cannot be recommended.

In many parts of the world, ivermectin is used as a heartworm preventive and microfilaricide. A new oral formulation of ivermectin (Heartgard: MSD Agvet) is given monthly PO at 0.006 mg/kg for heartworm prevention. Unapproved forms of ivermectin (Ivomec: MSD Agvet) have been used as a microfilaricide; 1 ml was diluted in 9 ml propylene glycol and given PO at 1 ml/20 kg (0.05 mg/kg) every other month, or alternatively at 0.02 mg/kg monthly PO. The microfilaricidal dosage of 0.05 mg/kg is also effective against hookworms, while higher dosages (0.2 mg/kg) are also effective against whipworms.

Amitraz

Amitraz (Mitaban: Upjohn) is an antiparasitic dip marketed for treatment of generalized demodectic mange. It is fairly safe but must be applied exactly as recommended by the manufacturer. Many veterinary dermatologists have found that the dosage often must be increased (doubled) or the treatment interval shortened (halved) to eradicate the mites in problem cases. This, however, is considered extralabel use and is at the veterinarian's and owner's risk, since it is not according to the manufacturer's recommendations. Since it first appeared in the marketplace with almost miraculous claims, amitraz has now been accepted in the veterinary community as a useful product but not one that effects cures in all cases. The product has also been used successfully in treatment of sarcoptic mange. Side effects are rare but may include sedation, bradycardia, hypotension, hypothermia, bloat, polyuria, vomiting and hyperglycemia.

Protocol for Use of Amitraz

1. Clip the hair as much as possible to facilitate penetration of the drug.

2. Use an antiseborrheic shampoo to remove crust and scales first. This should preferably be done the night before the dip.

3. Empty the contents of a Mitaban vial into 9 L (2 gal) of water. This amount may need to be doubled for very large or chronically affected dogs.

4. Slowly sponge on the entire amount of solution prepared, concentrating on problem areas.

5. Allow the animal to air dry; do not rinse or blow dry.

6. Do not allow the animal to get wet between treatments, or the dip must be repeated.

7. Repeat every 2 weeks (perhaps weekly) until the condition has been adequately controlled. Treated dog should not be stressed during the 24 hours following dipping.

8. Obtain skin scrapings before each dip. When scrapings are negative on 2 successive occasions, no further treatment is indicated.

9. For demodectic pododermatitis, mix 0.5 ml of Mitaban in 30 ml of mineral oil and apply every 3-4 days.

10. Outdated or opened bottles of Mitaban should not be used in treatment, since the breakdown products are more toxic than the Mitaban itself.

Additional Reading

1. Bennett, DG: Clinical pharmacology of ivermectin. *JAVMA* 189:100-104, 1986.

2. Pulliam, JD *et al:* Investigating ivermectin toxicity in Collies. *Vet Med* 80(6):33-40, 1985.

3. Calvert, CA: Ivermectin for treatment of internal parasitism and heartworms in dogs. *MVP* 66:307-308, 1985.

4. Folz, SD *et al*: Clinical evaluation of amitraz for treatment of canine scabies. *MVP* 65:597-600, 1984.

5. Hsu, WH and Schaffer, DD: Effects of topical application of amitraz on plasma glucose and insulin concentrations in dogs. *Am J Vet Res* 49:130-131, 1988.

6. Mason, KV *et al*: Fenthion for flea control on dogs under field conditions: Dose response efficacy studies and effect on cholinesterase activity. *JAAHA* 20:591-595, 1984.

7. Houston, DM *et al*: Ivermectin toxicosis in a dog. *JAVMA* 191:78-80, 1987.

8. Paul, AJ *et al*: Clinical observations in Collies given ivermectin orally. *Am J Vet Res* 48:684-685, 1987.

9. Garg, RC and Donahue, WA: Pharmacologic profile of methoprene, an insect growth regulator, in cattle, dogs, and cats. *JAVMA* 194:410-412, 1989.

10. Hsu, WH *et al:* The safety of ivermectin. *Comp Cont Ed Pract Vet* 11:584-588, 1989.

11. Dorman, DC: Pyrethrin poisoning in dogs and cats. *Compan Anim Pract* 2(8):12-13, 1988.

Antimicrobials

Antimicrobials are chemicals that exert a harmful effect on certain microorganisms. They may be of natural, semisynthetic or synthetic origin. Some antimicrobials are bactericidal (destroy bacteria), others are bacteriostatic (inhibit growth of bacteria) and some may be either, depending upon their concentration.

Beta-Lactam Antibiotics

The beta-lactam group of antibiotics includes penicillins and cephalosporins, important compounds not only in veterinary medicine but in human medicine as well. Clavulanic acid also belongs to this group and acts by inhibiting a group of enzymes (beta-lactamases) that would normally break down the active structure of the beta-lactam antibiotics. Thus, when antibiotics normally destroyed by beta-lactamases (produced by resistant bacteria) are combined with clavulanic acid, the antibiotic is protected from inactivation. Clavulanic acid is combined with amoxicillin in the human product Clavulin (Augmentin in the United States), marketed as Clavamox for animals and recently in combination form with ticarcillin (Ticillin: Beecham).

Penicillins and cephalosporins act by inhibiting formation of the cell wall in susceptible bacteria. When the integrity of the cell wall is compromised, the bacteria cannot survive and reproduce. This effect is termed bactericidal. Since *Staphylococcus intermedius*, the most common bacterium implicated in canine skin infections, is a frequent producer of beta-lactamases, many of the more basic penicillins (*eg,* ampicillin, amoxicillin, penicillin G) are quickly inactivated and unlikely to benefit the animal. Beta-lactamase-resistant penicillins, such as cloxacillin, oxacillin, dicloxacillin, flucloxacillin as well as amoxicillin or ticarcillin combined with clavulanic acid, are useful in cutaneous bacterial infections, as are the cephalosporins, such as cephalexin, cefadroxil and cephradine. New generations of cephalosporins and penicillins are constantly being formulated as organisms become resistant to existing varieties. Since these products are very important in human medicine, they should only be used when absolutely necessary in animals, since indiscriminate use will result in increased bacterial resistance. As with other forms of medication, beta-lactam antibiotics may cause toxicity and hypersensitivity reactions (*eg,* drug eruption, allergy).

Aminoglycosides

Aminocyclitol antibiotics, or aminoglycosides, comprise a large number of antibiotics, including streptomycin, gentamicin, neomycin, kanamycin, amikacin, tobramycin and spectinomycin. They are bactericidal by virtue of their ability to inhibit formation of proteins within bacteria. Spectinomycin acts by a different mechanism and is bacteriostatic (slows bacterial growth). Aminocyclitol antibiotics are ototoxic and nephrotoxic. Since skin diseases often require antibiotic therapy for weeks or months, these products are poor choices despite their excellent efficacy. These antibiotics are therefore usually prescribed only for dermatologic use in the form of topical solutions applied to the surface of the skin, where the risk of toxic side effects is greatly reduced.

Trimethoprim-Sulfas

Combinations of trimethoprim and sulfonamides (such as sulfamethoxazole or sulfadiazine) are bactericidal by virtue of their ability to block formation of an essential compound, folic acid, within bacteria. In combination, the products are much more effective than individually. This "synergism" means that each potentiates the effects of the other. In combination, the risk of bacterial resistance decreases. Side effects are few but include a slight risk of decreased tear production (keratoconjunctivitis sicca) and a lupus erythematosus-like syndrome in Doberman Pinschers. Whether this is a breed-related susceptibility to sulfa drugs has not been determined, but to be on the safe side it is best to avoid use of this product in Dobermans if another product will suffice.

Macrolides and Lincosamides

Macrolides, such as erythromycin, and lincosamides, such as lincomycin and clindamycin, are bacteriostatic antibiotics that inhibit formation of proteins in bacteria. They are effective in about 75% of cutaneous bacterial infections in dogs. With the wide exposure these drugs have, resistance is becoming more common. Though they do not function in exactly the same manner, it appears that animals resistant to erythromycin show cross-resistance for lincomycin and *vice versa*. The only real side effect is GI problems, such as vomiting and diarrhea with erythromycin but rarely with lincomycin. In people and in horses, lincomycin is rarely used because of its profound damaging effect on the colon; however, dogs do not appear to be affected this way. Lincomycin is currently the most commonly prescribed antibiotic for use in treating skin infections in dogs. Clindamycin (Antirobe: Upjohn) is used to treat abscesses or deep, infected wounds.

Chloramphenicol

Chloramphenicol is a bacteriostatic antibiotic that inhibits formation of proteins within bacteria. The antibiotic has been useful because of its activity against many different bacteria, its ability to penetrate tissues well and its infrequent toxic effects. Chloramphenicol is usually successful in treatment of simple bacterial infections, but creation of resistant organisms poses an ever-increasing problem.

Fluoroquinolones

Fluoroquinolones are bactericidal antimicrobials related structurally to nalidixic acid and inhibit the A subunit DNA gyrase, which appears to be essential for DNA replication. Fluoroquinolones, such as enrofloxacin (*eg,* Baytril: Haver), quickly reach serum levels and kill bacteria rapidly. They are partially metabolized in the liver and excreted in urine and bile at high concentrations of active drug. Fluoroquinolones have an excellent spectrum of activity but reach lower levels in the skin and subcutis than they do in most other tissues. Major trials have not yet been conducted to clearly define their applicability to cutaneous bacterial infections though they have excellent antibacterial activity *in vitro.* Use may be contraindicated during periods of active growth, as fluoroquinolones may cause lesions of the articular cartilage.

Rifampin

Rifampin, a semisynthetic hydrazine derivative of rifamycin B, is a macrocytic compound with a broad spectrum of antimicrobial activity mediated by selective inhibition of DNA-dependent RNA polymerase in bacterial mitochondria. Rifampin penetrates septic foci, granulomas and abscesses well and can enter phagocytic cells and kill intracellular bacteria. Because of the rapid onset of bacterial resistance, rifampin is usually used in combination with another bactericidal antibiotic, such as a potentiated penicillin or cephalosporin. Rifampin is probably the most potent antibiotic available for staphylococci but should not be used indiscriminantly. Indications for use of rifampin include bacterial granuloma (botryomycosis) and chronic deep-seated abscesses.

Table 1 lists the major families of antimicrobials used in treating skin diseases, some individual generic antimicrobials, and some common trade names. Table 2 lists some dosages. This is not a comprehensive listing of all antimicrobials available, nor an endorsement of those mentioned. Some antimicrobials, such as ampicillin, amoxicillin and tetracycline, have poor therapeutic value in treatment of skin infections, while others, such as gentamicin and kanamycin, are too toxic to be used for the long periods required for skin infections.

Appendix 1

Table 1. Antimicrobials used in skin disease.

Family	Generic Name	Example
Cephalosporins	Cefadroxil	Cefa-Tabs
	Cephalexin	Keflex
	Cephalothin	Keflin
	Cephradine	Velosef
Chloramphenicol	Chloramphenicol	Rogar-Mycine
Fluoroquinolones	Ciprofloxacin	Cipro
	Enrofloxacin	Baytril
	Norfloxacin	Noroxin
Lincosamides	Clindamycin	Antirobe
	Lincomycin	Lincocin
Macrolides	Erythromycin	E-Mycin
Penicillins	Amoxicillin-clavulanate	Clavulin, Clavamox
	Carbenicillin	Geopen
	Cloxacillin	Orbenin, Tegopen
	Dicloxacillin	Dynapen
	Oxacillin	Prostaphlin
Trimethoprim-sulfas	Trimethoprim-sulfadiazine	Tribrissen
	Trimethoprim-sulfamethoxazole	Septra, Apo-Sulfatrim

Table 2. Antimicrobial drug dosages.

Antimicrobial	Action	Dosage
Amoxicillin-clavulanate	Bactericidal	12-14 mg/kg BID
Cephalexin	Bactericidal	30 mg/kg BID
Chloramphenicol	Bacteriostatic	50 mg/kg TID
Ciprofloxacin	Bactericidal	11-22 mg/kg BID
Cloxacillin	Bactericidal	15 mg/kg TID
Enrofloxacin	Bactericidal	2.5 mg/kg BID
Erythromycin	Bacteriostatic	15 mg/kg TID
Flucloxacillin	Bactericidal	15 mg/kg TID
Lincomycin	Bacteriostatic	20 mg/kg BID
Norfloxacin	Bactericidal	22 mg/kg BID
Oxacillin	Bactericidal	15 mg/kg TID
Trimethoprim-sulfa	Bactericidal	30 mg/kg BID

Additional Reading

1. Ihrke, PJ: Therapeutic strategies involving antimicrobial treatment of the skin in small animals. *JAVMA* 185:1165-1168, 1984.

2. Riviere, JE: Calculation of dosage regimens of antimicrobial drugs in animals with renal and hepatic dysfunction. *JAVMA* 185:1094-1097, 1984.

3. Powers, TE and Garg, RC: Pharmacotherapeutics of newer penicillins and cephalosporins. *JAVMA* 176:1054-1060, 1980.

4. Burrows, GE: Aminocyclitol antibiotics. *JAVMA* 176:1280-1281, 1980.

5. Bushby, SRM: Sulfonamide and trimethoprim combinations. *JAVMA* 176:1049-1053, 1980.

6. Burrows, GE: Pharmacotherapeutics of macrolides, lincomycins, and spectinomycin. *JAVMA* 176:1072-1077, 1980.

7. Sisodia, CS: Pharmacotherapeutics of chloramphenicol in veterinary medicine. *JAVMA* 176:1069-1071, 1980.

8. Neer, TM: Clinical pharmacologic features of fluoroquinolone antimicrobial drugs. *JAVMA* 193: 577-580, 1988.

9. Wilcke, JR: Therapeutic application of sulfadiazine/trimethoprim in dogs and cats: A review. *Compan Anim Pract* 2(4):3-8, 1988.

10. Angarano, DW: Efficacy of cefadroxil in the treatment of bacterial dermatitis in dogs. *JAVMA* 194:57-59, 1989.

Antifungals

Topical antifungal therapy is useful if not too many areas of the animal are involved. Good products for "spot" treatment include miconazole (Conofite), naftifine hydrochloride (Naftin) and clotrimazole (Canesten). Nystatin (included in such products as Panolog) is not effective against ringworm fungi. Other products with at least some antifungal properties include chlorhexidine, povidone-iodine and thiabendazole (included in Tresaderm). Tolnaftate (Tinavet) is ineffective on haired skin and is thus a poor choice for any topical antifungal therapy on animals. A more comprehensive listing may be found in Chapter 3 and Appendix 2.

Captan

Captan and lime sulfur are products marketed to control garden fungi, and are safe and effective antifungal topical preparations for use on animals. Captan is relatively nontoxic to dogs but is a potent contact sensitizer to people; therefore, gloves should be worn by people applying the solution. A 0.25% solution can be formulated by adding 2 tbsp of the 50% powder to 1 gal of water, or adding 1 tsp of technical captan (45%) to 1 L of water. Dogs should be dipped once or twice a week until clinical improvement is seen and then for a few more treatments to ensure that all the fungi have been eradicated.

Lime Sulfur

Lime sulfur is marketed as an orchard spray. When diluted to a 2.5% solution, it also makes a useful dip to control ringworm fungi. This dilution can be obtained by adding 100 ml of the lime sulfur 29% concentrate to 1 L of water. Though lime sulfur is exceptionally safe, it has a markedly disagreeable odor and may stain white haircoats. The odor has been partially masked in the commercial product LymDip (DVM).

Griseofulvin

Griseofulvin (Fulvicin) is an antifungal used in treatment of ringworm (dermatophytosis). It may be overprescribed, since most cases of ringworm clear spontaneously within a few months with topical treatment only or even in spite of it. Griseofulvin may be given as a microsized (50-150 mg/kg) or ultramicrosized (25-75 mg/kg) preparation once daily with a fat meal or some corn oil for usually 6 weeks, but at least until 2 weeks beyond apparent clinical cure. The drug has an unpleasant taste and may cause vomiting. The product should never be given to pregnant animals, since it can cause birth defects.

Amphotericin B

Amphotericin B (Fungizone) is fungistatic and is the standard treatment for systemic mycoses against which all the newer antifungal agents are judged. The major side effects are nephrotoxicity, anemia and hypokalemia. The drug must be given IV and patients should be monitored weekly or biweekly to evaluate blood counts, liver and kidney function, urinalyses, and electrolytes (especially potassium). The material is extremely irritating and if injected perivascularly can cause phlebitis. Treatment is often lengthy (months) and must continue for 4 weeks beyond clinical cure. The suggested dosage is 0.15-0.25 mg/kg IV in 10 ml 5% dextrose given over a 5-minute period 3 times weekly and continued for 4 weeks beyond clinical cure. Compared with rapid bolus administration, slow infusion of amphotericin B with supplemental fluids causes less functional impairment, less severe systemic signs and less renal damage.

Flucytosine

Flucytosine (Ancobon: Ancotil) is an oral antifungal with activity against cryptococcosis and candidiasis. It is less toxic than amphotericin B but still has some mild adverse effects on the liver, bone marrow and GI tract. The main limiting feature is rapid development of fungal resistance, sometimes in as little as 3 weeks. Some of these problems can be offset by using a combination of flucytosine and amphotericin B in lesser doses. Blood counts as well as kidney and liver function tests should be performed about every 2 weeks. Though the drug is not toxic to the kidneys, it is excreted by them and the dose should thus be adjusted accordingly in patients with kidney disease. It is used PO at 60 mg/kg TID.

Ketoconazole

Ketoconazole (Nizoral) is an oral broad-spectrum antifungal, effective against dermatophytes (ringworm), *Candida* and systemic mycoses. Therapeutic levels of ketoconazole are reached in all body tissues except the brain, testes and eyes. At the dosages reported (5-15 mg/kg BID), ketoconazole is considered almost nontoxic, though activity of liver-specific enzymes may become slightly elevated. Coat color change may become evident in dogs following prolonged administration. The drug is excreted via the bile into the digestive tract and exits the body in the stool. Combinations of ketoconazole and amphotericin B may be advantageous in certain resistant fungal infections.

Itraconazole

Itraconazole is a new triazole with activity against blastomycosis, sporotrichosis, cryptococcosis and perhaps eumycotic mycetoma. It is better tolerated than ketoconazole in most patients and a preliminary dosage of 10 mg/kg/day is proposed. Itraconazole is better absorbed with food and does not suppress testosterone or cortisol synthesis as does ketoconazole. Like ketoconazole, the drug is teratogenic and should not be given to pregnant animals.

Garlic

A report from China documented use of garlic, by oral, IM or IV administration, in treatment of cryptococcosis in 21 people. They found it to be clinically effective and seemingly superior to amphotericin B. Side effects were minimal but included headache, vomiting and mild neurologic signs. North American studies have not yet been undertaken to compare results.

Additional Reading

1. Pyle, RL: Clinical pharmacology of amphotericin B. *JAVMA* 179:83-84, 1981.

2. Moriello, KA: Ketoconazole: Clinical pharmacology and therapeutic recommendations. *JAVMA* 188:303-306, 1986.

3. Hunan Medical College: Garlic in cryptococcal meningitis. *Chinese Med J* 93:123-126, 1980.

4. Rubin, SI *et al:* Nephrotoxicity of amphotericin B in dogs. A comparison of two methods of administration. *Can Vet J* 53:23-28, 1989.

Immunostimulants

Immunostimulants are a relatively recent addition to the drugs used by veterinarians. Their intention is to bolster a faltering immune system so that the animal mounts its own natural assault on the disease process. How immunostimulants work and their actual efficacy is still a matter of controversy. To benefit from an immunostimulant, an animal must already have a functional immune system. An animal with an impaired immune function likely will not respond. The most common immunostimulants are bacterial cell-wall products or compounds that exert some stimulatory effect as an adjunct to their primary function.

Bacterins

Toxoids are toxins treated in such a way that their poisonous properties have been modified without destroying their ability to stimulate formation of antibodies. The basic toxoid is prepared by growing the toxin-producing organism, filtering off the organisms and treating the filtrate with formaldehyde. These products are used in canine dermatology as general immunostimulants when the defective immune system needs bolstering to overcome disease. Such products as Staphoid-AB (Wellcome), Staphage Lysate (Delmont) and Lysigen (Boeringer Ingelheim) are derived from staphylococci and used in the hopes of stimulating the immune system to functional levels. Staphoid-AB is a staphylococcal cell-wall antigen and toxin mixture. Staphage

Table 3. Staphoid A-B dosage schedule (dilute 50:50 with saline).

Day	Intradermal Dose	Subcutaneous Dose	Total Dose
1	0.1 ml	0.15 ml	0.25 ml
2	0.1 ml	0.40 ml	0.50 ml
3	0.1 ml	0.65 ml	0.75 ml
4	0.1 ml	0.90 ml	1.00 ml
5	0.1 ml	1.15 ml	1.25 ml
12	0.1 ml	1.40 ml	1.50 ml
19	0.1 ml	1.65 ml	1.75 ml
26	0.1 ml	1.90 ml	2.00 ml
Monthly	0.1 ml	1.90 ml	2.00 ml

Table 4. Staphage Lysate dosage schedule.

Week	Dose for Superficial Pyoderma	Dose for Deep Pyoderma
1	0.1 ml SC	0.25 ml SC
2	0.2 ml SC	0.50 ml SC
3	0.3 ml SC	0.75 ml SC
4	0.5 ml SC	1.00 ml SC
Weekly	0.5 ml SC	1-2 ml SC

Lysate is produced by lysing cultures of *Staphylococcus aureus* with a *Staphylococcus* bacteriophage. After ultrafiltration the lysate contains both antigenic fractions of the bacteria and the active bacteriophage. Tables 3 and 4 are some suggested guidelines for use of these products. Presumably these products may act by either nonspecific immunostimulation or specific staphylococcal hyposensitization. In any case, protein A is likely the therapeutic component of these products.

A relatively new product (ImmunoRegulin: Immunovet) is derived from the bacterium *Propionibacterium acnes*, with claims of immunostimulation, activating macrophages, increasing proliferation of lymphoblasts, and stimulating resistance to bacterial infections. The manufacturer claims an 81% cure or control rate in dogs with chronic or recurrent pyoderma based on uncon-

Table 5. Dosage schedule for ImmunoRegulin administration.

Weight	Dose
<15 lb (<7 kg)	0.25 ml
15-45 lb (7-20 kg)	0.50 ml
46-75 lb (21-34 kg)	1.00 ml
>75 lb (>34 kg)	2.00 ml

trolled field trials, but no convincing studies have demonstrated the effectiveness of this product.

The therapeutic effect of ImmunoRegulin may be compromised if the drug is used in conjunction with large doses of glucocorticoids. The product should be used with caution in animals with any suspected cardiac condition. ImmunoRegulin should be given IV or IP (Table 5). Such adverse reactions as transient fever, chills and lethargy are infrequent, according to the manufacturer. It should be given twice per week for 1-2 weeks, followed by 1 injection per week until signs abate or stabilize.

A new product currently under investigation is Stimune S/A (Vetrepharm), a mycobacterial cell-wall extract similar to Equimune, marketed by the same pharmaceutical company. The product should be administered in a single IM dose as an immunostimulant. On an experimental basis, the dosage on the package insert is as follows:

Weight	Volume
<17 lb (<8 kg)	0.25 ml
17-33 lb (8-15 kg)	0.50 ml
34-88 lb (16-40 kg)	0.75 ml
>88 lb (>40 kg)	1.00 ml

Concrete data on efficacy are currently unavailable.

Levamisole

Levamisole, marketed as an anthelmintic for large animals, also potentiates the immune system in carefully regulated dosages of 2.2 mg/kg 3 times weekly. It is important to note that larger or smaller doses may actually suppress the immune response. The product reportedly causes a number of possible side effects in dogs, including depression, inappetence, GI disturbances, ataxia, cutaneous eruptions, hepatic degeneration, hemolytic anemia, cardiac arrhythmias, respiratory distress and convulsions due to its nicotine-like action. There is no specific antidote for levamisole toxicosis, but drugs of potential benefit include alpha-adrenergic, nicotinic and cholinergic receptor antagonists.

Cimetidine

Cimetidine has been used with some success as an immunostimulant. A dosage of 5 mg/kg has been suggested, but there are few controlled studies to document this. Cimetidine should not be used with other monoamine oxidase inhibitors, such as amitraz (Mitaban), which limit its usefulness in treatment of generalized demodicosis.

Thymus Gland Extracts

Another product currently under investigation in my office is a thymus gland extract (available from NutriSpecialties) derived from Australian lamb and combined with a variety of nutrients important to immune regulation, such as dimethyl glycine, zinc, and vitamins A and C. It contains no added synthetic growth hormones, drugs or toxic pesticides, and produces no known allergic reactions. The rationale for its use is that the thymus gland is the "master gland" of the immune system, producing several important hormones, including thymopoietin, thymosin and serum thymic factor. It aids in control of autoimmune and infectious diseases, and is the site of T-cell differentiation. The specific interrelationships between observed immune defects in animals and thymus gland function are potentially complex and poorly documented. Too few treated dogs have been evaluated to comment on the efficacy of this product, though it appears to have some merit.

Additional Reading

1. Degen, MA and Breitschwerdt, EB: Canine and feline immunodeficiency-Part I. *Comp Cont Ed Pract Vet* 8:313-323, 1986.

2. Degen, MA and Breitschwerdt, EB: Canine and feline immunodeficiency-Part II. *Comp Cont Ed Pract Vet* 8:379-386, 1986.

3. Pilarczyk, JP: Use of *Staphylococcus* lysate in treating bacterial hypersensitivity. *Canine Pract* 8(1):38-40, 1981.

4. Brunner, CJ and Muscoplat, CC: Immunomodulatory effects of levamisole. *JAVMA* 176:1159-1162, 1980.

5. Montgomery, RD and Pidgeon, GL: Levamisole toxicosis in a dog. *JAVMA* 189:684-685, 1986.

6. Pukay, BP: Treatment of canine bacterial hypersensitivity by hyposensitization with *Staphylococcus aureus* bacterin-toxoid. *JAAHA* 21:479-483, 1985.

7. Kent, S: Rejuvenating the immune system. *Geriatrics* 36(12):13-16, 1981.

Corticosteroids

Corticosteroids are cortisone-like products that have a profound effect on most tissues in the body. In a normal dog, cortisol is produced in the equivalent of a daily dosage of prednisone at 0.2 mg/kg or hydrocortisone at 1.0 mg/kg. When greater than physiologic doses of corticosteroids are given over a long period, the adrenal glands may atrophy and become incapable of responding to the body's need for cortisol production.

In the meantime, all of the other tissues of the body are subjected to the abnormally high levels of exogenous corticosteroids. This usually is first manifested by increased thirst (polydipsia), urination (polyuria) and hunger (polyphagia). Long-term corticosteroid use may result in diabetes mellitus, since corticosteroids are antagonistic to the effects of insulin. Additionally, corticosteroids promote gluconeogenesis and deposition of glycogen in the liver. Corticosteroids also lead to decreased resistance to infection. Thyroid and growth hormone levels may decrease, as well as the threshold for seizure activity. Finally, fluids may be retained and fat deposited in the liver. Muscle wasting is usually associated with gluconeogenesis. Acute pancreatitis has also been reported as a sequel to corticosteroid administration. Chronic elevation of corticosteroid levels results in iatrogenic hyperadrenocorticism (Cushing's disease). Because of all of these potential side effects, corticosteroids should be cautiously used, especially in the following situations: diabetes mellitus, pregnancy, young animals, epilepsy, heart or kidney disease, infectious diseases, osteoporosis and GI ulcers.

Why, then, are corticosteroids so commonly prescribed? In antiinflammatory doses, corticosteroids effectively suppress most forms of inflammation, from the pruritus of allergies to the joint pain of arthritis. In the proper hands and with the proper respect, corticosteroids are an important tool in management of many dermatologic conditions. In immunosuppressive doses, side effects are unavoidable but relatively acceptable, since the conditions being treated are often life-threatening or debilitating. Before the introduction of corticosteroids, many autoimmune disorders proved fatal. It now appears that the eventual death of many patients is directly attributable to the side effects of treatment, most notably susceptibility to infection. There is thus an important give-and-take situation if corticosteroids are to be used in therapy.

Corticosteroids are usually given in the form of a free base or as esters of acetate, diacetate, sodium phosphate and sodium succinate. The sodium phosphate and succinate esters are very water soluble, quickly attain high blood levels and are quickly excreted. The acetate and diacetate esters are poorly water soluble, and are slowly absorbed and slowly excreted.

When possible, alternate-day therapy should be instituted so that the adrenal glands have an opportunity during the "off" day to produce cortisol, thus making adrenal atrophy less likely. Only certain corticosteroids may be used on an alternate-day basis, and these should always be the first choice of therapy Table 6). Repository forms of corticosteroids (*eg,* Depo-Medrol or Depocoid 40) are a much less desirable alternative and have little or no place in maintenance therapy, unless the pet owner is completely unprepared to give safer medications in tablet form. Patients on long-term corticosteroid therapy should be evaluated twice yearly, including a thorough physical examination, CBC, blood chemistry profile and urinalysis. Patients that respond well initially may tend to become less responsive to the beneficial effects of corticosteroids in time (corticosteroid tachyphylaxis). This can usually be overcome by changing to another form of corticosteroid for 3 weeks, then returning to the former therapy.

Corticosteroids can be used in a safe manner if intelligently prescribed. Alternatives to corticosteroid use, however, should

Table 6. Corticosteroids and alternate-day therapy.

Form of Corticosteroid	Relative Potency	Equivalent dose (mg)	Suitable for Alternate-Day Therapy
Hydrocortisone	1	25	No
Prednisone	4	5	Yes
Methylprednisolone	5	4	Yes
Triamcinolone	5	4	Yes
Flumethasone	15	1.5	No
Dexamethasone	30	0.75	No
Betamethasone	30	0.60	No

Table 7. Corticosteroid dosages.

Form of Corticosteroid	Anti-inflammatory Dosage (mg/kg/day)	Immuno-suppressive Dosage (mg/kg/day)
Hydrocortisone	2.5-5.0	5.0-25.0
Prednisone/prednisolone	0.25-1.5	2.2-6.6
Methylprednisolone	0.25-1.5	2.2-6.6
Triamcinolone	0.25-1.25	2.0-6.0
Dexamethasone	0.05-0.08	0.1-1.0
Betamethasone	0.05-0.08	0.1-1.0

always be considered. Table 7 lists various forms of corticosteroids and their dosages.

Additional Reading

1. Ferguson, DC: Rational glucocorticoid therapy in small animals. Part 1. *MVP* 66:101-105, 1985.

2. Ferguson, DC: Rational glucocorticoid therapy in small animals. Part II. *MVP* 66:175-179, 1985.

3. Scott, DW: Dermatologic use of glucocorticoids. *Vet Clin No Am* 12(1):19-32, 1983.

4. Dillon, AR *et al*: Prednisolone induced hematologic, biochemical, and histologic changes in the dog. *JAAHA* 16:831-837, 1980.

5. Gallant, C and Kenny, P: Oral glucocorticoids and their complications. *J Am Acad Dermatol* 14:161-177, 1986.

6. Claman, HN: Anti-inflammatory effects of corticosteroids. *Clin Immunol Allergy* 4:317-329, 1984.

Antihistamines

The first antihistamine, Antergan, was marketed in France in 1942. Its first American counterpart, Benadryl (diphenhydramine hydrochloride) entered the picture 2 years later. Now there are almost 200 brands of antihistamines on the market. There are 6 classes of classic antihistamines, plus a miscellaneous group that contains some of the newest products on the market. The binding of antihistamines to the H1 receptor site is reversible and the number of receptors blocked is directly proportional to the concentration of the drug at the receptor site. Therefore, therapeutic failure results from an inability to achieve high enough concentrations of the drug to compete with histamine at the receptor sites.

Table 8. Antihistamines and their dosages.

Class	Generic	Example	Suggested Dosage
Alkylamines	Brompheniramine maleate	Dimetane	0.25-0.5 mg/kg BID-TID
	Chlorpheniramine maleate	Chlortripolon	0.25 or 1.0 mg/kg BID, TID
Ethanolamines	Clemastine	Tavist	0.25-1.0 mg/kg BID
	Diphenhydramine HCl	Benadryl	1-2 mg/kg BID or TID
Ethylenediamines	Pyrilamine maleate	Triaminic	1-2 mg/kg BID or TID
Phenothiazines	Trimeprazine tartrate	Temaril	1-2 mg/kg BID
Piperazines	Hydroxyzine HCl	Atarax	2.2-4.4 mg/kg TID
Piperidines	Astemizole	Hismanal	0.5-1 mg/kg SID or BID
	Cyproheptadine HCl	Periactin	0.1 mg/kg BID-TID
	Terfenadine	Seldane	2.5-5 mg/kg BID

The classic antihistamines are all similar in their effects, usually metabolized in the liver and excreted in the urine. Full human doses or even more must be given to most dogs to relieve pruritus. Table 8 contains a list of antihistamines and their suggested dosages. These products have not been approved for use in dogs, and standardized doses have not been calculated. These products should only be used with this express understanding. Veterinarians using these products do so at their own risk.

Additional Reading

1. Ackerman L: Antihistamines in the treatment of canine allergic skin diseases. *Vet Allergist* Fall:1-2, 1986.

2. Flowers, FP et al: Antihistamines. *Intl J Dermatol* 25:224-231, 1986.

3. Girard, JP et al: Double-blind comparison of astemisole, terfenadine and placebo in hay fever with special regard to onset of action. *J Int Med Res* 13:102-108, 1985.

Omega 3 and Omega 6 Fatty Acids

The omega 3 fatty acids include eicosapentanoic acid (EPA), docosapentanoic acid (DPA) and docosahexanoic acid (DHA). Their names are derived from their biochemical structure. All are derivatives of linolenate and originate in phytoplankton and algae, later to be consumed by larger marine life, such as fish. Some fish (*eg*, herring, mackerel, salmon) store these fatty acids in their muscles, while others (*eg*, cod) store them in their liver. Cod liver oil with 9-20% EPA and krill with 40% EPA are acceptable natural sources of the omega 3 fatty acids, but excessive supplementation of the diet with cod liver oil may result in vitamin D toxicity. Products that include EPA and that are suitable for veterinary use include Derm Caps (DVM), OFA Plus (Nutri-Specialties), EFA-Z Plus (Allerderm), Pet-F.A. Liquid (Beecham), Nutrisol (Norden), Opticoat II (Natural Animal Nutrition) and EfaVet (Efamol).

Eicosapentanoic acid is chemically similar to arachidonic acid and interferes with formation of leukotrienes, which are importtant mediators of inflammation. As such, they also block a proportion of the inflammation that causes pruritus in allergic dogs. In people, they also decrease serum cholesterol and the risk of developing hypertension, atherosclerosis, stroke and heart disease. Some benefit may also be derived for gout, rheumatoid arthritis, psoriasis and asthma. Their primary use has been in treatment of allergic dermatitis in dogs. This material is also discussed in Chapter 7.

The most important of the omega 6 fatty acids is gamma linolenic acid. Evening primrose oil, which contains 9% gamma linolenic acid, appears to be readily metabolized, despite the higher content of other products. Other important sources of gamma linolenic acid include black currant (*Ribes nigrum*) seed oil, fungal (*eg, Phycomycetes*) oil and borage (*Borago officinalis*) oil.

Defective enzyme function may be responsible for some clinical manifestations of atopic dermatitis in people (and dogs?). The positive effects of omega fatty acids are probably due to enyzme bypass rather than correction of any immune defect.

Such products as Derm Caps (DVM), OFA-Plus (Nutri-Specialties), EFA-Z Plus (Allerderm) and EfaVet (Efamol) contain a combination of omega 3 and 6 fatty acids. Nutrisol (Norden), Pet-F.A. Liquid (Beecham) and Opticoat II (Natural Animal Nutrition) contain only functional omega 3 fatty acids. Since almost all nutritional supplements contain cis-linoleic and alpha-linolenic acid (and neither has biologic activity on its own), it is important from a practical standpoint not to consider them as functional omega fatty acids.

Additional Reading

1. Ackerman, L: Omega 3 fatty acids. *Bull Can Acad Vet Dermatol* 3(2): 2, 1986.

2. Somer, E: The Omega 3 fatty acids: A review. *The Nutrition Report* 4(6): 42-48, 1986.

3. Ackerman, L: Fatty acid supplementation in the treatment of allergic inhalant dermatitis. *Vet Allergist* Fall:4, 1987.

4. Radha, E et al: Krill as a dietary source of EPA and DHA in the prevention of cardiovascular disease. *Fed Proc* 45:353, 1986.

Retinoids

Retinoids are synthetic derivatives of vitamin A. They were formulated to offer the beneficial effects of Vitamin A while minimizing the risks of toxicity. Retinoids inhibit keratinization and dramatically reduce sebum production. There is also some antineoplastic effect on keratinizing tumors. Their antiinflammatory actions are due to inhibition of neutrophil and eosinophil motility and migration.

The major retinoids used in people are isotretinoin (Accutane: Hoffmann-La Roche) and etretinate (Tegison: Hoffmann-La Roche). Isotretinoin has a more profound effect on sebaceous gland secretion and is principally prescribed in people for severe nodulocystic acne. I have used it experimentally in sebaceous-gland hyperplasia, vitamin A-responsive dermatosis, periappendageal dermatitis (sebaceous adenitis), acne and perianal pyoderma in dogs, with some success. Etretinate is most commonly prescribed for psoriasis in people and I have used it in a small group of dogs with keratinization defects and generalized intracutaneous cornifying epitheliomas, also with some success. Etretinate would also be indicated for ichthyosis and T-cell lymphomas but I have not yet confirmed this. Acitretin is the presumed active metabolite of etretinate and in all likelihood will soon replace commercial etretinate in the marketplace.

The major side effect appears to be drying of the lips, nose and mucocutaneous junctions and some elevation of liver-specific enzyme activity. Expense appears to be a major limiting factor. In animals that do respond, treatment for several months often leads to prolonged remission (2-6 months). Empirically, I have used isotretinoin at 0.5-1.0 mg/kg/day and etretinate at 0.25-1.0 mg/kg/day.

Additional Reading

1. Dicken, CH: Retinoids: A review. *J Am Acad Dermatol* 11:541-552, 1984
2. Roenigk, Jr., HH: Liver toxicity of retinoid therapy. *J Am Acad Dermatol* 19:199-208, 1988.
3. Ellis, CN and Voorhees, JJ: Etretinate therapy. *J Am Acad Dermatol* 16:267-291, 1987.

Chemotherapy

Azathioprine, 6-mercaptopurine, cyclophosphamide, chlorambucil, doxorubicin, methotrexate, vincristine and cisplatin are chemotherapeutic agents that, because of their potent suppression of the immune system, are sometimes used in management of autoimmune diseases and some skin cancers. Unfortunately, their potent activities are accompanied by similarly dramatic side effects, and treated patients must be carefully monitored to prevent serious consequences.

Handling of chemotherapeutic agents poses problems to veterinarians, in that even minute quantities of these drugs may be an occupational health hazard. For this reason, they should be segregated in a safe cabinet and used only in dust-free areas away from ventilation ducts and other personnel. Two pairs of surgical gloves should be used when handling these cytotoxic drugs, and careful attention paid to technique during injection. Gowns and face masks are also recommended. Technicians should wear gloves when counting out antineoplastic tablets or capsules, and clients should be advised to wear rubber gloves when giving the medication to their animal. Finally, all materials used to administer antineoplastic drugs and empty containers should be carefully disposed of.

Azathioprine

Azathioprine is probably the chemotherapeutic treatment of choice for autoimmune skin diseases in dogs, given at 1.1-2.2 mg/kg on alternating days with prednisone. It interferes with DNA and RNA synthesis, inhibits coenzyme formation and mitosis, and influences humoral and cell-mediated immune functions in people. There is a lag period of 3-5 weeks before its beneficial effects are seen. Toxic side effects include bone marrow suppression, GI disturbances and hepatic dysfunction. These are usually reversible on discontinuation of therapy. Blood counts and liver-specific enzyme assays (serum alanine transaminase and alkaline phosphatase) should be performed regularly to minimize the risk of serious side effects. A moderate elevation of alkaline phosphatase is to be anticipated in all animals and need not necessitate discontinuation of therapy unless accompanied by other evidence of liver dysfunction. Azathioprine is converted rapidly to 6-mercaptopurine in the liver and therefore doses should be reduced in animals with impaired liver function. When a xanthine oxidase inhibitor, such as allopurinol, is used to prevent uric acid formation, the dose of azathioprine should be reduced to one-third or one-fourth of the usual dose.

Six-mercaptopurine, the presumed active metabolite of azathioprine, may be given initially at 50 mg/m^2 body surface (about 1.5 mg/kg) daily, also with prednisone (Table 9).

Table 9. Conversion table of weight to body surface area.

Weight kg	Body Surface Area m^2	Weight kg	Body Surface Area m^2	Weight kg	Body Surface Area m^2
1	0.10	21	0.76	41	1.19
2	0.15	22	0.78	42	1.21
3	0.20	23	0.81	43	1.23
4	0.25	24	0.83	44	1.25
5	0.29	25	0.85	45	1.26
6	0.33	26	0.88	46	1.28
7	0.36	27	0.90	47	1.30
8	0.40	28	0.92	48	1.32
9	0.43	29	0.94	49	1.34
10	0.46	30	0.96	50	1.36
11	0.49	31	0.99	51	1.38
12	0.52	32	1.01	52	1.40
13	0.55	33	1.03	53	1.41
14	0.58	34	1.05	54	1.43
15	0.60	35	1.07	55	1.45
16	0.63	36	1.09	56	1.47
17	0.66	37	1.11	57	1.48
18	0.69	38	1.13	58	1.50
19	0.71	39	1.15	59	1.52
20	0.74	40	1.17	60	1.54

Cyclophosphamide, Chlorambucil

Cyclophosphamide (Cytoxan: Mead Johnson) and chlorambucil (Leukeran: Wellcome) are synthetic alkylating agents used in cancer chemotherapy. They are now only infrequently used in treatment of autoimmune diseases. Cyclophosphamide has a number of severe side effects, including hemorrhagic cystitis, leukopenia, thrombocytopenia, GI disturbances, nephrotoxicity, hepatotoxicity, carcinogenicity and hair loss.

Cyclophosphamide may be given at 50 mg/m^2 (1.5- 2.5 mg/kg) on alternating days with prednisone, or on 4 consecutive days each week (Table 9).

The incidence of cyclophosphamide-induced cystitis can often be dramatically lessened by concurrent administration of furosemide (Lasix) twice daily on days when cyclophosphamide is given. Since cyclophosphamide is metabolized by the liver and excreted by the kidneys, kidney and liver function should also be assessed, in addition to monitoring for leukopenia.

If the WBC count drops below 4000/μl or the platelet count drops below 100,000/μl, the dosage should be reduced by 25%. Hair loss is most common in breeds with continuous hair growth (*eg,* Poodles, Old English Sheepdogs, Schnauzers) and the effects are often reversible on discontinuation of therapy.

Chlorambucil (Leukeran: Wellcome) is the least toxic of synthetic mechlorethamines but also the least effective in autoimmune disorders. It may cause lymphopenia and thrombocytopenia, GI signs and hepatotoxicity. It is given at 0.1-0.2 mg/kg on alternate days.

Doxorubicin

Doxorubicin HCl (Adriamycin: Adria Labs) is a relatively new product useful in treatment of many skin tumors. The drug is metabolized by the liver and excreted by the kidneys; the animal's urine may temporarily turn a red-orange color. It is given IV and is highly irritating if injected perivascularly. One side effect is a hypersensitivity reaction. These may be lessened by slow administration of the drug or pretreatment with an antihistamine, such as diphenhydramine HCl (Benadryl: Parke-Davis) IV at 0.50-1.1 mg/kg or cimetidine (Tagamet: SKF) at 10 mg/kg TID. Hemorrhagic diarrhea may also be noted and is frequently lessened by antihistamine administration. Cardiac toxicity is a very important adverse effect of the drug and may be anticipated at cumulative dosages of >250 mg/m^2 (Table 9).

Methotrexate

Methotrexate (Lederle) is an antimetabolite that penetrates most tissues well (except the nervous system) and is excreted in bile and urine. It is commonly used in treatment of lymphoma. Side effects include GI irritation. Profound toxicities can be reversed with leucovorin (citrovorum factor), which is expensive.

Vincristine, Vinblastine

The vinca alkaloids, vincristine and vinblastine, are rarely used in treatment of autoimmune skin diseases other than idiopathic thrombocytopenia, but do find some application in treatment of skin cancers, especially lymphoid and hematopoietic neoplasms. Vincristine is also effective in treatment of transmissible venereal tumor in dogs.

The cytotoxic activity of the vinca alkaloids is considered cell-cycle specific and is a result of their ability to bind to tubulin and inhibit mitosis. Vincristine causes little myelosuppression at usual doses, and therefore can be used in combination with chemotherapies that cause myelosuppression. Vinblastine differs from vincristine in that it causes leukopenia. There is no specific therapy for vincristine or vinblastine toxicosis but most toxic effects are temporary and resolve on discontinuation of therapy or with dose/frequency reduction. A dosage for vincristine is 0.5-0.7 mg/m^2 (0.025-0.05 mg/kg) by slow IV injection or infusion of isotonic saline on a weekly basis (Table 9). It is highly irritating to tissues if injected perivascularly. Vinblastine is used less frequently in treatment of lymphoreticular neoplasms and disseminated mast-cell tumors in dosages of 2 mg/m^2 administered every 7-14 days by slow IV infusion. Because vinblastine is myelosuppressive, blood counts should be closely monitored.

Cisplatin

Cisplatin (Platinol: Bristol) has been used in treatment of a number of neoplasms in people, but in dogs it appears to be at least somewhat beneficial in management of squamous-cell carcinoma, osteosarcoma, and nasal adenocarcinoma. It is given IV at dosages of 60 mg/m^2 at 3-week intervals (Table 9). Saline diuresis immediately before and after administration may help avoid renal toxicity. Toxic side effects are primarily gastrointestinal and include vomiting, diarrhea and anorexia. Additional clinical trials are warranted to delineate further the potential value of platinum therapy in veterinary medicine.

Additional Reading

1. Scott, DW et al: Observations on the immunopathology and therapy of canine pemphigus and pemphigoid. *JAVMA* 180:48-52, 1982.

2. McDonald, CJ: Cytotoxic agents for use in dermatology. I. *J Am Acad Dermatol* 12:753-775, 1985.

3. McDonald, CJ: Use of cytotoxic drugs in dermatologic diseases. II. *J Am Acad Dermatol* 12:965-975, 1985.

4. Dantzig, PI: Immunosuppressive and cytotoxic drugs in dermatology. *Arch Dermatol* 110:393-406, 1974.

5. Beale, KM: Azathioprine for treatment of immune-mediated diseases of dogs and cats. *JAVMA* 192: 1308-1318, 1988.

6. Stanton, ME and Legendre, AM: Effects of cyclophosphamide in dogs and cats. *JAVMA* 188:1319-1322, 1986.

7. Golden, DL and Langston, VD: Uses of vincristine and vinblastine in dogs and cats. *JAVMA* 193: 1114-1117, 1988.

8. Rosenthal, RC: Clinical application of vinca alkaloids. *JAVMA* 179:1084-1086, 1981.

9. Knapp, DW *et al:* Cisplatin therapy in 41 dogs with malignant tumors. *J Vet Int Med* 2: 41-46, 1988.

10. Rogers, KS: L-asparaginase for treatment of lymphoid neoplasia in dogs. *JAVMA* 194:1626-1630, 1989.

Chrysotherapy

Such gold compounds as aurothioglucose (Solganal) or gold sodium thiomalate (Myochrysine) have been used more commonly to treat autoimmune disease over the last few years. An oral gold compound, triethylphosphine gold (Auranofin or Ridaura), is currently undergoing evaluation and used at 0.1-0.2 mg/kg every 12 hours. The mechanism of action has not been completely elucidated. Effects include decreased activity of lysosomal enzymes containing sulfhydryl groups, as well as decreased immunoglobulin and prostaglandin synthesis.

Therapy is initiated by giving 2 test doses a week apart by IM injection. Cats and small dogs (<10 kg) are given 1-mg then 2-mg injections, while larger dogs receive 5 mg, then 10 mg a week later. If no adverse reactions are encountered, gold therapy is continued at 1 mg/kg weekly until the condition responds, then tapered to alternate weeks, then monthly.

Toxic side effects may include skin rashes, oral ulcers, nephrotic syndrome, blood dyscrasias, thrombocytopenia and allergic reactions. Therefore, patients must be routinely monitored at scheduled intervals. Complete blood counts and urinalyses should be performed before each injection. Eosinophilia or proteinuria may signal impending toxicosis. Treatment usually commences with corticosteroids at the same time, since there is a lag period of many weeks until the effects of the gold can be realized. Unlike the situation of combining corticosteroids with azathioprine and cyclophosphamide, side effects do not appear to be additive with chrysotherapy and corticosteroids.

Additional Reading

1. Long, RE: Potential of chrysotherapy in veterinary medicine. *JAVMA* 188:539-542, 1986.

2. Serra, DA and White, SD: Oral chrysotherapy with auranofin in dogs. JAVMA 194:1327-1330, 1989.

Dapsone

Dapsone is a sulfone used for treatment of leprosy in people. It is also effective in immune-mediated disorders and in noninfectious diseases characterized by infiltration of neutrophils.

Dapsone is used in veterinary medicine to treat cutaneous vasculitis, subcorneal pustular dermatosis and (if it actually occurs in dogs) dermatitis herpetiformis. It is used at 1.1 mg/kg, initially TID and slowly tapered to SID, then on alternate days, and then perhaps even less frequently. It is not licensed for use in animals and side effects, including death, have been reported in the veterinary literature. Therefore, the product should only be used when a diagnosis is confirmed. The patient must be routinely monitored via blood tests during dapsone treatment.

Additional Reading

1. Piamphongsant, T: Dapsone for the treatment of vesiculo bullous and pustular diseases. *Intl J Dermatol* 21:512, 1982.

2. Lees, GE *et al*: Fatal thrombocytopenic hemorrhagic diathesis associated with dapsone administration to a dog. *JAVMA* 175:49-52, 1979.

Plasmapheresis

Plasmapheresis or plasma exchange involves removing blood from patients, separating the plasma from the cellular elements, and then reintroducing the cellular elements back into the patient together with saline, fresh plasma or the patient's own immunoadsorbed (filtered) plasma. Because of its speed, effectiveness and prevention of protein deficiencies, it has become useful in treatment of a number of conditions, including immunologic diseases (SLE), diseases of excessive serum components (paraproteinemia) and removal of blocking factors in some neoplasms.

The procedure must be repeated several times to effectively reduce antibody levels. Prednisone or other immunosuppressive drugs must be given to prevent a rebound in antibody levels. Thus, the main uses of plasmapheresis are initially to achieve rapid improvement or to augment therapy when the disease is not controlled by large prednisone doses alone. Plasmapheresis does not remedy the underlying factors causing production of antibodies; it only lessens their numbers and, thereby, their clinical effects. Plasmapheresis has been used in veterinary medicine in treatment of SLE and hyperviscosity syndrome, and experimentally in therapy of FeLV infection.

Additional Reading

1. Matus, RE *et al*: Plasmapheresis-immunoadsorption for the treatment of systemic lupus erythematosus in a dog. *JAVMA* 182:499-502, 1983.

2. Lockwood, CM: Plasma exchange: An overview. *Plasma Ther* 1:1-12, 1979.

3. Matus, RE *et al*: Plasmapheresis and chemotherapy of hyperviscosity syndrome associated with monoclonal gammopathy in the dog. *JAVMA* 183:215-218, 1983.

Cyclosporine A

Cyclosporine A has recently received worldwide attention as an immunosuppressive agent used in tissue transplants. In people, it has also been used in treatment of psoriasis, alopecia areata, psoriatic arthritis, pemphigus, pemphigoid, pyoderma gangrenosum, atopic dermatitis, lichen planus, scleroderma and epidermolysis bullosa aquisita. It is a cyclic polypeptide metabolite of the fungus *Tolypocladium inflatumgams* and acts by blocking a substance responsible for proliferation of T-lymphocytes. Veterinary applications in treatment of autoimmune disorders using dosages of 10-30 mg/kg/day have yielded disappointing results. Side effects have included vomiting and lymphoplasmacytoid dermatitis in some animals.

Topical cyclosporine may have some ophthalmic applications in immune-mediated disorders, such as keratoconjunctivitis sicca, Sjogren's disease and cicatricial pemphigoid.

Additional Reading

1. White, JV: Cyclosporine: Prototype of a T-cell selective immunosuppressant. *JAVMA* 189:566-570, 1986.

2. Rosenkrantz, WS *et al*: Cyclosporine and cutaneous immune-mediated disease. *J Am Acad Dermatol* 14:1088-1089, 1986.

Appendix 2

Topical Products

Topical preparations are commonly prescribed for dogs with localized cutaneous lesions. Some of these products are very well formulated, while others are ineffective but are marketed well. The premise involved in topical therapy is a simple one: "primum non nocere" (first, do no harm). Therefore, select the mildest product that will accomplish the task. When choosing a topical agent, the dosage form should be selected using the following rule of thumb: When treating a condition, if the skin is wet, dry it. If the skin is dry, wet it.

Creams and ointments lubricate the skin and form a protective covering that maintains hydration. Creams or ointments should be applied as a thin film several times a day. Since they form an almost occlusive covering, it is unwise to use these products in oozing lesions in that they effectively seal in the infection. They are best used in treatment of dry skin conditions, for which it is desirable to increase hydration of the skin.

Lotions are liquids in which are suspended therapeutic agents. They tend to be drying, cooling and helpful in relieving some pruritus. They are ideally suited for oozing lesions that must be dried up.

Gels are clear, colorless nonoily vehicles that, when rubbed into the skin, are absorbed almost completely and are not overly messy to apply.

The stratum corneum is the major barrier to drug penetration. Therefore, factors reducing the integrity of this layer enhance drug penetration. Drugs may penetrate through the pilosebaceous units and sweat ducts, as well as through the unbroken stratum corneum. Drug penetration is influenced by the drug's concentration, vehicle solubility, partition coefficient, particle size, viscosity and effect of the vehicle on the skin. Lipid-soluble drugs tend to penetrate better than water-soluble drugs.

Topical Antibacterials

Antibacterials were all originally formulated from products produced by a variety of bacteria and fungi. Such agents as neomycin, polymixin B, bacitracin, gramicidin and nitrofurazone are commonly used in topical preparations. Antiseptics are substances that kill or prevent the growth of microorganisms, especially on living tissue. They are often classified as germicides and subclassified as to their specific spectrum of action (bactericide, fungicide, virucide, sporicide, etc). Such antiseptics as chlorhexidine, povidone-iodine, polyhydroxydine complex (Xenodine: Solvay) and benzoyl peroxide are frequently employed for their antibacterial action.

As a general rule, one should not use the same antibacterial topically and systemically because of the potentially increased incidence of drug hypersensitivity. Thus, the antibacterials most commonly marketed in topical form are only rarely used systemically. Penicillin, streptomycin and the sulfanilamides have a very high incidence of sensitization and are only infrequently found in topical preparations.

Nitrofurazone, neomycin and cetrimide commonly cause contact sensitivity in people. Sulfathiazole, povidone-iodine, bacitracin and gentamicin sulfate only occasionally cause contact sensitivity, and chlorhexidine hydrochloride, mupirocin and fucidic acid very rarely. Cross-sensitivity among neomycin, framycetin, gentamicin and bacitracin has been observed. Therefore, the less sensitizing the antibacterial agent and the fewer compounds present in a formulation, the better off the patient is likely to be. In my opinion, the simpler the formulation, the safer.

Tables 1, 2, 8 and 9 list a number of topical antibacterials and antibacterial combinations. Most of the products listed in these tables are available by prescription only.

Topical Antifungals

Topical antifungals are commonly used individually and in combination with antibacterials and corticosteroids. Such products as clotrimazole (Canesten, Lotrisone, Mycelex), miconazole (Conofite), econazole (Ecostatin, Spectazole), oxiconazole (Oxi-

Table 1. Topical antibacterials.

Antibacterial	Examples
Bacitracin	Bacitracin
Chloramphenicol	Anispray
Erythromycin	Ilotycin, Staticin
Fucidic acid	Fucidin
Furazolidone	Topazone
Mupirocin	Bactoderm, Bactroban
Neomycin	Myciguent, Mycifradin
Nitrofurazone	Furacin, Furazone, Nifulidone
Sulfathiazole	Alphadol Ointment

Table 2. Topical antibacterial combinations.

Antibacterial	Examples
Neomycin sulfate, chloramphenicol	Zoomycetin Cream
Polymixin B, bacitracin,	Polysporin Ointment
Polymixin B, bacitracin, neomycin sulfate	V-Sporin Aerosol
Polymixin B, gramicidin	Polysporin Cream
Polymixin B, gramicidin, lidocaine	Lidosporin
Sulfanilamide, sulfathiazole	Sulfurea

stat), sulconazole (Exelderm), tioconazole (Trosyd), naftifine hydrochloride (Naftin), haloprogin (Halotex), ciclopiroxolamine (Loprox) and ketoconazole (Nizoral) are effective against dermatophytes, *Candida* and *Malassezia* (*Pityrosporum*).

Enilconazole is available in spray and smoke forms in Europe and will soon become available in North America.

Nystatin (Nadostine) is only effective for *Candida* infections, which are relatively rare in animals. Tolnaftate (*eg,* Tinavet) is ineffective on haired skin and is thus a poor choice for treating any fungal disorder on animals.

Chlorhexidine acts as a broad-spectrum antibacterial and antifungal agent with rapid microbial "kill," good residual activity and little potential for sensitization. It is nonirritating, nontoxic and more effective than either hexachlorophene or povidone-iodine, and does not dry the skin or stain the haircoat.

Captan and lime sulfur are marketed to control garden fungi but are safe and effective antifungals for topical use on dogs.

Captan is relatively nontoxic to dogs but is a potent contact sensitizer to people. For this reason, gloves should be worn when applying captan to dogs. A 0.25% solution can be formulated by adding 2 tbsp of the 50% powder to 1 gal of water, or adding 1 tsp of 45% technical captan concentrate to 1 L of water. Dogs should be dipped twice a week until clinical improvement is seen, then a few more times to be sure the fungi have been eradicated.

Lime sulfur is marketed as an orchard spray but is useful in controlling ringworm in dogs. A 2.5% solution can be made by adding 100 ml of 29% lime sulfur concentrate to 1 L of water. Though lime sulfur is very safe, it has a disagreeable odor and may stain white haircoats.

Cuprimyxin, sulfur, povidone-iodine and thiabendazole are other safe topicals suitable for treatment of superficial fungal infections.

Topical Antiseptics

Antiseptics tradionally have been underused in topical therapy, but they have applications in treatment of bacterial and fungal skin infections (Tables 3, 4).

Chlorhexidine (Nolvasan) is a broad-spectrum antibacterial and antifungal with quick killing action, good residual activity and little potential for sensitization. It is nonirritating, nontoxic and more effective than either hexachlorophene or povidone-iodine, and does not dry the skin or stain the haircoat. In people, chlorhexidine gluconate has caused ototoxicity and deafness when applied to the middle ear.

Povidone-iodine solutions are commonly used to flush wounds. Dilute solutions (0.1-1%) are more effective than full-strength solutions (10%). Since its bactericidal activity lasts only for 4-6 hours, povidone-iodine must be used several times daily

Table 3. Topical antiseptics.

Ingredients	Examples
Benzoyl peroxide	Benoxyl, H_2Oxyl, Oxydex, Pyoban, Vetoxyl
Cetyl alcohol, coal tar, crude coal tar, sulfur, salicylic acid	Pragmatar Ointment
Chlorhexidine	Hibitane Ointment
Povidone-iodine	Poviodine Ointment
Resorcinol	Pellitol
Triclosan	Tersaseptic

Table 4. Antiseptic washes.

Ingredients	Examples
Benzalkonium chloride	Zephiran
Benzethonium chloride	V-Tergent 8X
Cetrimide	Cetrimide
Chlorhexidine	Hibitane
Chlorhexidine, cetrimide	Savlon
Hexachlorophene	Phisohex, Septisol
Phenoxetol	Lanohex
Povidone-iodine	Betadine

for best results. Blood and other organic debris should be removed from wounds before povidone-iodine flushing.

Benzoyl peroxides have considerable antimicrobial effect and are discussed in the section on shampoos.

Hydrogen peroxide (3%) is commonly used to irrigate wounds but is damaging to tissues. It has some sporicidal effects and should be reserved for use in wounds with suspected clostridial contamination.

Topical Corticosteroids

Topical corticosteroids act by a number of mechanisms to suppress inflammation and the results of inflammation. Unfor-

Appendix 2

Table 5. Mild topical corticosteroids.

Ingredients	Example	Form	Manufacturer
Alclometasone dipropionate 0.05%	Aclovate	O,Cr	Glaxo
Cortisol acetate 1%	Corticreme	Cr	Rougier
Desonide 0.05%	Desowen	Cr	Owen
	Tridesilon	O,Cr	Miles
Fluocinolone acetonide 0.01%	Synalar	Sol	Syntex
Hydrocortisone 0.5%	Cortate	O,Cr	Schering
	Unicort		Allen& Hanburys
	Sarna	L	Stiefel
Hydrocortisone 1%	Cortate	O,Cr	Schering
	Hyderm	Cr	MTC
	Hydrocortisone	O,Cr	Quantum
	Hytone	O,Cr,L	Dermik
	Sarna	L	Steifel
	Unicort	Cr	Allen& Hanburys
	PTD-HC	L	Vet Rx
Hydrocortisone 1%, salicylic acid 2%, sulfur 3%	Sterodex	Cr,L	Upjohn
Hydrocortisone 2.5%	Hytone	O,Cr,L	Dermik
Hydrocortisone acetate 1%, urea 10%	Calmurid-HC	Cr	Pharmacia
	Uremol-HC	Cr,L	Trans Canada Dermapeutics
Methylprednisolone 0.25%	Medrol	Cr	Upjohn
Triamcinolone acetonide 0.025%	Aristocort D	Cr,O	Lederle
	Cremocort	Cr	Pharmacia
	Kenalog E	Cr,O	Solvay
Mometasone furoate	Elocon	O,Cr	Schering

Key
O — Ointment Cr — Cream Sol — Solution L — Lotion Emol — Emollient cream

tunately, corticosteroids are often prescribed for conditions that benefit little from their use (Tables 5-9). Potent topical corticosteroids may cause a number of side effects, including hair loss, allergic sensitization and even iatrogenic hyperadrenocorticism (Cushing's disease) due to corticosteroid absorption through the skin. Adrenocortical suppression may occur with use of topical triamcinolone acetate (Panolog), betamethasone valerate (Topa-

Table 6. Intermediate-strength topical corticosteroids.

Ingredients	Example	Form	Manufacturer
Beclomethasone dipropionate 0.025%	Propaderm	O	Allen & Hanburys
Betamethasone valerate 0.05%	Betnovate	Cr,O,L	Glaxo
Betamethasone valerate 0.1%	Betnovate	Cr,O,L	Glaxo
Clobetasone butyrate 0.05%	Eumovate	O,Cr	Glaxo
Desoximetasone 0.05%	Topicort	Emol	Hoechst
Difluocortolone valerate 0.01%	Nerisone	O,Cr	Stiefel
Fluocinolone acetonide 0.025%	Synalar	Cr	Syntex
Fluocinonide 0.01%	Lidex Mild	O,Cr	Syntex
Halcinonide 0.025%	Halog	Cr	Solvay
Hydrocortisone acetate 2.5%	Cortamed	O	Pentagone
Hydrocortisone butyrate 0.1%	Locoid	O,Cr	Owen
Hydrocortisone valerate 0.2%	Westcort	O,Cr	Westwood
Triamcinolone acetonide 0.1%	Aristocort	O,Cr	Lederle
	Cremocort	Cr	Pharmacia
	Kenalog	O,Cr	Solvay

Table 7. Potent topical corticosteroids.

Ingredients	Example	Form	Manufacturer
Amcinonide 0.01%	Cyclocort	O,Cr,L	Lederle
Betamethasone	Diprolene	O,Cr,L	Schering
	Diprosone	O,Cr,L	Schering
	Maxivate	O,Cr,L	Westwood
Clobetasol propionate 0.05%	Dermovate	O,Cr,L	Glaxo
	Temovate	O,Cr	Glaxo
Desoximetasone 0.25%	Topicort	Emol	Hoechst
Diflorasone diacetate 0.05%	Florone	O,Cr	Dermik
	Psorcon	O	Dermik
Fluocinonide 0.05%	Lidex	O	Syntex
Halcinonide 0.1%	Halog	O,Cr,Sol	Solvay

gen), dexamethasone (Tresaderm), 1% prednisolone acetate (Pred Forte) and fluocinolone (Lidex, Synotic). It is often best to begin therapy with a potent preparation if needed for 1-2 weeks

Appendix 2

Table 8. Topical antibacterial-corticosteroid combinations.

Ingredients	Examples
Gentamicin sulfate, betamethasone valerate	Topagen, Valisone, Diprogen
Kanamycin sulfate, calcium amphomycin, hydrocortisone acetate	Amphoderm
Neomycin palmitate, hydrocortisone acetate, trypsin/chymotrypsin	Kymar
Neomycin sulfate, fluocinolone acetonide	Neo-Synalar
Neomycin sulfate, methylprednisolone acetate	Neo-Medrol
Neomycin sulfate, polymixin B sulfate, procaine penicillin G, hydrocortisone acetate, hydrocortisone sodium succinate	Forte-Topical Suspension
Polymixin B sulfate, zinc bacitracin, hydrocortisone	Cortisporin
Procaine penicillin G, dihydrostreptomycin sulfate, dexamethasone, chlorampheniramine maleate, procaine hydrochloride	Dexotic

Table 9. Topical antibacterial-antifungal-corticosteroid combinations.

Ingredients	Examples
Neomycin sulfate, dexamethasone, thiabendazole	Tresaderm (MSD)
Neomycin, gramicidin, nystatin, triamcinolone	Kenacomb (Squibb)
Neomycin sulfate, gramicidin, nystatin, triamcinolone acetonide	Combilean
Neomycin sulfate, thiostrepton, nystatin, triamcinolone acetonide	Panolog (Squibb)
Neomycin sulfate, triamcinolone acetonide, bacitracin, nystatin lidocaine	Oribiotic (MTC)

until the condition is under control, then continue treatment with a less potent product, such as hydrocortisone, which has fewer potential side effects.

Intermediate- (triamcinolone) to long-acting (betamethasone, dexamethasone) corticosteroids have a longer half-life than the short-acting corticosteroids, such as hydrocortisone. Significantly, the addition of a fluorine atom, methyl or hydroxyl group to the steroid molecule increases the potency and antiinflammatory activity, while addition of an acetate, acetonide or phosphate group to the molecule prolongs its activity. The characteristics of the vehicle also influence potency since some (propylene glycol, occlusive ointments and creams, urea) enhance penetration of the corticosteroid molecule into the skin. Trade name pharmaceuticals are also often more potent than their generic substitutions.

Combinations of antibacterials and corticosteroids are occasionally indicated for chronic dry inflammatory skin conditions and ear conditions (otitis externa) in which relieving inflammation is an important part of medical management (Tables 8, 9). Unfortunately, multi-drug topical preparations are overused in veterinary medicine, often when a single-drug product would suffice. This overuse increases the risk of sensitization and side effects.

Medicated Shampoos

Shampoos are an important component of dermatologic treatment in that they remove scales, crusts, microorganisms and debris from the skin and haircoat. Shampoo suds should remain in contact with the skin for 10-15 minutes to allow adequate hydration of the stratum corneum and penetration of the active ingredients. Affected animals should be bathed as often as necessary to maintain a normal haircoat and skin.

Though many human shampoos are available, veterinary preparations are formulated for the different characteristics of animal skin. The pH of canine skin is 5.5-7.2 vs 5.5 in human skin.

Most medicated shampoos are designed to be antiseborrheic, that is, to remove dandruff. The 2 mechanisms by which this may be achieved have the same result: removing the top layers of the stratum corneum, the shingle-like covering of the epidermis. Keratolytics decrease the thickness of the stratum corneum by hydrating, softening and peeling, while keratoplastics have a "normalizing" effect on the keratinization process.

Sulfur

Sulfur has been used for thousands of years as a topical remedy. It is remarkably safe, even on newborn animals, and is keratolytic, keratoplastic, antibacterial, antifungal, antiparasitic and antipruritic. The action of sulfur depends on direct interaction with the skin; the smaller the particle size, the greater the area available for sulfur-cutaneous interaction and the greater the efficacy. Sublimed sulfur is prepared by direct conversion of crude sulfur from solid phase to gas, the vapor then condensed to yield a fine yellow powder. Precipitated sulfur is prepared by further modifying sublimed sulfur by adding hydrochloric acid. Colloidal sulfur consists of particles even smaller than those of precipitated sulfur. Precipitated sulfur with a smaller particle size is more effective than sublimed sulfur, and colloidal sulfur is considered the most active form of sulfur available.

Sulfur can be used in a 1-5% concentration in powders, shampoos and dips (Tables 10, 12). One disadvantage of sulfur products is that they are not degreasing; therefore, animals with a greasy coat benefit little from bathing with sulfur. The other disadvantage is that sulfur-based products often have a disagreeable odor and may dry the skin. The antiparasitic effect includes some mites and lice but unfortunately sulfur has little effect on fleas. The antibacterial effect is not profound but in higher concentrations sulfur is a good remedy for dermatophyte infections.

Selenium

Selenium sulfide is a mildly keratolytic shampoo that also has some degreasing action. Because it does not have a very dramatic

Table 10. Sulfur-based shampoos.

Product	Mfr	Sulfur	Salicylic Acid	Hexachlorophene	Triclosan
Fosteen	Rogar/STB	2%	2%	1%	—
SebaLyt	DVM	2%	2%	—	0.5%
Sebbafon	Winthrop	5%	0.5%	—	—
Sterodex	Upjohn	2%	2%	—	—
Sultex	Dermavet	3%	1%	—	—
Sebolux	Allerderm	2%	2.3%	—	—

Table 11. Tar shampoos.

Product	Manufacturer	Tar	Salicylic Acid
Clear Tar	Veterinary Prescription	2%	—
Dermolar	Fort Dodge	9%	—
Pragmatar	Norden	0.1%	—
Sulfur Tar	Adams	3%	2%
Thiomar	Evsco	0.5%	—

effect on the skin, it is rarely prescribed but is a safe medicated shampoo. Examples are Seleen (Ceva), which contains 0.9% selenium sulfide, and Selenium Sulfide Shampoo (Vet-Derm).

Salicylic Acid

Salicylic acid is mildly antibacterial, astringent and somewhat antipruritic. It is rarely used alone (*eg*, Soothing Medicated Shampoo: Vet-Derm, Medi-Clean: Lambert Kay, Cerbinol: Pitman-Moore) but is commonly incorporated with sulfur as a combination product (Tables 10-12).

Coal Tar

Tar is a residue remaining after organic matter is heated in the absence of oxygen.

Therapeutic tars are derived from 3 sources. Coal tar is produced in coking ovens as a byproduct in the manufacture of coke. Crude coal tar contains about 10,000 compounds, and can be modified to yield liquor carbonis detergens and a variety of other distillates. Wood tar is derived from such trees as pine, juniper and beech. Bituminous tar is obtained from rock formations containing fish fossils.

Tar is quite keratoplastic and keratolytic, somewhat antipruritic and commonly prescribed in human medicine for problem dandruff and psoriasis. Because tar is sometimes harsh on sensitive skin and can cause contact sensitivity, gloves should always be worn when using such products. In general, as the tar concentration increases, the chances for excessive drying, staining and follicular irritation also increase. Tars may also stain haircoats, especially in white dogs.

One cannot judge a product's strength or efficacy by its tar content in that different tar constituents differ markedly in those regards. For example, since a coal tar solution is 20% tar, a product containing 2.5% coal tar solution actually contains only 0.5% coal tar (Tables 11, 12).

Despite many investigations into the ability of tars to induce certain types of skin cancer, no firm conclusions have been drawn that tars pose any real danger. Time and continued research will tell.

Benzoyl Peroxide

Benzoyl peroxide is extemely keratolytic and antibacterial (Table 13). It has the additional advantages of follicular flushing activity and degreasing, which are desirable in treating dogs with cutaneous bacterial infections and/or greasy coats. It is also mildly antipruritic. Disadvantages of benzoyl peroxide are that it dries the skin, may irritate sensitive skin, and bleach a variety of fabrics. A Japanese research team claimed that benzoyl peroxide may increase the incidence of some cancers, but this has not been validated in North American studies.

Hypoallergenic Shampoos

Hypoallergenic shampoos are not strictly nonallergenic but are mild shampoos that lack many of the potentially irritating properties of medicated shampoos. In addition, they often include such moisturizing agents as sodium lactate, glycerin, essential fatty acids, lactic acid, urea and aloe vera. Such products as Hylyt EFA (DVM), Allergroom (Allerderm), Micro Pearls Skin

Table 12. Tar and tar-sulfur-based shampoos.

Product	Manufacturer	Tar	Sulfur	Salicylic Acid
Allerseb T	Allerderm	3%	2%	2%
Dermaquel	Tech America	2.5%	5%	1%
LyTar	DVM	2%	2%	2%
Mycodex	Beecham	0.5%	5%	1%
Sastar	Vetrepharm	1%	2%	2%
Sebtar	Daniels	3%	2%	2%
Sebutone	Westwood	0.5%	2%	2%
Tar & Sulfur	Vet-Kem	0.5%	5%	1%

Table 13. Benzoyl peroxide shampoos.

Product	Manufacturer	Form	Concentration
Ben A Derm	Rogar/STB	Shampoo	2.5%
Benoxyderm	Coopers	Shampoo	2.5%
Oxydex	DVM	Shampoo/Gel	2.5%/5%
Oxydex HP	DVM	Shampoo	5%
Pyoben	Allerderm	Shampoo/Gel	3%/5%
Sulf/Oxydex	DVM	Shampoo/Sulfur	2.5% 2%
Vet-Derm	Vet-Derm	Shampoo	3%
Vetoxyl	Vetrepharm	Shampoo/Gel	2.5%/5%

& Coat Moisturizing Shampoo (Evsco), Vet-Derm Hypoallergenic (Vet-Derm), Shampoo/Conditioner (Veterinary Prescription), Olilanol-H (Langford), Vetaderm H (Winthrop) and Outright (Bramton) have been formulated not for animals that might require a medicated shampoo, but rather for animals that cannot tolerate more irritating products. Shampoos containing perfumes, astringents and medication may be poorly tolerated by individuals with sensitive skin. Dishwashing detergents that contain emollients are often good products because they are mild, degreasing and cleansing; however, care should be taken when ethyl alcohol is a component, since dogs may become intoxicated following bathing with such products.

Moisturizers

Moisturizers are designed to rehydrate the skin in dry, scaly conditions or following shampooing with drying agents, such as benzoyl peroxide. Moisturizers may be applied directly to the coat (Humilac: Allerderm, Hylyt EFA: DVM, Micro Pearls Humectant Spray: Evsco, Sesame Oil Emulsion Spray: Veterinary Prescription, Vet-Derm Hypoallergenic Dermal Spray:Vet-Kem, Replenische: Grand Island) or applied as a final rinse following bathing (Micro Pearls Cream Rinse: Evsco, Sesame Oil Rinse: Veterinary Prescription, Alpha Keri: Westwood, Skin-So-Soft: Avon). Final rinses must not be overdone, since these products, if not diluted properly (*eg*, 1 capful per gallon of water), can leave a slick, oily coat. Therefore, apply these agents in moderation.

A new concept involves microencapsulation of moisturizers within multiple concentric lipid bilayers and inclusion in a number of different topical products. These liposomes (novasomes) are included in the Micro Pearls system of dermatologic shampoos, sprays and cream rinse (Evsco).

Aloe Vera

Aloe vera contains various pharmacologically active ingredients, plus a substance that inhibits thromboxane formation. It is a common ingredient in a variety of products. Aloe gel purportedly has emollient, moisturizing and healing effects. Conditions that may benefit from aloe vera include burns, wounds and frostbite.

Additional Reading

1. Ihrke, PJ: Topical therapy: uses, principles and vehicles. Dermatologic therapy (Part I). *Comp Cont Ed Pract Vet* 2:28-35, 1980.

2. Ihrke, PJ: Topical therapy: specific topical pharmacologic agents. Dermatologic therapy (Part II). *Comp Cont Ed Pract Vet* 2:156-164, 1980.

3. Tan, PL *et al:* Current topical corticosteroid preparations. *J Am Acad Dermatol* 14:79-93, 1986.

4. Del Mar, E: Apparent ethanol poisoning in puppies shampooed in dishwashing detergent. *Vet Med* 79: 318-319, 1984.

5. Swaim, SF and Lee, AN: Topical wound medication: a review. *JAVMA* 190:1588-1593, 1987.

6. Zenoble, RD and Kempainen, RJ: Adrenocortical suppression by topically applied steroids in healthy dogs. *Proc 1st Ann Mtg Am Acad Vet Dermatol*, 1987. p 72.

7. Moriello, KA *et al:* Adrenocortical suppression associated with topical otic administration of glucocorticoids in dogs. *JAVMA* 193:329-331, 1988.

8. Eichenbaum, JD *et al:* Effect in large dogs of ophthalmic prednisolone acetate on adrenal gland and hepatic function. *JAAHA* 24:705-709, 1988.

9. Lee, AN *et al:* Effects of chlorhexidine diacetate, povidone- iodine and polyhydroxydine on wound healing in dogs. *JAAHA* 24:77-84, 1988.

10. Lin, AN *et al:* Sulfur revisited. *J Am Acad Dermatol* 18:553-558, 1988.

11. Lin, AN and Moses, H: Tar revisited. *Intl J Dermatol* 24:216-218, 1985.

12. Klein, AD and Penneys, NG: Aloe vera. *J Am Acad Dermatol* 18:714-720, 1988.

13. Cera, LM *et al:* The therapeutic efficacy of aloe vera cream in thermal injuries: two case reports. *JAAHA* 16:768-772, 1985.

Appendix 3
Pharmaceutical Companies

Abbott Laboratories
5400 Cote de Liesse
Montreal, Quebec H4P 1A5
(416) 447-7211
(514) 341-6880
(902) 469-5906
(403) 451-6613
(604) 524-2251
(204) 633-1094

Abbott Laboratories
Abbott Park
North Chicago, IL 60064
(800) 622-2688
(312) 937-6161

Adams Veterinary Research
Laboratories
3270 Pineda Ave
Melbourne, FL 32935
(800) 327-9002 in US

Addison Biological Laboratory
507 Cleveland Ave
Fayette, MO 65248
(816) 248-2215
(800) 331-2530

Adria Laboratories
5000 Post Rd
Dublin, OH 43017
(614) 764-8100

Agrivet
150 Signet Dr
Weston, Ontario M9L 1T9
(416) 749-6320

Allen & Hanburys
1025 The Queensway
Toronto, Ontario M8Z 5S6
(416) 252-2281
(514) 631-9049
(604) 731-6574
(204) 772-9348
(506) 382-4014

Allerderm / Virbac
PO Drawer 277
Hurst, TX 76053
(817) 589-1700
(800) 338-3659

Allerpet
PO Box 1076
Lenox Hill Station
New York, NY 10021
(212) 861-1134

Allervet
858 N Country Club Dr
Mesa, AZ 85201
(602) 833-7330

ARC Laboratories
PO Box 18884
Irvine, CA 92713
(800) 999-3111 in US
(714) 832-1960

Austin Laboratories
675 St-Pierre Sud
Joliette, Quebec J6E 3Z1
(514) 759-3600

Appendix 3

Ayerst Laboratories
1025 Laurentien Blvd
Montreal, Quebec H3C 3J1
(416) 447-2421

Ayerst Laboratories
685 Third Ave
New York, NY 10017
(212) 878-5900

Bayvet Division Chemagro
77 Belfield Rd
Etobicoke, Ontario M9W 1G6
(416) 248-0771
(800) 268-0666 in Ontario & Quebec
(800) 268-1331

BDH Chemicals Canada
Microbiology materials
350 Evans Ave
Toronto, Ontario M8Z 1K5
(800) 268-2129
(416) 255-8521

Beecham Laboratories
115 Brunswick Blvd
Pointe Claire, Quebec H9R 1A4
(800) 361-2280
(514) 695-6551

Beecham Laboratories
501 Fifth St
Bristol, TN 37620
(800) 251-7040
(605) 764-5141

Bencard Allergy Laboratories
Allergy materials
1345 Fewster Dr
Mississauga, Ontario L4W 2A5
(800) 268-2038
(416) 624-6250
(514) 695-6551

Bio-Ceutic Laboratories
PO Box 999
St. Joseph, MO 64502
(816) 233-2804

Boehringer Ingelheim
977 Century Dr
Burlington, Ontario L7L 5J8
(416) 639-0333

Boehringer Ingelheim
2621 N Belt Hwy
St. Joseph, MO 64502
(816) 233-2571

The Bramton Co
PO Box 688480
Dallas, TX 76265
(214) 438-0397
(800) 527-9919 Ext. 0397
(800) 442-7950 Ext. 0397 in TX

Bristol-Myers Animal Health
Evansville, IN 47721-0001
(800) 535-2353

Care Veterinary Pharmaceuticals
(CARE VET)
212-1940 Lonsdale Ave
North Vancouver, BC
V7M 2K2
(604) 987-5453

Center Laboratories
Port Washington, NY 11050
(516) 767-1873
(516) 767-1800
(800) 645-6335 in US

CEVA Laboratories
100551 Barkley, Suite 500
Overland Park, KS 66212
(800) 255-6144 in US

Chesapeake Biological Laboratories
6000 Metro Dr
Baltimore, MD 21215
(301) 358-9600

Ciba Pharmaceuticals
6860 Century Ave
Mississauga, Ontario L5N 2W5
(416) 821-4420

Coopers Agropharm
270 Dreyer Dr West
Ajax, Ontario L1S 3C5
(416) 427-2737

Coopers Animal Health
520 West 21st St
PO Box 419167
Kansas City, MO 64141-6167

Dade Diagnostics
Aguada, PR 00602

Daniels Pharmaceuticals
2517 25th Ave North
St. Petersburg, FL 33713
(800) 237-7427
(800) 331-4831 in Florida

Delmont Laboratories
PO Box AA
Swarthmore, PA 19081
(215) 543-3365
(215) 543-2747

Dermatologic Lab and Supply
201 Ridge
Council Bluffs, IA 51501
(712) 325-0719

Dermatologics for Veterinary
Medicine (DVM)
8785 NW 13th Terrace
Miami, FL 33172
(305) 591-8577

Dormer Laboratories
6600 Trans-Canada Hwy, Suite 750
Pointe Claire, Quebec H9R 4S2
(514) 697-0519

Eli Lilly
3650 Danforth Ave
Scarborough, Ontario M1N 2E8
(416) 694-3221

Eli Lilly
307 E McCarty St
Indianapolis, IN 46285
(317) 276-3714

Evsco Pharmaceuticals
PO Box 209
Harding Hwy
Buena, NJ 08310
(609) 691-2577
(800) 225-0270

Fisons Animal Health
80 Melford Dr
Scarborough, Ontario M1B 2G3
(416) 292-8700

Fisons Corporation
Rochester, NY 14603
(617) 275-1000

Fort Dodge Laboratories
800 5th St
Fort Dodge, IA 50501
(800) 247-1776
(800) 362-2898

Glaxovet
1025 The Queensway
Toronto, Ontario M8Z 5S6
(416) 252-2281

Gordon Piller
2175 Dunwin Dr, Unit 2
Mississauga, Ontario L6L 1X2
(416) 828-6600

Grand Island Research &
Development
2323 Whitehaven Rd
Grand Island, NY 14072
(716) 773-7352

Greer Laboratories
Allergy materials
315 Willow St NW
Lenoir, NC 28645
(800) 438-0088 in USA
(800) 524-7337 in NC

Haver
55 Oakmount Rd, Suite 1212
Toronto, Ontario M6P 2M5
(800) 268-7934
(416) 669-1060

Haver
PO Box 390
Shawnee, KS 66201
(800) 255-6517
(913) 631-4800

Herbert Laboratories
2525 Dupont Dr
Irvine, CA 92713
(714) 752-4500

Appendix 3

Hermal Pharmaceutical Laboratories
Route 145
Oak Hill, NY 12460
(518) 239-6485
(800) HERMAL1

Hoechst Canada
4045, boul Cote Vertu
Montreal, Quebec H4R 1R6
(514) 333-3500

Hoechst-Roussel Agri-Vet
Animal Health Division
Route 202-206 North
Somerville, NJ 08876
(800) 554-6782

Hoffmann-La Roche
1000, Boulevard Roche
Vaudreuil, Quebec J7V 6B3
(416) 456-3800
(514) 487-8000
(204) 633-6510
(403) 253-8221
(604) 437-4481

Hoffmann-La Roche
340 Kingsland St
Nutley, NJ 07110
(201) 235-5000

Hollister-Stier
Allergy materials
77 Belfield Rd
Rexdale, Ontario M9W 1G6
(416) 247-6191

Hollister-Stier
PO Box 3145
Spokane, WA 99220-3145
(509) 489-5656

ICN Canada
1956 Bourdon St, St. Laurent
Montreal, Quebec H4M 1V1
(416) 767-8416
(514) 744-6792

Immunovet
5910-G Breckenridge Pkwy
PO Box 30125
Tampa, FL 33610
(813) 621-9447

International Vaccine & Supply
Rt 1, Box 115
Jourdanton, TX 78026
(512) 769-3382

Janssen Pharmaceutica
6535 Mill Creek Dr
Mississauga, Ontario L5N 2M2
(800) 387-2112
(800) 387-8209
(800) 387-8251
(416) 821-9161

Janssen Pharmaceutica
40 Kingsbridge Rd
Piscataway, NJ 08854
(201) 524-9881

Jensen Salsbery Laboratories
520 W 21st St
Kansas City, MO 64141

Kenvet
100 Elm St
Walpole, MA 02081-1898
(508) 660-3300
(800) 338-7953

Langford
400 Michener Road
Guelph, Ontario N1K 1E4
(519) 837-2040

Lederle Products
2255 Sheppard Ave East
Willowdale, Ontario M2J 4Y5
(416) 293-8181
(514) 457-2110
(403) 253-0924

Lederle Products
Pearl River, NY 10965
(914) 735-2815

Leo Laboratories
1305 Sheridan Mall Pkwy
Pickering, Ontario L1V 3P2
(416) 831-2332

Pharmaceutical Companies

Maurry Biological
6109 S Western Ave
Los Angeles, CA 90047
(213) 759-1128
(213) 759-1127

Mead Johnson Pharmaceuticals
2404 W Pennsylvania St
Evansville, IN 47721
(812) 429-5000

Merrell Dow Pharmaceuticals
7777 Keele St, Unit 10
Concord, Ontario L4K 1Y7
(416) 669-6941

Merrell Dow Pharmaceuticals
2110 E Galbraith Rd
Cincinatti, OH 43215
(513) 948-6040

3M Canada
155 Lesmill Rd
PO Box 1500
North York, Ontario M3C 2V3
(800) 268-7770
(416) 449-8010

3M Animal Care Products
255-58 3M Center
St. Paul, MN 55144
(612) 733-8771

Mobay Corp
Animal Health Division
Shawnee, KS 66201
(800) 633-8405

MSD Agvet
PO Box 1005
Pointe Claire, Quebec H9R 4P8
(800) 361-0260

MSD Agvet
PO Box 2000
Rahway, NJ 07065
(800) 325-9034

MTC Pharmaceuticals
Canada Packers Chemicals
5100 Timberlea Blvd
Mississauga, Ontario L4W 2S5
(800) 268-2331
(416) 624-7000

Natural Animal Nutrition
2214 Old Emmorton Rd
Bel Air, MD 21014
(301) 879-7474

Norden Laboratories
6581 Kitimat Rd, Unit #8
Mississauga, Ontario L5N 3T5
(800) 387-8218

Norden Laboratories
PO Box 80809
Lincoln, NE 68521
(800) 228-4025
(800) 742-7588 in NE

Novopharm
1290 Ellesmere Rd
Scarborough, Ontario M1P 2Y1
(416) 291-8876
(604) 687-2016
(514) 739-4136

NutriSpecialties
175 Dunwin Dr, Unit 2
Mississauga, Ontario L6L 1X2
(416) 828-6600

Omega Laboratories
11,450 Rue Hamon
Montreal, Quebec H3M 3A3
(514) 335-0310
(416) 233-5849

Organon Canada
565 Coronation Dr
West Hill, Ontario M1E 4S2
(416) 284-6131
(514) 336-2800
(604) 437-4481

Organon Pharmaceuticals
375 Mt Pleasant Ave
West Orange, NJ 07052
(201) 325-4500

Osborn
PO Box 459
Fort Dodge, IA 50501
(515) 576-4225
(800) 328-4862

Oxoid Canada
217 Colonnade Rd
Nepean, Ontario K2E 7K3
(800) 267-1007
(416) 270-7763

Pan American Veterinary
Pharmaceuticals
4156 Danvers Ct
Grand Rapids, MI 49508
(616) 949-4531
(800) 942-0986

Pentagone Pharmaceuticals
2260 32nd Ave, Lachine
Montreal, Quebec H8T 3H4
(514) 631-7400
(403) 253-8221

Pfizer Canada
Pharmaceutical Division
17,300 Trans-Canada Hwy
Kirkland, Quebec H9J 2M5
(416) 671-2130

Pfizer
235 E 42nd St
New York, NY 10017
(212) 573-2422

Pharmaderm
60 Baylis Rd
Melville, NY 11747
(516) 454-7677

Pitman-Moore
421 E Hawley St
Mandeleia, IL 60060
(800) 541-7459

PRA Research International
12772 Valley View, Suite 3
Garden Grove, CA 92645
(714) 898-3082
(800) 821-0111

PRN Pharmacal
5830 McAllister
Pensacola, FL 32504
(904) 476-9462
(800) 874-9764

Prozyme Products
6600 N Lincoln Ave
Lincolnwood, IL 60645
(800) 522-5537

Purepet
1399 Bockman Rd
San Lorenzo, CA 94580
(415) 481-8174

PVU
345 boul Labbe
Victoriaville, Quebec G6P 1B1
(519) 823-5496
(819) 758-0506

Quantum
140 Milner Ave, Unit 18
Scarborough, Ontario M1S 3R3
(416) 291-2281

A.H. Robins
Richmond, VA 23220-6609
(804) 257-2000

Rogar/STB
6560 Northwest Dr
Mississauga, Ontario L4V 1P2
(800) 268-9932
(416) 671-4275

Rougier
8480 Blvd, St. Laurent
Montreal, Quebec H2P 2M6
(800) 361-6114
(416) 675-5527
(514) 381-5631

Schering
3535 Trans-Canada Hwy
Pointe Claire, Quebec H9R 1B4
(800) 268-4937
(416) 675-5527

Pharmaceutical Companies

Schering
Animal Health Division
Kenilworth, NJ 07033
(800) 442-5034

SmithKline & French
1940 Argentia Rd
Mississauga, Ontario L5N 2V7
(416) 821-2200

SmithKline & French
PO Box 7929
Philadelphia, PA 19101
(215) 251-7400

Solvay Veterinary
PO Box 7348
Princeton, NJ 08540
(800) 524-1645
(609) 987-2600

Squibb
2365 Cote de Liesse Rd
Montreal, Quebec H4N 2M7
(514) 331-7423

Sterivet
3909 Nashua Dr, Unit 5
Mississauga, Ontario L4V 1R3
(800) 268-4702 in Canada
(800) 268-4711 in Quebec
(416) 678-6800

Stiefel Canada
6635 Henri Bourassa Blvd West
Montreal, Quebec H4R 1E1
(416) 226-6949
(514) 332-3800

Syntex Animal Health
2100 Syntex Ct
Mississauga, Ontario L5N 3X4
(416) 821-1082

Syntex Animal Health
PO Box 653
Des Moines, IA 50303
(515) 262-9341

Upjohn Veterinary Division
TUCO Products
40 Centennial Rd
Orangeville, Ontario L9W 3T3
(800) 265-9122

Upjohn Veterinary Division
7000 Portage Rd
Kalamazoo, MI 49001
(800) 246-1146

Vedco
St. Joseph, MO 64504

Vet-A-Mix
604 West Thomas Ave
Shenandoah, IA 51601
(712) 246-3763
(800) 831-0004

Veterinary Insecticide Products
Terminix Animal Health
855 Ridge Lake Blvd
Memphis, TN 38119
(800) 426-4104

Veterinary Prescription
1656 W 240th St
Harbor City, CA 90710
(213) 326-2720

Veterinary Products Laboratories
PO Box 34820
Phoenix, AZ 85067-4570
(602) 285-1667

Vet-Kem
12200 Denton Dr
Dallas, TX 75234
(214) 243-2321
(800) 263-3774 in Canada

Vetrepharm
69 Bessemer Rd, Unit 27
London, Ontario N6E 2V6
(800) 265-5464
(519) 685-5800

Vetrepharm
119 Rowe Rd
Athens, GA 30601
(404) 549-4503

Appendix 3

Vita Plus Industries
953 E Sahara Ave #21B
Las Vegas, NV 89104
(702) 733-8805

Willamette Animal Bacteriological &
Central Labs
9108 NE Sandy Blvd
Portland, OR 97220

Winthrop Animal Health Products
Yonge St South
Aurora, Ontario L4G 3H6
(800) 263-2040
(800) 663-3759

Winthrop Animal Health Products
90 Park Ave
New York, NY 10016
(212) 907-2592
(800) 446-6267

Zinpro
1107 Hazeltine Blvd
Chaska, MN 55318
(612) 448-3751

Appendix 4
Diagnostic Laboratories

The following is not a complete list of diagnostic laboratories, and inclusion of a laboratory on this list does not constitute an endorsement.

A & M Biosciences RAST allergy test
6350 E Main, Suite 206
Mesa, AZ 85205
(800) 225-2857
(602) 464-9282

Advanced Veterinary Laboratories Diagnostic laboratory
PO Box 68
North Aurora, IL 60542
(800) 323-0623

Animal Diagnostic Laboratory Diagnostic laboratory
2802 El Barito
Tucson, AZ 85721
(602) 622-4377

Animal Health Diagnostic Laboratory Endocrine diagnostic laboratory
Endocrine Diagnostic Section
PO Box 30076
Lansing, MI 48909-7576
(517) 353-0621

Animal Reference Pathology Diagnostic laboratory
390 Wakara Way
Salt Lake City, UT 84108
(801) 583-2787

APL Veterinary Laboratories Diagnostic laboratory
4230 S Burnham Ave, Ste 250
Las Vegas, NV 89119
(800) 433-2750

Auburn University Endocrine diagnostic laboratory
College of Veterinary Medicine
Department of Physiology & Pharmacology
Auburn, AL 36849
(205) 844-5400

Appendix 4

Bioproducts for Medicine AREST allergy test
2330 South Industrial Park Dr
Tempe, AZ 85282
(602) 966-7248
(800) 528-4401 in US or
(800) ALLERGY
(800) 544-1455 in Canada

California Veterinary Diagnostics Diagnostic laboratory
3911 West Capitol Ave
West Sacramento, CA 95691
(916) 372-4200

Canam Diagnostics Company Canine allergy services
81 Finchdene Square
Scarborough, Ontario M1X 1B4
(416) 293-4955

Carson City Veterinary Laboratory Diagnostic laboratory
1477 North Saliman
Carson City, NV 89701
(702) 883-5630

Central Laboratory for Veterinarians Diagnostic laboratory
5645 199th St
Langley, BC V3A 1H9
(604) 533-4884
(800) 242-5871 in British Columbia
(800) 663-1425 in Alberta

Cenvet Diagnostic laboratory
1676 First Ave
New York, NY 10128
(212) 534-4900
(800) 221-3025

Clinical Endocrinology Laboratory Endocrine diagnostic laboratory
Department of Environmental Practice
Veterinary Teaching Hospital, Rm A105
College of Veterinary Medicine
Knoxville, TN 37916
(615) 546-9240, Ext. 173

Colorado State University Diagnostic laboratory
Veterinary Diagnostic Laboratory
Fort Collins, CO 80523
(303) 491-6128
(303) 491-1281

Colorado Veterinary Laboratory Diagnostic laboratory
2150 West Sixth Ave, Unit F
Broomfield, CO 80020
(800) 321-2418

Diagnostic Laboratories

Daryl Laboratories Diagnostic testing (titers)
2220 Martin Ave
Santa Clara, CA 95050
(408) 988-3793

Diagnostic Veterinary Medical Laboratory Diagnostic laboratory
17 Sylvan St
Rutherford, NJ 07070
(800) 624-2594

Diagnostic Veterinary Systems Diagnostic laboratory
10 Gateway Blvd
Don Mills, Ontario M3C 2A1
(416) 429-1633

Illinois Veterinary Laboratory Diagnostic laboratory
650 Grand Ave, Ste 206
Elmhurst, IL 60126
(800) 433-6928

Immunologic Diagnostic Services Diagnostic laboratory
2519 W Peterson Ave
Chicago, IL 60659
(312) 878-5200

Inter Veterinary Services Diagnostic laboratory
12401 E Washington Blvd
Whittier, CA 90606
(213) 698-0721

Iowa State University Diagnostic laboratory
Veterinary Diagnostic Laboratory
Ames, IA 50010
(515) 294-1950

Kemptville Vet Diagnostics Service Diagnostic laboratory
c/o Mailbag 2005
Kemptville, Ontario K0G 1J0
(613) 258-8323

Laboratories of Veterinary Diagnostic Diagnostic laboratory
Medicine
University of Illinois
Urbana, IL 61801
(217) 333-1620

Labstat Diagnostic laboratory
262 Manitou Drive
Kitchener, Ontario N2C 1L3
(519) 893-3571

Appendix 4

Louisiana Veterinary Medical   Diagnostic laboratory
Diagnostic Laboratory
Louisiana State University
Baton Rouge, LA 70803
(504) 346-3193

Medical Express Laboratories   Diagnostic laboratory
1265 Union Ave
Memphis, TN 38104
(901) 726-7182

Minneapolis/St. Paul VeterinaryPathology   Diagnostic laboratory
Lowry Medical Arts Bldg, Ste 532
St. Paul, MN 55102
(612) 228-1619

Minnesota Veterinary Diagnostic Lab   Diagnostic laboratory
University of Minnesota
1943 Capter Ave
St. Paul, MN 55108
(612) 625-8787

Mississippi Veterinary   Diagnostic laboratory
PO Box 4389
Jackson, MS 39216
(601) 354-6091

Montana Veterinary Diagnostic Lab   Diagnostic laboratory
PO Box 997
Bozeman, MT 59771

New Hampshire Vet Diagnostic Lab   Diagnostic laboratory
University of New Hampshire
Durham, NH 03824

New York State College of Veterinary Diagnostic laboratory
Medicine
Diagnostic Laboratory
Cornell University
PO Box 786
Ithaca, NY 14851-0786
(607) 253-3900

North America Veterinary Laboratory   Diagnostic laboratory
180 NW 40th St
Boca Raton, FL 33431
(305) 391-4886

Oregon State Veterinary Diagnostic   Diagnostic laboratory
Laboratory
Oregon State University
Corvallis, OR 97339
(503) 754-3261

Diagnostic Laboratories

Provincial Veterinary Laboratory   Diagnostic laboratory
4840 Wascana Pkwy
Regina, Saskatchewan S4S 0B1
(306) 787-6426

Radionuclide & Hormone RIA Laboratory   Diagnostic laboratory
University of Wisconsin
School of Veterinary Medicine
2015 Linden Dr West
Madison, WI 53706
(608) 263-5863
(608) 263-4908

Riverside Veterinary Laboratories   Diagnostic laboratory
PO Box 3889
Richmond, VA 23235
(800) 522-0100

Sommer Laboratories   Endocrine laboratory
RR 1
Mount Albert, Ontario L0G 1M0
(416) 473-5100

Sonora Laboratory Sciences   Diagnostic laboratory
1500 South Dobson, Suite 217
Mesa, AZ 85202
(602) 833-5224
(800) 231-9510

Southeast VetLab   Diagnostic laboratory
18131 SW 98th Ct
Miami, FL 33157

Southwest Veterinary Diagnostics   Diagnostic laboratory
13633 N Cave Creek Rd
Phoenix, AZ 85023
(317) 494-7564

Specialized Assays   Various assays
206 12th Ave South
Nashville, TN 37202
(800) 433-3648

Texas Vet Med Diagnostic Lab System   Diagnostic laboratory
Drawer 3040
College Station, TX 77841
(409) 845-3414

Tox/Path Service   Diagnostic laboratory
650 Salfordville Rd
Harleysville, PA 19438

Appendix 4

Tufts University Diagnostic Laboratory 305 South St Jamaica Plain, MA 02130	Diagnostic laboratory
Veterinary Diagnostic Laboratory University of Arizona Room 102, Bldg 90 Tucson, AZ 85721 (602) 621-2356	Diagnostic laboratory
Diagnostic Assistance Laboratory University of Georgia Athens, GA 30602 (404) 542-5568	Diagnostic laboratory
Veterinary Medical Diagnostic Laboratory University of Missouri Columbia, MO 65211 (314) 882-6811	Diagnostic laboratory
Veterinary Diagnostic Laboratory University of New Hampshire Durham, NH 03824 (603) 862-2726	Diagnostic laboratory
Endocrine Diagnostic Laboratory University of Pennsylvania Philadelphia, PA 19104	Endocrine diagnostic laboratory
Veterinary Diagnostic Services Maryland Medical Labs 1901 Sulphur Spring Rd Baltimore, MD 21227 (301) 247-9100, Ext 440	Diagnostic laboratory
Veterinary Laboratory Services Branch Ontario Ministry of Agriculture & Food Guelph Agriculture Centre PO Box 1030 Guelph, Ontario N1H 6N1 (519) 767-3116	Diagnostic laboratory
Veterinary Lab Branch 99-762 Moanalua Rd Aiea, HI 96701	Diagnostic laboratory
VetPath Division 5516 Nicholson La Kensington, MD 20895 (800) 638-6587	Diagnostic laboratory

Diagnostic Laboratories

Vet-Pro Labs
PO Box 33001
Tulsa, OK 74153
(800) 999-8387
    Diagnostic laboratory

Veterinary Diagnostic Laboratory
College of Veterinary Medicine
Manhattan, KS 66506
(913) 532-5650
    Diagnostic laboratory

Veterinary Reference Laboratory
1871 Chris La
Anaheim, CA 92805
(714) 937-0161
(800) 854-7133 in US
(800) 422-7328 in California
(800) 432-7305 in southern California
    Diagnostic laboratory

Veterinary Reference Laboratory
3191 Commonwealth Dr
Dallas, TX 75247
(214) 263-5503
(800) 347-6300 in US
    Diagnostic laboratory

Veterinary Reference Laboratory
14796 Wicks Blvd
San Leandro, CA 94577
(415) 352-7960
(800) 736-5151 in US
(800) 528-2050 in northwestern states
(800) 228-3591 in northern California
    Diagnostic laboratory

Vet Tech Labs
909 Old Fern Hill Rd
Box 2315
West Chester, PA 19380
(215) 436-5648
    Diagnostic laboratory

Vitamin Diagnostics
Rt 35 & Industrial Dr
Cliffwood Beach, NJ 07735
(201) 583-7773
    Vitamin detection

Vita-Tech
151 Esna Park Dr, Unit 13
Markham, Ontario L3R 3B1
(416) 475-6499
(416) 242-3816
    Diagnostic laboratory

Appendix 5
Board-Certified Veterinary Dermatologists

Dr. Lowell Ackerman
Mesa, Arizona
Tucson, Arizona
Markham, Ontario

Dr. Richard Anderson
South Weymouth, Massachusetts
Dedham, Massachusetts

Dr. Donna Walton Angarano
Auburn, Alabama

Dr. Victor Austin
Westlake Village, California

Dr. Benjamin Baker
Pullman, Washington

Dr. Karin Beale
Gainesville, Florida

Dr. Diane Bevier
Raleigh, North Carolina

Dr. James Blakemore
West Lafayette, Indiana

Dr. Patrick Breen
Cincinnati, Ohio
Richfield Village, Ohio
Columbus, Ohio
Louisville, Kentucky
Lexington, Kentucky

Dr. Robert Buerger
Baltimore, Maryland

Dr. Paul Caciolo
St. Louis, Missouri

Dr. Karen Campbell
Urbana, Illinois

Dr. David Chester
College Station, Texas

Dr. James Conroy
Mississippi State, Mississippi

Dr. Douglas DeBoer
Madison, Wisconsin

Dr. George Doering
Walnut Creek, California

Dr. Anne Evans
North Grafton, Massachusetts

Dr. Valerie Fadok
Denver, Colorado

Dr. Carol Foil
Baton Rouge, Louisiana

Dr. Craig Griffin
Garden Grove, California
Santa Monica, California
San Diego, California
Alta Loma, California
Las Vegas, Nevada
Anchorage, Alaska

Dr. Richard Halliwell
Scotland

Dr. Peter Ihrke
Davis, California

Appendix 5

Dr. Robert Kirk
Ithaca, New York

Dr. Gail Kunkle
Gainesville, Florida

Dr. Kenneth Kwochka
Columbus, Ohio

Dr. John MacDonald
Auburn, Alabama
Kansas City, Missouri

Dr. Thomas Manning
Raleigh, North Carolina

Dr. Patrick McKeever
St. Paul, Minnesota

Dr. Linda Medleau
Athens, Georgia

Dr. William Miller
Ithaca, New York

Dr. Karen Moriello
Madison, Wisconsin

Dr. George Muller
Stanford, California

Dr. Alan Mundell
Davis, California

Dr. Gene Nesbitt
West Caldwell, New Jersey

Dr. Susan Reinke
Corte Madera, California

Dr. Karen Helton Rhodes
New York, New York

Dr. Lloyd Reedy
Dallas, Texas

Dr. Wayne Rosenkrantz
Garden Grove, California
Santa Monica, California
San Diego, California
Alta Loma, California
Las Vegas, Nevada
Anchorage, Alaska

Dr. Edmund Rosser
East Lansing, Michigan

Dr. Vicki Scheidt
Lyme, New Hampshire

Dr. Robert Schick
Roswell, Georgia

Dr. Lynn Schmeitzel
Knoxville, Tennessee

Dr. Robert Schwartzman
Philadelphia, Pennsylvania

Dr. Danny Scott
Ithaca, New York

Dr. Kevin Shanley
Philadelphia, Pennsylvania

Dr. Erwin Small
Urbana, Illinois

Dr. Candace Sousa
Sacramento, California

Dr. Anthony Stannard
Davis, California

Dr. Stephen White
Fort Collins, Colorado

Canada

Dr. Lowell J. Ackerman
Denison Veterinary Services
1151 Denison St, Suite 2
Markham, Ontario L3R 3Y4
(416) 477-4660

Great Britain

Dr. Richard E.W. Halliwell
Department of Veterinary
    Clinical Studies
Royal (Dick) School of Vet Studies
Veterinary Field Station
Easter Bush, ROSLIN
Midlothian, EH25 9RG Scotland
031 445 2001

Board-Certified Veterinary Dermatologists

United States

Alabama

Dr. Donna Walton Angarano
College of Veterinary Medicine
Auburn University
Auburn, AL 36849
(205) 826-4690

Dr. John M. MacDonald
College of Veterinary Medicine
Auburn University
Auburn, AL 36849
(205) 826-4690

Alaska

Dr. Craig Griffin
Dr. Wayne Rosenkrantz
Northern Lights Animal Hospital
2002 W Benson Blvd
Anchorage, AK 99517
(907) 248-2111

Arizona

Dr. Lowell Ackerman
Mesa Veterinary Hospital
858 N Country Club Dr
Mesa, AZ 85801
(608) 833-7330

Dermatology and Allergy Service
1717 N Swan Road
Tucson, AZ 85712
(602) 326-6363

California

Dr. Victor Austin
Westlake Village, CA 91361

Dr. George Doering
1411 Treat Blvd
Walnut Creek, CA 94598
(415) 934-8051

Dr. Craig E. Griffin
Animal Dermatology Clinic
13132 Garden Grove Blvd, #B
Garden Grove, CA 92643
(714) 971-6211

Animal Dermatology Clinic
13240 Evening Creek Dr, Suite 302
San Diego, CA 92128

Animal Dermatology Clinic
1304 Wilshire Blvd
Santa Monica, CA 90403
(714) 971-6211

Baseline Animal Hospital
9350 Baseline Rd, Suite A
Alta Loma, CA 91701
(714) 987-4788

Dr. Peter Ihrke
School of Veterinary Medicine
University of California
Davis, CA 95616
(916) 752-1363

Dr. George H. Muller
Dermatology Department
Stanford University Medical School
Stanford, CA 94305

Dr. Alan Mundell
Davis, CA 95616

Dr. Susan I. Reinke
Madera Pet Hospital
5796 Paradise Dr
Corte Madera, CA 94925
(415) 924-1271

Dr. Wayne Rosenkrantz
Animal Dermatology Clinic
13132 Garden Grove Blvd, #B
Garden Grove, CA 92643
(714) 971-6211

Animal Dermatology Clinic
13240 Evening Creek Dr, Suite 302
San Diego, CA 92128

Animal Dermatology Clinic
1304 Wilshire Blvd
Santa Monica, CA 90403
(714) 971-6211

Baseline Animal Hospital
9350 Baseline Rd, Suite A
Alta Loma, CA 91701
(714) 987-4788

Appendix 5

Dr. Candace A. Sousa
Animal Dermatology Clinic
5701 H St
Sacramento, CA 95819
(916) 451-6445

Dr. Anthony Stannard
School of Veterinary Medicine
University of California
Davis, CA 95616
(916) 752-1363

Colorado

Dr. Valerie Fadok
Denver, CO

Dr. Stephen White
College of Vet Med and Biomed Sci
Colorado State University
Ft. Collins, CO 80523
(303) 221-4535

Florida

Dr. Karin Beale
College of Veterinary Medicine
University of Florida
Gainesville, FL 32610
(904) 392-4751

Dr. Gail Kunkle
College of Veterinary Medicine
University of Florida
Gainesville, FL 32610
(904) 392-4751

Georgia

Dr. Linda Medleau
College of Veterinary Medicine
University of Georgia
Athens, GA 30602
(404) 542-3221

Dr. Robert Schick
Atlanta Animal Allergy &
 Dermatology Clinic
408 S Atlanta St, Suite 155
Roswell, GA 30075

Illinois

Dr. Erwin Small
College of Veterinary Medicine
Universtiy of Illinois
1008 West Hazelwood Dr
Urbana, IL 61801
(217) 333-5300

Dr. Karen Campbell
College of Veterinary Medicine
University of Illinois
1008 West Hazelwood Dr
Urbana, IL 61801
(217) 333-5300

Indiana

Dr. James C. Blakemore
School of Veterinary Medicine
Purdue University
West Lafayette, IN 47907
(317) 494-1107

Kentucky

Dr. Patrick Breen
Louisville Animal Emergency Clinic
4306 Bishop La
Louisville, KY 40218
(502) 456-6102

AA Small Animal Emergency Service
509 Southland Dr
Lexington, KY 40503
(606) 276-2505

Louisiana

Dr. Carol Foil
School of Veterinary Medicine
Louisiana State University
Baton Rouge, LA 70803
(504) 346-3333

Maryland

Dr. Robert G. Buerger
Veterinary Dermatology Center
PO Box 24032
5230 Washington Blvd
Baltimore, MD 21227
(301) 242-5536

Board-Certified Veterinary Dermatologists

Massachusetts

Dr. Richard K. Anderson
South Shore Veterinary Associates
595 Columbian St
South Weymouth, MA 02190
(617) 337-6622

Bruce Veterinary Clinic
326 Bridge St
Dedham, MA 02026
(617) 326-2800

Dr. Anne Evans
Tufts School of Veterinary Medicine
200 Westboro Rd
North Grafton, MA 01536
(508) 839-5395

Michigan

Dr. Edmund J. Rosser, Jr.
Department of Vet Clinical Sciences
College of Veterinary Medicine
Michigan State University
East Lansing, MI 48823
(517) 355-7721

Minnesota

Dr. Patrick J. McKeever
C-342 Veterinary Hospital
University of Minnesota
St. Paul, MN 55108
(612) 625-9229

Mississippi

Dr. James D. Conroy
College of Veterinary Medicine
Mississippi State University
PO Box 5204
Mississippi State, MS 39762
(601) 325-3432

Missouri

Dr. Paul L. Caciolo
Dermatology Consultant
St. Louis, MO 63105
(314) 997-0920

Dr. John MacDonald
Brookside Animal Clinic
210 W 85th St
Kansas City, MO 64114
(816) 363-2115

Nevada

Dr. Craig Griffin
Dr. Wayne Rosenkrantz
Tropicana Veterinary Clinic
2385 E Tropicana Ave
Las Vegas, NV 89109
(702) 736-4944

New Jersey

Dr. Gene H. Nesbitt
Animal Dermatology Clinic
700 Bloomfield Ave
West Caldwell, NJ 07006
(201) 228-7756

New Hampshire

Dr. Vicki Scheidt
Lyme, NH

New York

Dr. Karen Helton-Rhodes
Animal Medical Center
510 E 62nd St
New York, NY 10021
(212) 838-8100

Dr. Robert W. Kirk
College of Veterinary Medicine
Cornell University
Ithaca, NY 14853

Dr. William H. Miller, Jr.
College of Veterinary Medicine
Cornell University
Ithaca, NY 14853
(607) 253-3060

Dr. Danny W. Scott
College of Veterinary Medicine
Cornell University
Ithaca, NY 14853
(607) 253-3060

North Carolina

Dr. Diane Bevier
School of Veterinary Medicine
North Carolina State University
Raleigh, NC 27606
(919) 821-9500

Dr. Thomas O. Manning
School of Veterinary Medicine
North Carolina State University
Raleigh, NC 27606
(919) 821-9500

Ohio

Dr. Patrick Breen
Veterinary Dermatology
4725 Cornell Rd
Cincinnati, OH 45241
(513) 489-4644

Veterinary Specialty Clinic
4050 Broadview
Richfield Village, OH 44286
(216) 659-4169

Med Vet/Columbus
6813 Flags Center Dr
Columbus, OH 43229
(614) 891-2070

Dr. Kenneth W. Kwochka
College of Veterinary Medicine
Ohio State University
1935 Coffey Rd
Columbus, OH 43210
(614) 292-3551

Pennsylvania

Dr. Kevin Shanley
School of Veterinary Medicine
University of Pennsylvania
Philadelphia, PA 19104
(215) 898-8861

Dr. Robert M. Schwartzman
School of Veterinary Medicine
University of Pennsylvania
Philadelphia, PA 19104
(215) 898-8861

Tennessee

Dr. Lynn P. Schmeitzel
Department of Urban Practice
College of Veterinary Medicine
University of Tennessee
PO Box 1071
Knoxville, TN 37901
(615) 546-9240

Texas

Dr. David K. Chester
College of Veterinary Medicine
Texas A&M University
College Station, TX 77843
(409) 845-2351

Dr. Lloyd M. Reedy
Dallas Animal Dermatology Referral Clinic
2353 Royal La
Dallas, TX 75229
(214) 241-6266

Washington

Dr. Benjamin B. Baker
106 McCoy Hall
College of Veterinary Medicine
Washington State University
Pullman, WA 99164
(509) 335-0711

Wisconsin

Dr. Douglas de Boer
School of Veterinary Medicine
University of Wisconsin
2015 Linden Dr West
Madison, WI 53706
(608) 263-9967

Dr. Karen A. Moriello
School of Veterinary Medicine
University of Wisconsin
2015 Linden Dr West
Madison, WI 53706
(608) 263-9970

Appendix 6
Dermatologic Terms, Conversion Tables

Abscess	A cavity filled with pus.
Acral	Relating to the peripheral parts of the body, especially the limbs.
Agar	A medium derived from seaweed, used in the growth of microorganisms.
Albinism	An inherited absence of pigment in the skin, hair and eyes.
Alkaline	The property of being basic, as opposed to acidic.
Allergen	A substance capable of causing an allergy.
Allergy	A heightened sensitivity to substances.
Alopecia	Hair loss.
Anemia	A condition in which red blood cells are present in subnormal numbers.
Anthropophilic	Pertaining to organisms adapted specifically to people.
Antibody	A substance, produced by lymphocytes (actually plasma cells) that protects the body, as part of the immune system.
Antigen	A substance that elicits antibody production.
Antimicrobial	A substance that inhibits the growth of microorganisms.
Antinuclear antibody	A group of substances that show antibody activity toward the nucleus or other cellular constituents.
Antiseptic	A substance that inhibits or destroys microorganisms, usually on living tissue.
Apocrine	The most common form of sweat gland in animals.
Autoantibody	An antibody directed against an animal's own tissue.
Autogenous	Originating from the animal's own body, such as an autogenous vaccine made up of bacteria harvested directly from the animal to be treated.
Autoimmune	A process whereby the body directs antibodies against its own tissues.
Basal cells	The deepest row of cells in the epidermis.
Biopsy	Removing tissue from living patients for diagnostic evaluation.
Bulla	A large blister.

Appendix 6

Cellulitis	Inflammation of the connective tissue that fails to come to a "head," instead travelling along tissue planes.
Cerumen	A wax-like secretion found in the ear canal.
Chemotherapy	Treatment of disease by chemical substances or drugs.
Chrysotherapy	Treatment of disease with gold compounds.
Collagen	The fibrous connective tissue of the dermis.
Complement	A group of 9 components, triggered by combinations of antigen and antibody, that act in sequence to bring about the destruction of foreign substances.
Congenital	A feature, present at birth, that may or may not be hereditary.
Crust	A dried exudate on the surface of the skin (scab).
Cryosurgery	Surgery using very cold temperatures, such as those produced by liquid nitrogen or carbon dioxide.
Cutis	Another name for the skin.
Cytologic examination	The diagnostic evaluation of individual cells, rather than tissue.
Cytoplasm	The liquid part of a cell surrounding the nucleus.
Depigmentation	Loss of color (pigment) from the skin.
Dermal-epidermal junction	The interface between the dermis and epidermis.
Dermal papilla	A structure formed by the dermis to provide nutrition and a blood supply to a developing hair follicle.
Dermatology	The study of skin disorders.
Dermatophyte	An organism capable of causing a superficial fungal infection.
Dermis	That fibrous part of the skin located between the epidermis and subcutaneous fat.
Eccrine	An uncommon type of sweat gland in animals, located only on the footpads and nose.
Eczema	A poorly defined term commonly referring to inflammatory rashes with various other clinical features.
Electrosurgery	Cutting and cautery provided by an electric current.
Emollient	An agent that softens the skin or soothes irritation.
Eosinophil	A type of white blood cell often conspicuous in parasitic and allergic conditions.
Epidermal	A peeling edge of scale surrounding what once was a fluid-filled structure, such as a pustule or blister.
Epidermis	The most superficial layer of the skin.
Endocrinology	The study of hormones.
Erosion	A shallow defect in the skin that does not penetrate as far as the dermis.
Erythema	Redness.
Erythroderma	An inflammatory reaction in the skin often accompanied by redness and scaling.
Exfoliate	To shed.

Dermatologic Terms, Conversion Tables

Exudation	The oozing of material through the skin, such as pus or seru...
Fistula	An abnormal passage leading from a site of infection to the surface of the skin.
Folliculitis	Infection of hair follicles.
Fomites	Objects, such as bedding and grooming instruments, capable of transmitting infections.
Furunculosis	Pronounced folliculitis resulting in rupture of the hair follicle.
Geophilic	Pertaining to organisms that have become adapted specifically to live in the soil.
Granuloma	A type of dermal inflammatory reaction in which the histiocyte (macrophage) is prominent and often tries to "wall off" the invading matter.
Guard hairs	The long, primary hairs of animals.
Hematoma	The confined collection of blood within a tissue.
Heritable	A trait that can be inherited; transmitted by genetic material.
Histopathologic examination	Microscopic examination of abnormal tissue.
Hyperpigmentation	Increased pigmentation in the skin.
Hypodermis	Same as subcutis, the fat layer underlying the dermis.
Hyposensitization	A form of immunotherapy whereby allergic sensitivity to substances is alleviated by a series of injections (allergy shots).
Iatrogenic	Disorder caused by medical intervention.
Immunofluorescence	A diagnostic procedure whereby autoantibodies are identified by substances that glow and act as markers.
Immunopathology	The study of immune-mediated diseases using substances that identify autoantibodies in tissues, including immunofluorescence and immunoperoxidase studies.
Immunoperoxidase	A diagnostic procedure whereby autoantibodies are identified by peroxidase, an enzyme marker.
Immunotherapy	Treatment directed at the production of protective immunity.
Induration	Thickening of the skin.
Infection	A condition involving multiplication of microorganisms on or within the body.
Infestation	A condition in which parasites dwell on the surface of the skin.
Inflammation	A type of tissue reaction usually manifesting pain, redness, heat and sometimes loss of function.
Intradermal	Within the dermis.
Keratin	The proteins forming the basis of the shingle-like stratum corneum.
Keratinization	The process of forming the stratum corneum.
Keratinocyte	An epidermal cell that eventually dies to contribute to the stratum corneum.
Langerhans cell	An epidermal cell important in immune regulation.
Lesion	Any abnormal tissue.
Leukotrichia	Whitening of the hair.

Appendix 6

Leukotriene	A byproduct of arachidonic acid metabolism.
Lichenification	A thickening and hardening of the skin with exaggerated folding. Often referred to as resembling the skin of an elephant.
Lymphocyte	A type of white blood cell. B-lymphocytes become plasma cells, which produce antibodies. T-lymphocytes patrol the body, guarding against invasion.
Macrophage	A tissue cell important in immune regulation. In a different form (histiocyte), this cell is important in formation of granulomas.
Macule	A small (<1 cm) flat, colored spot on the skin.
Mange	A disease caused by mites.
Mast cell	A mesenchymal cell found in the dermis which contains a number of bioactive substances such as histamine and heparin.
Metastasis	Spreading of disease from one part of the body to another, especially neoplasia.
Monocyte	A white blood cell belonging to the same family as the tissue macrophage and histiocyte.
Mycosis	A disease caused by fungi.
Myiasis	Invasion of tissues by maggots.
Necrolysis	A breakdown of tissue due to cell death.
Necrosis	The death of cells or tissues in a living animal.
Neoplasia	Cancer, either benign or malignant.
Neoplasm	Literally, a "new growth"; usually synonymous with tumor.
Neutrophil	A white blood cell often prominent in bacterial infections.
Nodule	A solid mass extending deeply into the dermis.
Nucleus	A rounded or oval mass of genetic material (DNA) maintained separate from the surrounding cytoplasm.
Onychomycosis	Fungal infection of the nail beds.
Otoscope	An instrument designed to allow visualization of the ear canal for examination.
Panniculitis	An inflammatory reaction in the subcutaneous fat.
Panniculus	Another name for subcutis, the fat layer underlying the dermis.
Papule	A small (<1 cm) solid elevation of the skin.
Parasite	A life form that draws its nourishment from living in or on another life form.
Patch	A large (>1 cm) macule or colored area on the skin.
Photodermatitis	An inflammatory reaction in the skin due to exposure to sunlight.
Plaque	A large (>1 cm) papule.
Plasma	The fluid portion of the blood.
Poliosis	Depigmentation of the hairs.
Polydipsia	Increased thirst.
Polyphagia	Increased hunger.
Polyuria	Increased urination.

Prognosis	A forecast of the probable outcome of a disease.
Pruritus	Itchiness.
Pustule	A small, solid elevation of skin filled with pus; a pimple.
Pyoderma	A bacterial infection of the skin in which pus may be produced. May be a primary or secondary event.
Resistance	In bacteriology, a state whereby microorganisms are not adversely affected by an antimicrobial.
Ringworm	Colloquial term for a superficial fungal infection of the skin.
Scale	Accumulation of loose fragments of stratum corneum on the skin surface.
Scar	Fibrous tissue that replaces damaged dermis.
Sclerosis	Hardening or thickening.
Seborrhea	A general term denoting an increase in scaling on the skin surface.
Sebum	The waxy, oily product of the sebaceous glands excreted into the hair follicles.
Sensitivity	In bacteriology, a state whereby microorganisms are adversely affected by an antimicrobial.
Serum	The fluid portion of the blood remaining after the clot of blood cells has been removed.
Stratum	A layer.
Stratum corneum	The shingle-like covering of the epidermis.
Subcutis	The layer of fat underlying the dermis.
Tardive	An inherited trait not manifested at birth but appearing at some later time.
Thermoregulation	The ability to regulate temperature.
Titer	Serum levels of antibodies against specific entities.
Topical	Applied to the surface of the skin.
Toxin	A poisonous substance.
Tumefaction	A swelling.
Tumor	A swelling, usually pertaining to a form of neoplasia.
Ulcer	A local erosion that penetrates into the dermis.
Urticaria	Hives.
Vellus hairs	The soft down undercoat of animals.
Vesicle	A blister.
Vibrissae	Sensory hairs; whiskers.
Vitiligo	Localized loss of pigment on the skin.
Wheal	A hive.
Xerosis	Dryness.
Zone of inhibition	In bacteriology, the area of "no growth" surrounding an antimicrobial disc.
Zoonosis	A disease that may be transmitted from animals to people.

Appendix 6

Root Words

Root	Definition	Example
aden-	gland	lymphadenitis
arthr-	joint	arthritis
carcin-	malignant cancer	adenocarcinoma
cardi-	heart	cardiology
caud-	hind end; tail	caudal
cephal-	head	encephalitis
cerebr-	brain	cerebrum
chondr-	cartilage	osteochondrosis
cis-	to cut	incision
crani-	head; front end	cranial; cranium
crin-	to secrete	endocrine
cut-	skin	subcutaneous
cyt-	cell	cytology
dermat-	skin	dermatology
dors-	back	dorsal
electr-	electricity	electrocardiogram
enter-	intestines	enteritis
fluor-	to glow	immunofluorescence
gastr-	stomach	gastroenteritis
gynec-	woman	gynecology
hemat-	blood	hematology
hepat-	liver	hepatitis
immun-	immune	immunology
later-	side	lateral
mast-	mammary gland	mastitis
my-	muscle	myositis
myc-	fungus	mycology; mycosis
nephr-	kidney	nephritis
neur-	nerve	neurology
onc-	cancer	oncology
ophthalm-	eye	ophthalmology
onych-	nail	onychomycosis
oste-	bone	osteoarthritis
ot-	ear	otoscope
pannicul-	subcutaneous fat	panniculitis
path-	disease	pathology
phleb-	vein	phlebitis
phot-	light	photodermatitis
physi-	nature	physiology

pneum-	air; lung	pneumonia
rad-	rays	radiology
rhin-	nose	rhinotracheitis
sarcoma-	malignant cancer	osteosarcoma
scler-	thicken; harden	scleroderma
scop-	to examine	microscope
strat-	layer	stratum corneum
thromb-	clot	thrombophlebitis
ventr-	the underside	ventral; ventrum
xer-	dry	xerosis

Prefixes

Root	Definition	Example
anti-	against	antibody
a-, an-, ab-	not	abnormal
auto-	self	autoimmune
chemo-	chemical	chemotherapy
chryso-	gold	chrysotherapy
cry-	cold	cryosurgery
ecto-	outside	ectoparasite
endo-	inside	endocrine
epi-	above	epithelium
eu-	normal	euthyroid
ex-, exo-	out	exocrine
geno-	birth	genodermatosis
hetero-	different	heterozygous
homo-	same	homozygous
hyper-	above; over	hyperpigmentation
hypo-	below; under	hypopigmentation
meso-	middle	mesothelium
norm-	normal	normothermic
peri-	around	perivulvar
pheno-	to display	phenotype
pro-	before	prodromal
pyo-	pus	pyoderma
retro-	behind	retrospective
thermo-	temperature	thermoregulation
trans-	across	transect
zoo-	pertaining to animals	zoonosis

Suffixes

Root	Definition	Example
-ac, -al	pertaining to	cardiac; medical
-algia	pain	analgesic
-cyte	cell	melanocyte
-ectomy	to cut out	tonsillectomy
-emia	blood condition	anemia
-gram	record	electrocardiogram
-graph	graph; record	radiograph
-ia	condition	hemophilia
-ic	pertaining to	dermatologic
-ist	a specialist	dermatologist
-itis	inflammation	dermatitis
-lysis	breakdown of	hemolysis
-megaly	large	hepatomegaly
-meter	measure	thermometer
-ology	study of	dermatology
-oma	benign tumor	lipoma
-opsy	to view	biopsy
-osis	degenerative condition of	dermatosis
-scope	to examine	microscope
-tomy	to cut into	osteotomy
-type	model	genotype

Conversion Tables

Fahrenheit to Centigrade

degrees C = (°F-32) 9/5
degrees F = 9/5° x 32
1 degree F = 0.56 degree C

F	C
0	-17.8
32	0
98	36.7
99	37.2
100	38.3
101	38.3
102	38.9
103	39.4
104	40.0
105	40.6
106	41.1
212	100

Grains to Milligrams

1 mg = 1/60 gr
1 gr = 60 mg

gr	mg
1/600	0.1
1/100	0.6
1/60	1
1/30	2
1/10	6
1/6	10
1/4	15
1/2	30
1	60
2	120
5	300
10	600

Dermatologic Terms, Conversion Tables

Pounds to Kilograms

1 lb = 0.454 kg
1 kg = 2.2 lb

lb	kg
50	23
100	45
200	91
500	230
600	273
700	318
800	364
900	409
1000	455
1250	568
1500	682
1750	795
2000	909

Fluid Ounces, Teaspoons and Tablespoons to Milliliters

fl oz	tsp	tbsp	ml
1/6	1	1/3	5
1/2	3	1	5
1	6	2	30
2	12	4	60
5	30	10	150
10	60	20	300
20	120	40	600
50	300	100	1500

Imperial Gallons to Liters

gal	L
0.5	2.3
1	4.5
2	9.0
10	45

Pints, Quarts and Imperial Gallons to Milliliters and Liters

pt	qt	gal	ml	L
0.5	0.25	—	285	0.28
1	0.5	—	570	0.57
1.5	0.75	—	850	0.85
2	1	0.25	1140	1.14
4	2	0.5	2275	2.3
8	4	1	4545	4.545

Ounces to Grams

1 oz = 28.4 g (approximately 30 g)

oz	g
0.5	15
1	30
2	60
4	120

Inches and Feet to Centimeters and Meters

in	ft	cm	m
3	0.25	7.6	0.076
6	0.5	15.2	0.152
12	1	30.5	0.305
36	3	91.5	0.915
60	5	152	1.52

Appendix 6

Metric to SI Units

Component	Present Units	Conversion Factor	SI Units
Hematology			
Hemoglobin	g/dl	10	g/L
PCV	%	0.01	L/L
WBC	/μl	1,000,000	/L
Platelets	/μl	1,000,000	/L
Biochemistry			
ACTH	pg/ml	0.1913	pmol/L
ALAT (SGPT)	U/L	1.00	U/L
Albumin	g/dl	10.0	g/L
Alkaline phosphatase	U/L	1.0	U/L
Ammonia	μg/dl	0.5871	μmol/L
Amylase	U/L	1.85	U/L
ASAT (SGOT)	U/L	1.00	U/L
Bilirubin	mg/dl	17.10	μmol/L
Calcium	mg/dl	0.2495	mmol/L
Cholesterol	mg/dl	0.02586	mmol/L
Cortisol	μg/dl	27.59	nmol/L
Creatinine	mg/dl	88.40	μmol/L
Estradiol	pg/ml	3.671	pmol/L
Glucose	mg/dl	0.05551	mmol/L
Insulin	μU/ml	7.175	pmol/L
Progesterone	ng/ml	3.180	nmol/L
Protein	g/dl	10.0	g/L
Testosterone	mg/ml	3.467	nmol/L
Thyroxine (T_4)	μg/dl	12.87	nmol/L
Triiodothyronine (T_3)	ng/dl	0.01536	nmol/L
TSH	μU/ml	1.0	IU/L
Urea	mg/dl	0.3570	mmol/L
Zinc	μg/dl	0.1530	μmol/L

Color Plates

Figure 1. Typical appearance of chronic flea bite hypersensitivity.

Figure 2. Generalized demodicosis in a puppy.

Figure 3. Excoriations secondary to infestation with *Sarcoptes scabiei* var *canis*.

Figure 4. *Cheyletiella* mite recovered on skin scrapings.

Figure 5. Pododermatitis due to *Pelodera strongyloides*.

Figure 6. Superficial pyoderma with features of pyotraumatic dermatitis and fold pyoderma.

Figure 7. Somewhat atypical circular lesions of intermediate pyoderma, which may be confused with dermatophytosis (ringworm).

Figure 8. Typical circular lesion of intermediate pyoderma on the ventrum, with hyperpigmentation centrally and a peeling rim of stratum corneum (epidermal collarette) peripherally.

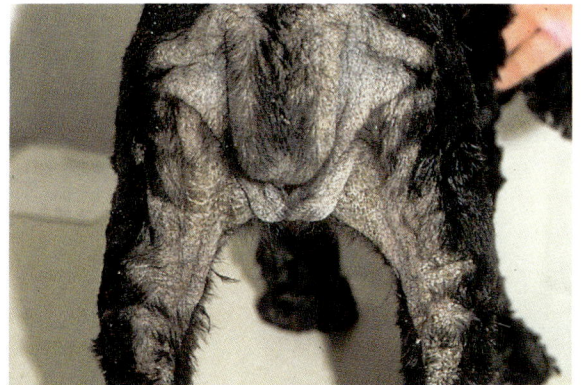

Figure 1

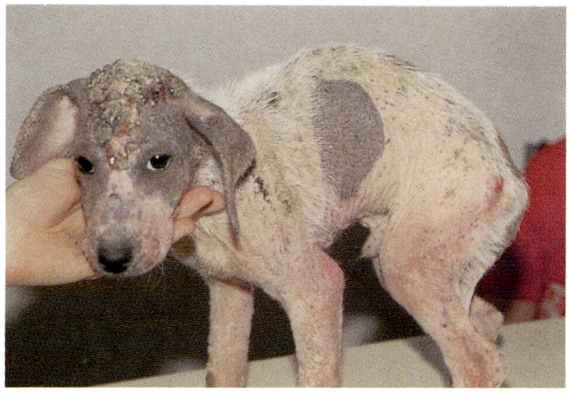

Figure 2

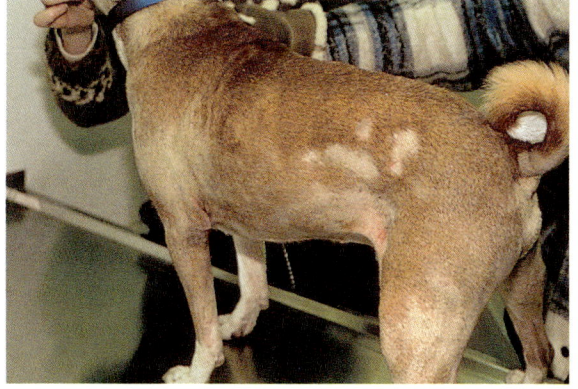

Figure 3

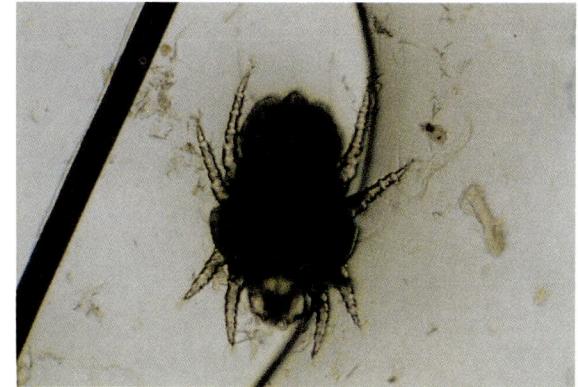

Figure 4

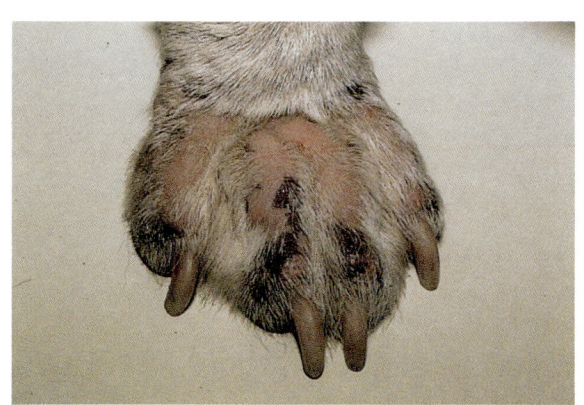

Figure 5

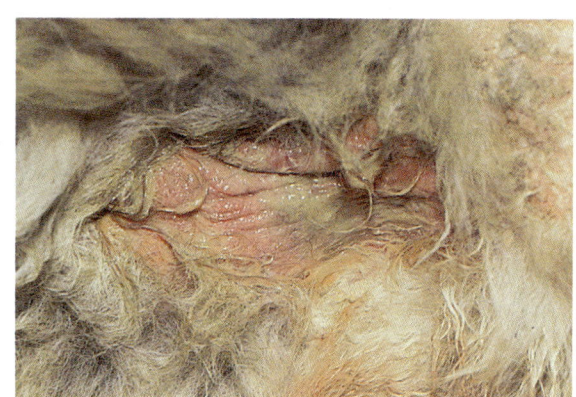

Figure 6

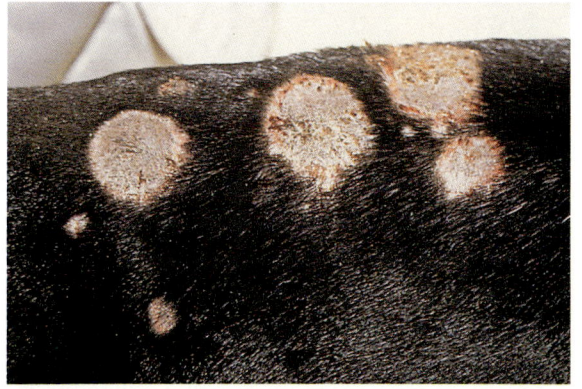

Figure 7

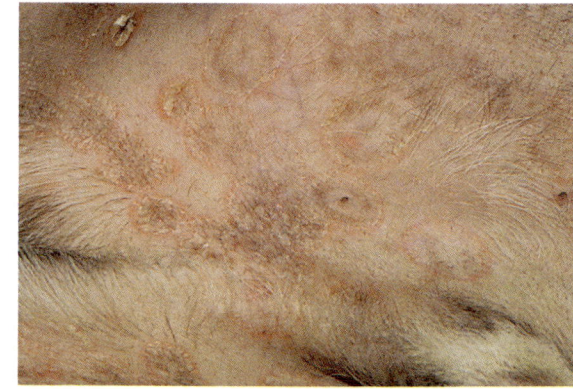

Figure 8

353

Figure 9. Deep pyoderma and cellulitis on the lateral aspect of the thigh of a German Shepherd.

Figure 10. Perianal fistulae, an atypical pyoderma in a German Shepherd. This dog responded to isotretinoin, a vitamin A derivative.

Figure 11. Bacterial granuloma (botryomycosis) in a 4-year-old Pit Bull Terrier.

Figure 12. A dermatophyte kerion, which is a granulomatous response to the fungi.

Figure 13. Nodular lesions of the cutaneolymphatic form of sporotrichosis.

Figure 14. Cutaneous nodule that, on cytologic examination of aspirates, contained numerous budding yeasts typical of *Blastomyces dermatitidis.*

Figure 15. Mucocutaneous lesions of histoplasmosis. (Courtesy of Dr. David Chester)

Figure 16. Intradermal allergy testing to detect inhalant allergies.

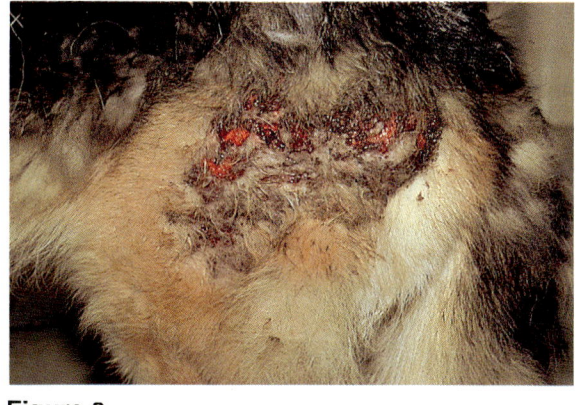

Figure 9

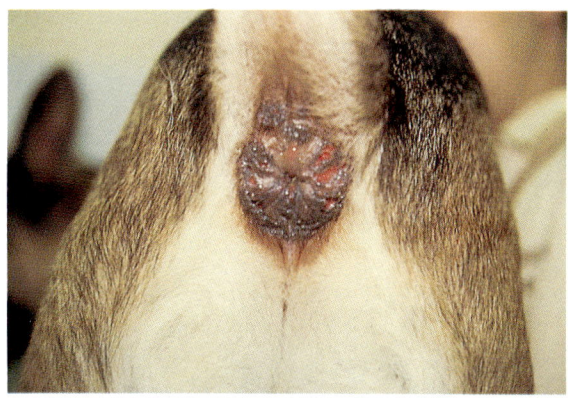

Figure 10

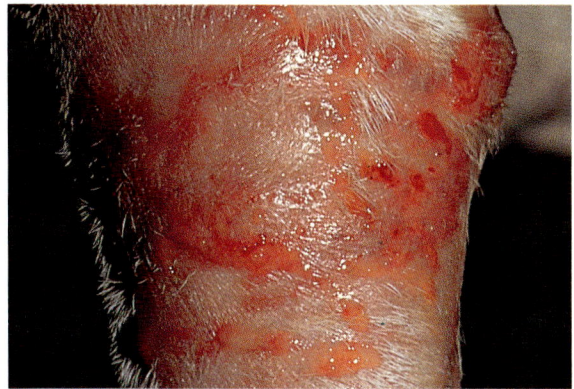

Figure 11

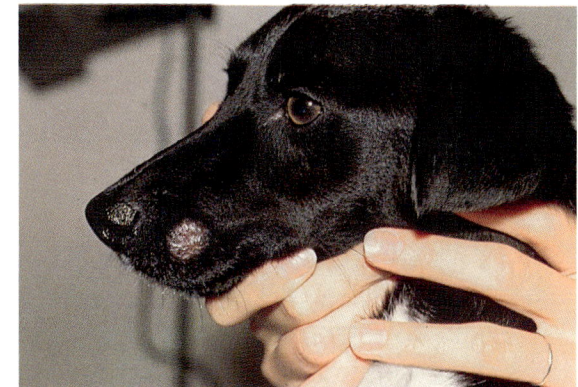

Figure 12

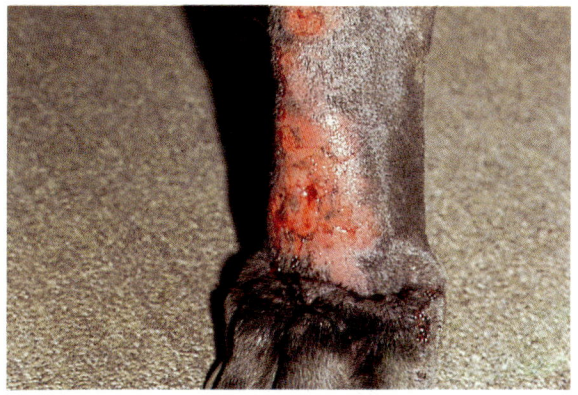

Figure 13

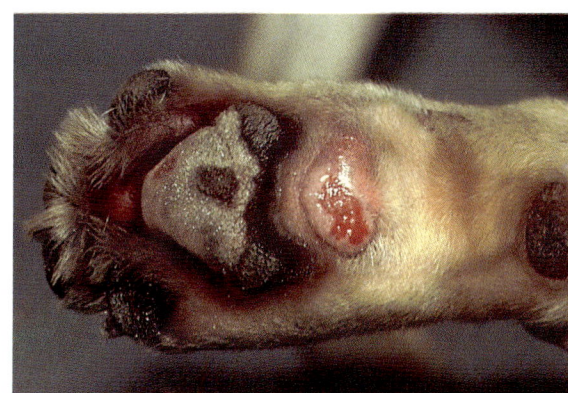

Figure 14

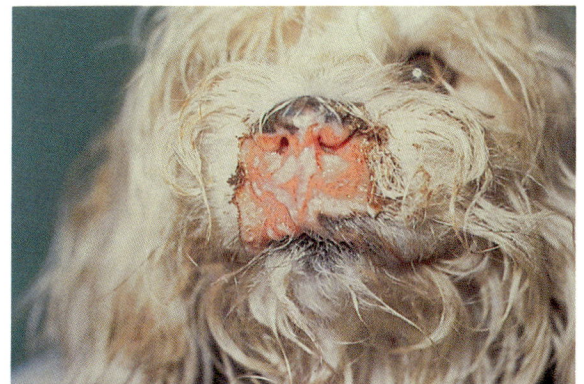

Figure 15

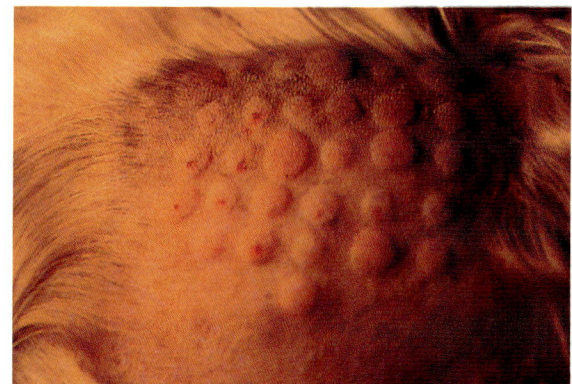

Figure 16

Figure 17. Facial erythema associated with food hypersensitivities.

Figure 18. Drug eruption secondary to an injection of penicillin.

Figure 19. Nasal dermatitis associated with systemic lupus erythematosus.

Figure 20. Nasal depigmentation and inflammation associated with cutaneous (discoid) lupus erythematosus.

Figure 21. Oral lesions associated with pemphigus vulgaris.

Figure 22. Multifocal lesions of pemphigus vegetans in an elderly Schnauzer.

Figure 23. Exfoliative facial dermatitis due to pemphigus foliaceus.

Figure 24. Inguinal lesions of bullous pemphigoid.

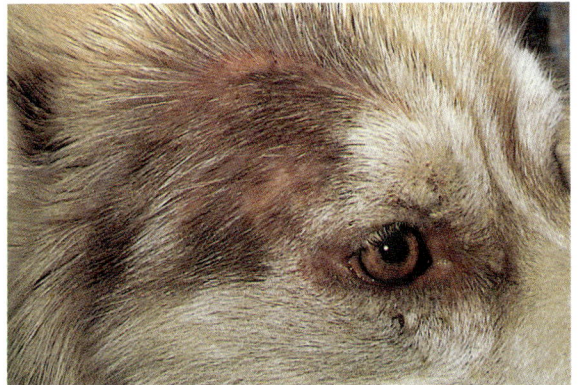

Figure 17

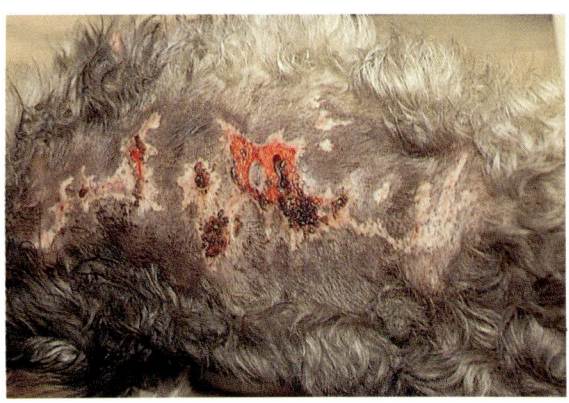

Figure 18

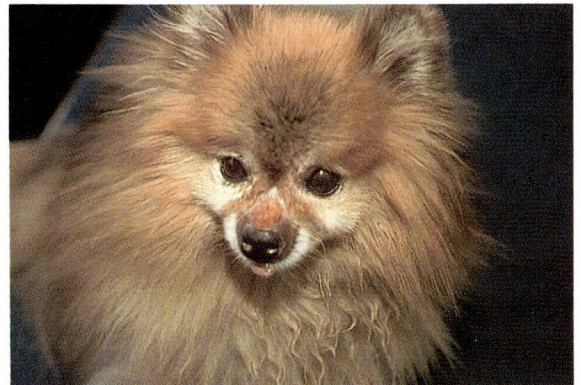

Figure 19

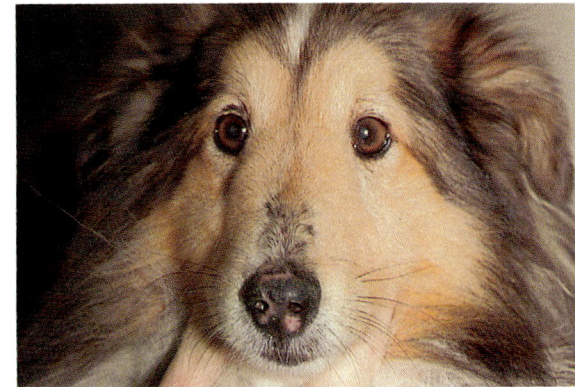

Figure 20

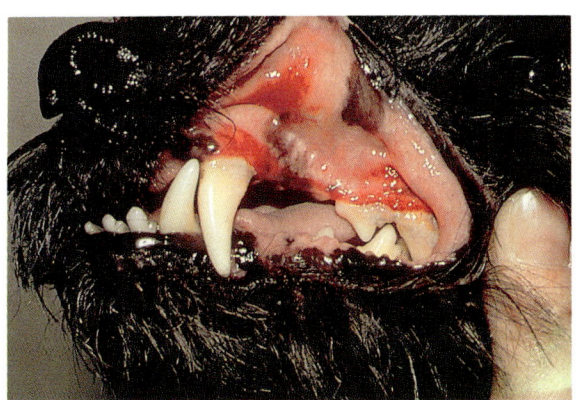

Figure 21

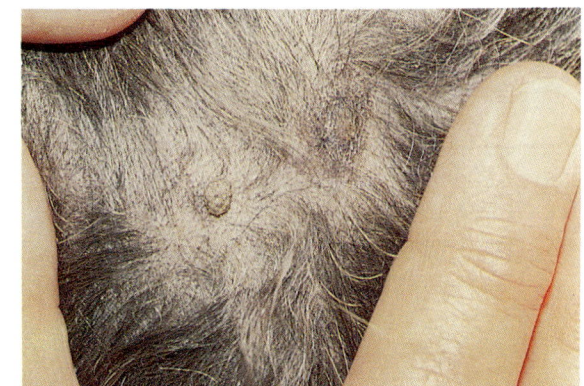

Figure 22

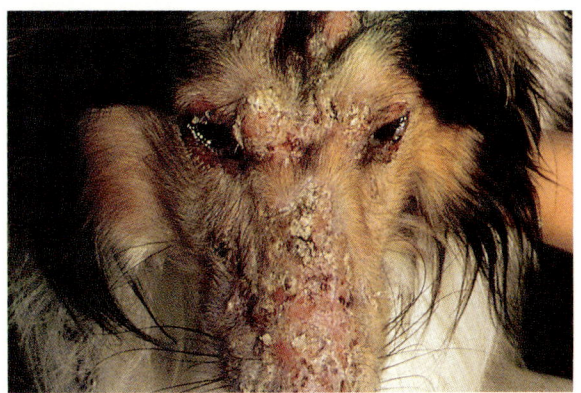

Figure 23

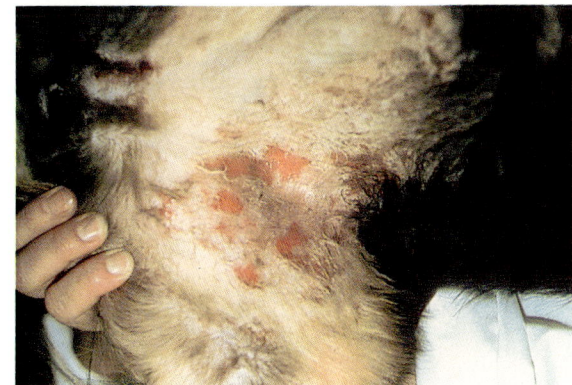

Figure 24

Figure 25. Depigmentation and photophobia in an Akita with uveodermatologic (Vogt-Koyanagi-Harada-like) syndrome.

Figure 26. Focal noninflammatory hair loss in a dog with alopecia areata.

Figure 27. Bilaterally symmetric alopecia in a dog with hypothyroidism.

Figure 28. Bilaterally symmetric alopecia in a dog with pituitary-dependent hyperadrenocorticism (Cushing's disease).

Figure 29. Hair loss and intense hyperpigmentation in a young dog with suspected growth hormone-responsive dermatosis.

Figure 30. Feminization in a male dog with a testicular Sertoli-cell tumor.

Figure 31. Exfoliative nasal dermatitis associated with zinc-responsive dermatosis.

Figure 32. Crusting dermatosis apparently from feeding generic dog food. The condition responded to dietary change.

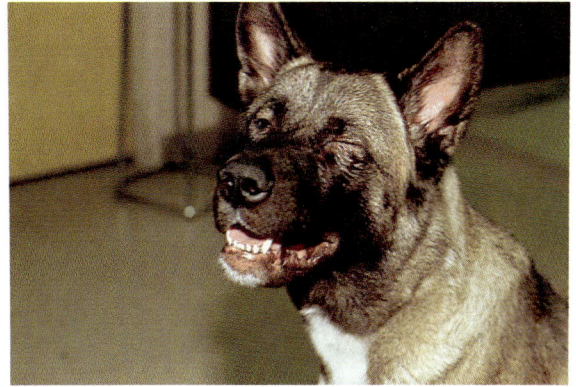

Figure 25

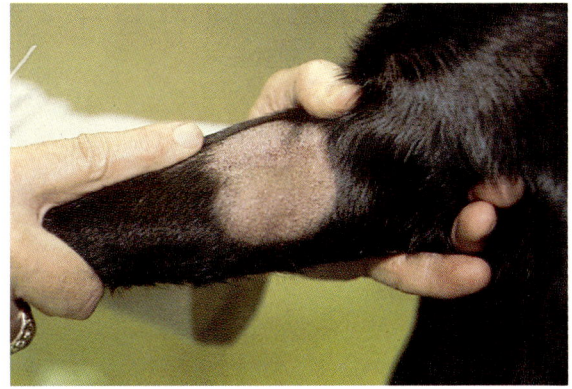

Figure 26

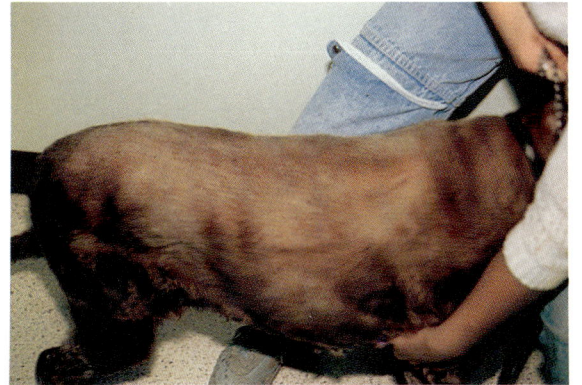

Figure 27

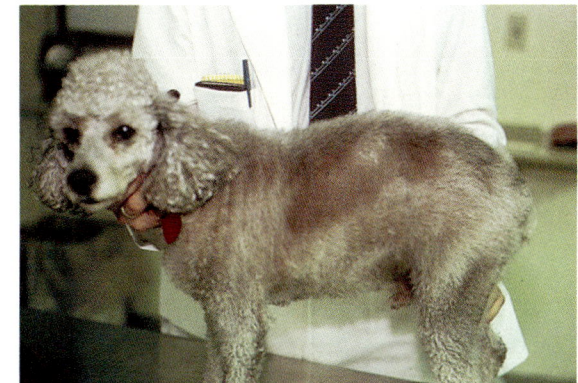

Figure 28

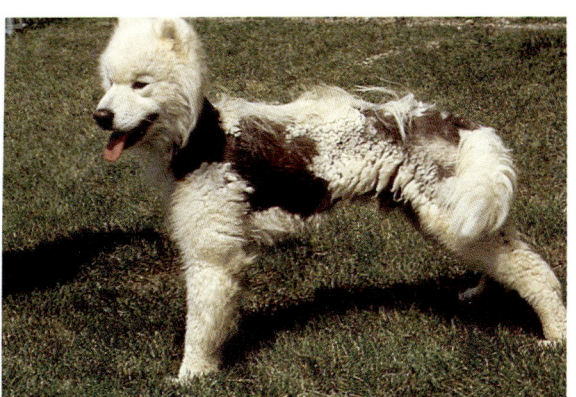

Figure 29

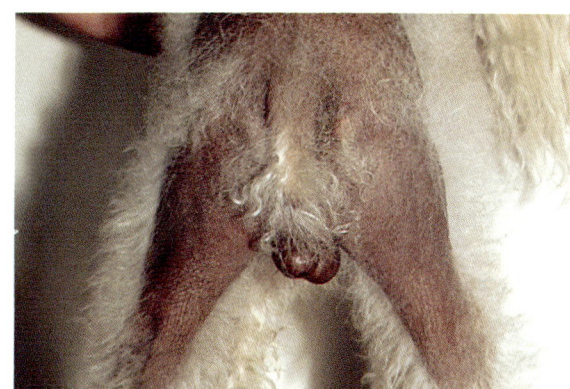

Figure 30

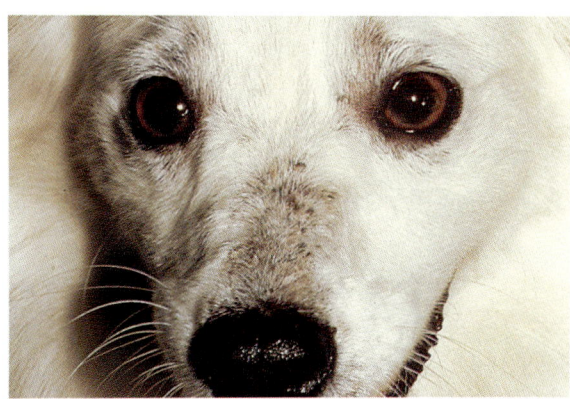

Figure 31

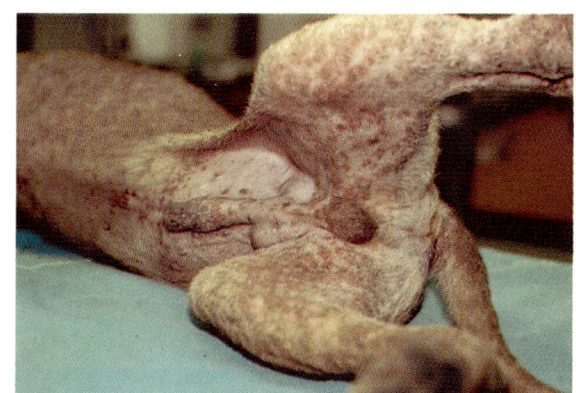

Figure 32

Figure 33. Follicular keratosis in a Spaniel with vitamin A-responsive dermatosis.

Figure 34. Dorsal discoloration of the haircoat in Dalmatian bronzing syndrome.

Figure 35. Color mutant alopecia in a Blue Doberman Pinscher.

Figure 36. Facial lesions of dermatomyositis.

Figure 37. Large hemangiopericytoma on the lateral aspect of the thigh.

Figure 38. Small, well-demarcated histiocytoma on the foot of a dog.

Figure 39. Erythroderma and ulceration in a Bouvier with cutaneous T-cell lymphoma.

Figure 40. Mast-cell tumors on the leg of a Doberman Pinscher.

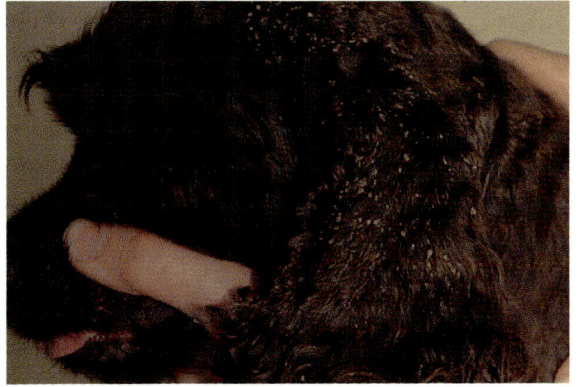

Figure 33

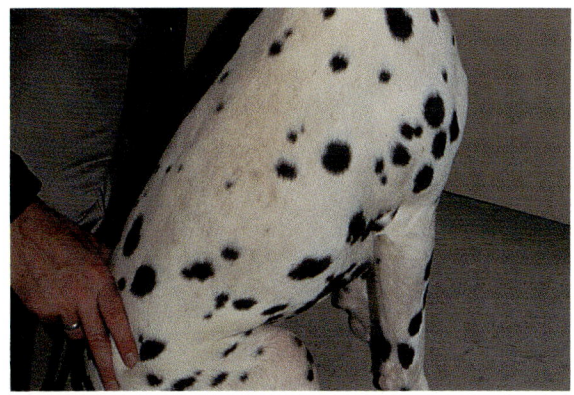

Figure 34

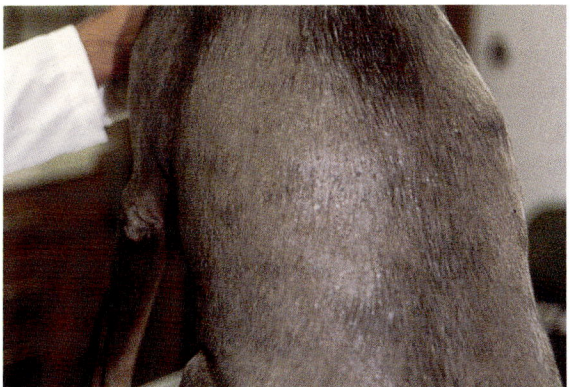

Figure 35

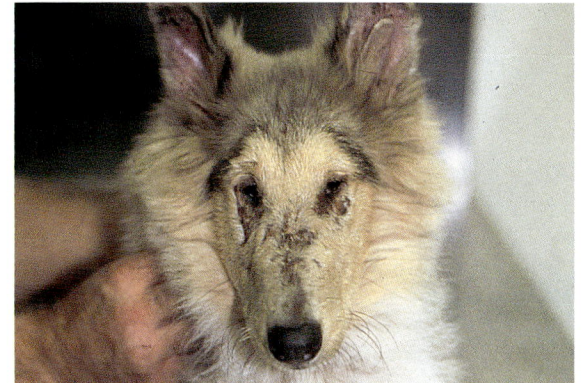

Figure 36

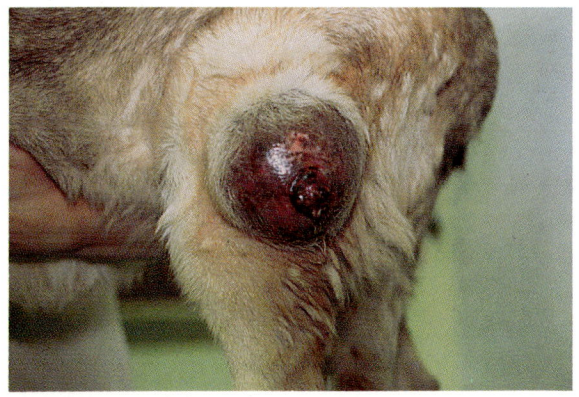

Figure 37

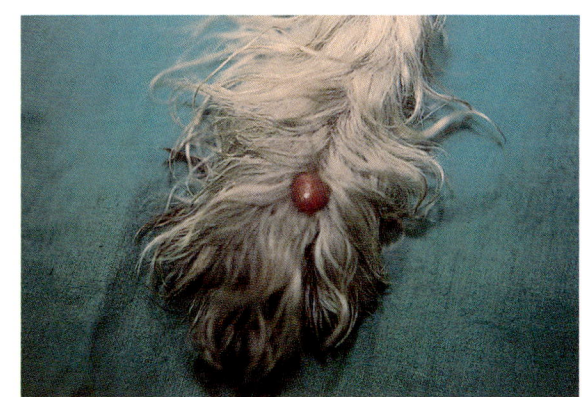

Figure 38

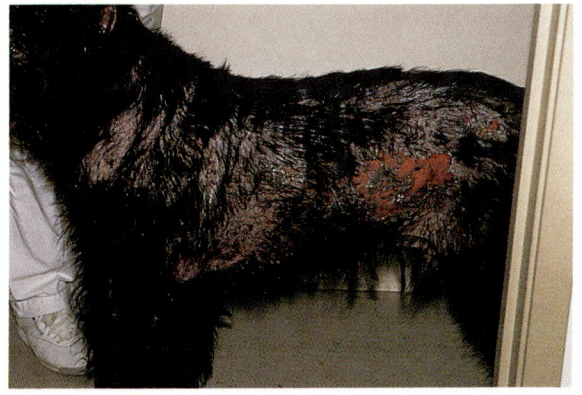

Figure 39

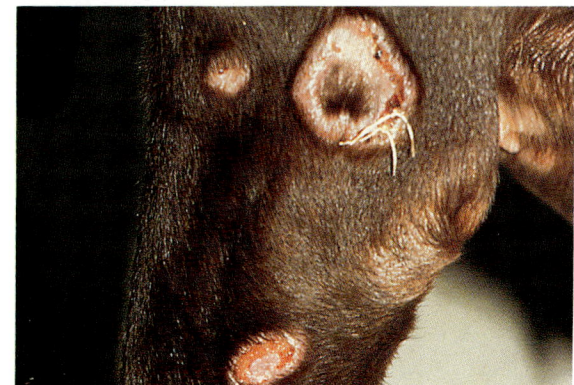

Figure 40

Figure 41. Axillary hyperpigmentation consistent with acanthosis nigricans in a Dachshund.

Figure 42. Extensive damage to the front leg in a dog with acral lick dermatitis.

Figure 43. Necrotic ear tips in a dog with cutaneous vasculitis.

Figure 44. Polycyclic patterns associated with erythema multiforme.

Figure 45. Juvenile cellulitis in a puppy.

Figure 46. Psoriasiform lichenoid dermatitis in a young Springer Spaniel.

Figure 47. Recurrent nodular panniculitis in an elderly Golden Retriever.

Figure 48. Pruritic papulopustular dermatitis in suspected subcorneal pustular dermatitis.

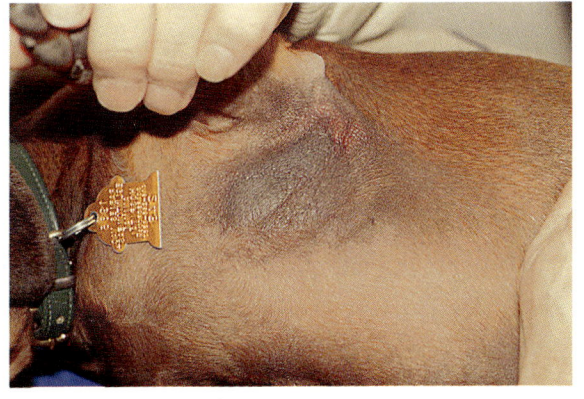

Figure 41

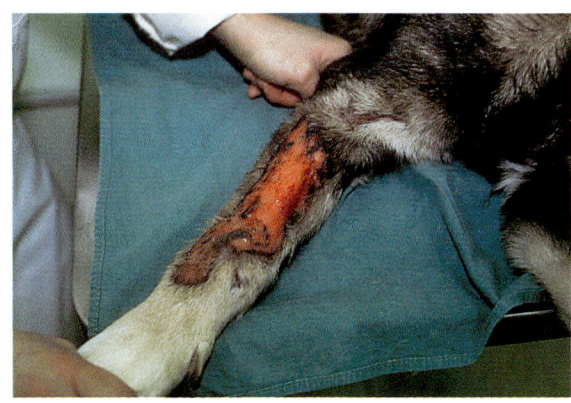

Figure 42

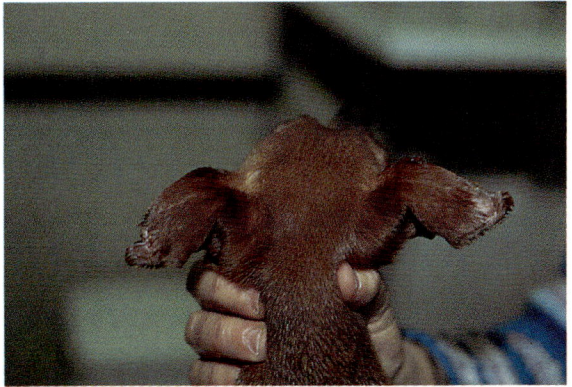

Figure 43

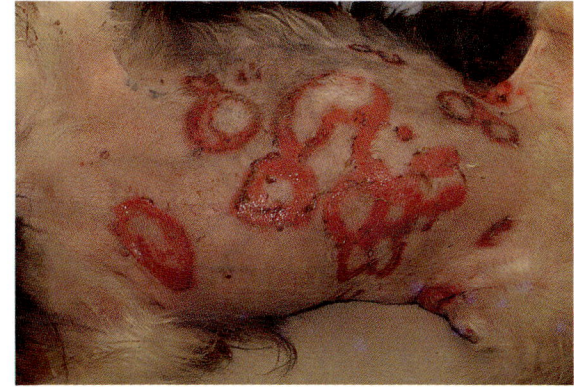

Figure 44

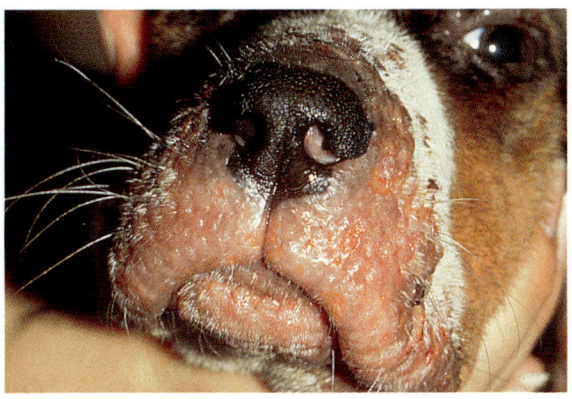

Figure 45

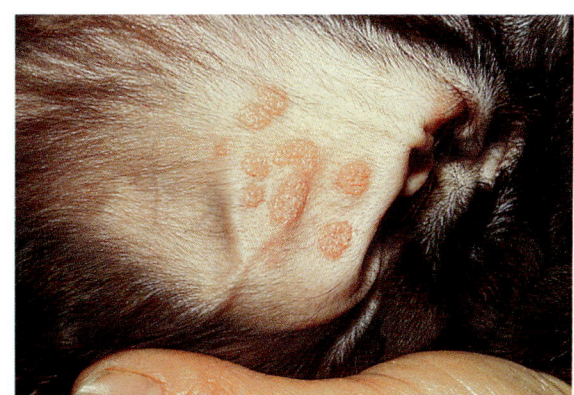

Figure 46

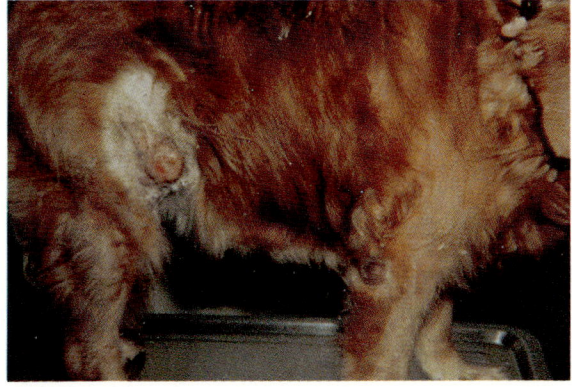

Figure 47

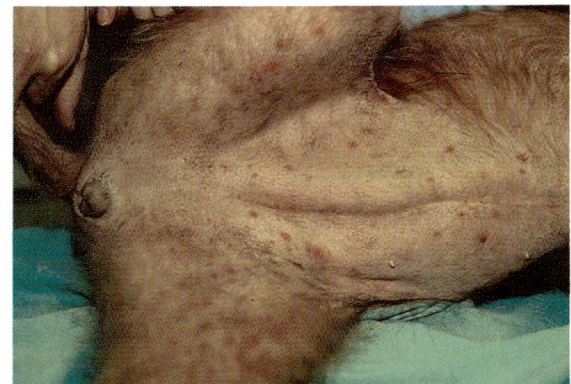

Figure 48

Index

A
Abscesses, 69
Acanthosis nigricans, 237, 238
Acne, 70, 71
Acral lick dermatitis, 238, 239
Acral mutilation syndrome, 200, 256
Acrodermatitis, lethal, 199, 256
Actinomycotic mycetoma, 74
Albinism, 195
Allergens, 100-114
Allergic disorders, 99-133
    allergy shots, 122, 123
    allergy tests, 30, 31, 100-114
    atopy, 99-124
    contact dermatitis, 129-131
    drug eruption, 131, 132
    food hypersensitivity, 124-130
    hormonal hypersensitivity, 132
    inhalant allergies, 99-124
    intradermal allergy tests, 30, 31, 100-114
    skin tests, 30, 31, 100-114
    therapy, 114
Allergy shots, 122, 123
Allergy tests, 30, 31, 100-114
Aloe vera, 318
Alopecia, 146, 147, 239-241
Alopecia areata, 146, 147
Amitraz, 279, 280
Anal sac disorders, 241, 242
Anatomy, skin, 1, 2
Antibacterial selection, 76-79
Antibacterials, systemic, 280-285
    topical, 306
Antifungals, systemic, 285-288
    topical, 306-308
Antihistamines, 118, 119, 294, 295
Antimicrobials, systemic, 280-285
    topical, 306
Antinuclear antibody tests, 42, 43
Antiparasitics, 275-280
Antiseptics, 308, 309
Apocrine-gland tumors, 232, 233
Aspergillosis, 87, 88
Atopy, 99-124
Atypical pyodermas, 70-76

B
Bacterial granuloma, 74
Bacterial hypersensitivity, 71
Basal-cell tumor, 202
Biopsy, 31-39
Black hair follicular dysplasia, 197
Blastomycosis, 91-93
Breed predispositions, 183-191
Bromelain, 180

C
Calcinosis circumscripta, 273
Callus pyoderma, 72
Carbamates, 275, 276
Cellulitis, 69
Chemotherapy, 297-301
Cheyletiellosis, 57
Chigger infestation, 58
Chlorinated hydrocarbons, 277
Chrysotherapy, 302
Circulating immune complex assay, 45
Claws, diseases of, 263, 264
Coccidioidomycosis, 93, 94
Collie nose, 264, 265
Color mutant alopecia, 192
Complement fixation, 44
Congenito-hereditary disorders, 183-200
    acral mutilation syndrome, 200, 256
    albinism, 195
    black hair follicular dysplasia, 197
    breed predispositions, 183-191
    color mutant alopecia, 192
    cutaneous asthenia, 192, 193
    dermatomyositis, 193, 194
    dermoid sinus, 195
    Ehlers-Danlos syndrome, 192, 193
    epidermolysis bullosa simplex, 193, 194
    follicular dysplasia, 197
    gray Collie syndrome, 196
    hair follicle defects, 196-198
    hypotrichosis, 196, 197
    ichthyosis, 198
    lentigo, 196
    lethal acrodermatitis, 199, 256
    pigmentation disorders, 195, 196
    spiculosis, 198

vitiligo, 195
Contact dermatitis, 130, 131
Corticosteroids, systemic, 292-294
    topical, 309-312
Cryptococcosis, 94, 95
Culture and sensitivity tests, 76-79
Cultures, 27-30
Cushing's disease, 156-162
Cutaneous asthenia, 192, 193
Cyclosporine A, 304
Cysts, 202, 203
Cytologic examination, 41

D

Dalmatian bronzing syndrome, 174, 175
Dapsone, 302, 303
Deep pyodermas, 69, 70
Demodectic mange, 52-56
Dermatitis herpetiformis, 244, 245
Dermatomyositis, 193, 194
Dermatophytosis, 81-85
Dermoid sinus, 195
Diagnosis, 7-46
Dietary supplements, 175-181
Dimethylglycine, 178, 179
Distribution, lesions, 18-25
    breeds, 25
    dorsum, 22
    ears, 21
    eyelids, 20, 21
    feet, 23, 24
    females, 25
    genitalia, 22, 23
    head, 21
    legs, 23
    males, 24
    mucocutaneous junctions, 24
    neck, 21
    perineum, 22
    ventrum, 22
    young dogs, 25
Dracunculiasis, 60
Drug eruption, 131, 132

E

Ear mite infestation, 57, 58
Ear problems, 245-252
Ehlers-Danlos syndrome, 192, 193
Endocrine disorders, 151-166
    Cushing's disease, 156-162
    estrogen-responsive dermatosis, 165
    growth hormone-responsive dermatosis, 162-164
    hyperadrenocorticism, 156-162
    hyperestrogenism, 164
    hyperthyroidism, 156-162
    hypothyroidism, 151-156
    Sertoli-cell tumors, 165
    sex hormone disorders, 164-166
Eosinophilic granuloma, 253

Eosinophilic pustulosis, sterile, 270
Epidermolysis bullosa simplex, 193, 194
Epithelioma, intracutaneous cornifying, 210
Erythema multiforme, 253, 254
Erythroderma, 257-260
Estrogen-responsive dermatosis, 165
Eumycotic mycetoma, 86, 87

F

Facial dermatoses, 18, 20
Fatty acid deficiency, 168, 169
Fibroma, 203
Fibronectin assay, 45, 46
Fibrosarcoma, 204
Flea infestation, 47-51
Fly-related dermatoses, 58, 59
Follicular dysplasia, 197
Folliculitis, 67, 68
Food hypersensitivity, 124-130
Footpad diseases, 255-257
Fungal dermatoses, 81-97
    aspergillosis, 87, 88
    blastomycosis, 91-93
    coccidioidomycosis, 93, 94
    cryptococcosis, 95
    dermatophytosis, 81-85
    eumycotic mycetoma, 86, 87
    histoplasmosis, 96, 97
    intermediate mycoses, 85
    penicillinosis, 87, 88
    phaeohyphomycosis, 88
    phycomycosis, 89
    rhinosporidiosis, 89, 90
    ringworm, 81-85
    sporotrichosis, 90, 91
    superficial mycoses, 81-85
    systemic mycoses, 91-97
    zygomycosis, 89
Furunculosis, 69

G

Generic dog food disease, 171
Germanium, 179, 180
Giant-cell tumor, 209
Gold salt therapy, 302
Granuloma, bacterial, 74
    eosinophilic, 253
Gray Collie syndrome, 196
Growth hormone-responsive dermatosis, 162-164

H

Hair analysis, 46
Hair follicle defects, 196-198
Heartworm dermatitis, 60
Hemangioma, 205
Hemangiopericytoma, 206, 207
Hemangiosarcoma, 205, 206
Hematomas, aural, 252

Index

Hepatoid-gland adenoma, 227
Histiocytoma, 207, 209
Histiocytosis, 208
Histoplasmosis, 96, 97
Hookworm dermatitis, 60
Hormonal hypersensitivity, 132
Hot spots, 67
Hyperadrenocorticism, 156-162
Hyperestrogenism, 164
Hyperthyroidism, 156-162
Hypothyroidism, 151-156
Hypotrichosis, 196, 197

I

Ichthyosis, 198
Immune-mediated dermatoses, 135-149
    alopecia areata, 146, 147
    LE cell test, 43, 136, 137
    lupus erythematosus, 135-149
    pemphigoid, 144, 145
    pemphigus, 139-143
    scleroderma, 147, 148
    Sjogren's syndrome, 148, 149
    uveodermatologic syndrome, 146
    Vogt-Koyanagi-Harada-like syndrome, 146
Immune system, function, 1-7
    immune-mediated dermatoses, 135-149
    immunotherapy, 122-124, 288-291
    tests, 30, 31, 39-46, 100-114
Immunodiffusion, 44
Immunopathologic examination, 39
Immunostimulants, 122-124, 288-291
Impetigo, 66
Inhalant allergies, 99-124
Insect growth regulators, 277
Interdigital pyoderma, 72
Intermediate pyodermas, 67, 68
Intradermal allergy tests, 30, 31, 100-114
Ivermectin, 278

J

Juvenile cellulitis, 257
Juvenile pustular pyoderma, 66

K

Keratinization disorders, 257-260
Keratoacanthoma, 210
Keratoses, 210, 211

L

Latex agglutination, 44, 45
LE cell test, 43, 136, 137
Leishmaniasis, 61-63
Lentigo, 196
Lesions, 8-19
Lethal acrodermatitis, 199, 256
Lice infestation, 52
Lichenoid dermatoses, 260, 261
Lipoma, 211

Lipomatosis, infiltrating, 212
Liposarcoma, 212
Lupus erythematosus, 135-139
Lymphosarcoma, 212-215

M

Mammary tumors, 215-217
Mange, demodectic, 52-56
    otodectic, 57, 58
    sarcoptic, 56
Mast-cell tumor, 217-219
Mastocytosis, 217-219
Melanoma, 219, 220
Metabolic dermatosis, 261, 262
Moisturizers, 317, 318
Mucinosis, focal, 254, 255
Mycobacterial pyoderma, atypical, 75, 76
Mycoses, see Fungal dermatoses
Mycosis fungoides, 214
Myxoma, 220, 221
Myxosarcoma, 221

N

Nail and nailbed diseases, 263, 264
Nasal dermatitis, 264, 265
Nasal pyoderma, 72, 73
Nasal tumors, 221, 222
Nasodigital hyperkeratosis, 256, 257
Neoplasia, see Tumors, skin
Nevi, 223, 224
Nikolsky's sign, 143
Nodular dermatofibrosis, 204, 205
Nodular panniculitis, 265-267
Nutritional supplements, 175-181
Nutritionally related disorders, 167-181
    bromelain, 180
    Dalmatian bronzing syndrome, 174, 175
    dietary supplements, 175-181
    dimethylglycine, 178, 179
    fatty acid deficiency, 168, 169
    generic dog food disease, 171
    germanium, 179, 180
    omega fatty acids, 177, 178, 295, 296
    protein deficiency, 167
    vitamin A-responsive dermatosis, 172, 173
    vitamin E deficiency, 173
    zinc-responsive dermatosis, 169-171

O

Omega fatty acids, 177, 178, 295, 296
Oral tumors, 224-226
Organophosphates, 276, 277
Otitis externa, 245-252
Otodectic mange, 57, 58

P

Papillomas, 226
Papillomatosis, viral, 226

Index

Parasitic disorders, 47-63
   cheyletiellosis, 57
   chigger infestation, 58
   demodectic mange, 52-56
   dracunculiasis, 60
   ear mite infestation, 57, 58
   flea infestation, 47-51
   fly-related dermatoses, 58, 59
   hookworm dermatitis, 60
   leishmaniasis, 61-63
   lice infestation, 52
   otodectic mange, 57, 58
   Pelodera dermatitis, 59, 60
   sarcoptic mange, 56
   tick infestation, 51, 52
   trombiculiasis, 58
Paronychia, 263, 264
Pelodera dermatitis, 59, 60
Pemphigoid, 144, 145
Pemphigus, erythematosus, 141
   foliaceus, 141
   vegetans, 141
   vulgaris, 140
Penicillinosis, 87, 88
Perianal fistulae, 73
Perianal tumors, 227
Periappendageal dermatitis, 269, 270
Periocular tumors, 228
Phaeohyphomycosis, 88
Phycomycosis, 89
Pigmentation disorders, 195, 196
Pilomatrixoma, 228, 229
Plasma-cell tumor, 229, 230
Plasmacytoma, 229, 230
Plasmapheresis, 303
Pododermatitis, 268
Protein deficiency, 167
Puppy strangles, 257
Pustular dermatosis, subcorneal, 271, 272
Pustulosis, eosinophilic, 270
Pyodermas, 65-79
   abscesses, 69
   acne, 70-71
   actinomycotic mycetoma, 74
   atypical, 70-76
   atypical mycobacterial, 75, 76
   bacterial granuloma, 74
   bacterial hypersensitivity, 71
   callus, 72
   cellulitis, 69
   cutaneous tuberculosis, 76
   deep, 69, 70
   folliculitis, 67, 68
   furunculosis, 69
   hot spots, 67
   impetigo, 66
   interdigital, 72
   intermediate, 66, 67
   juvenile pustular, 66
   nasal, 72, 73
   perianal, 73
   pyotraumatic, 67
   skin fold, 66
   superficial, 66, 67
Pyogranuloma, sterile, 271
Pyotraumatic dermatitis, 67
Pyrethrins, 275

R

Retinoids, 297
Rhinosporidiosis, 89, 90
Ringworm, 81-85

S

Sarcoptic mange, 56
Scleroderma, 147, 148
Scrapings, skin, 26
Sebaceous-gland tumors, 230, 231
Seborrhea, 257-260
Sensitivity testing, 27-30
Serologic tests, 42-46
Sertoli-cell tumors, 165
Sex hormone disorders, 164-166
Shampoos, 313-317
Sjogren's syndrome, 148, 149
Skin fold pyoderma, 66
Skin tests, 30, 31, 100-114
Spiculosis, 198
Sporotrichosis, 90, 91
Squamous-cell carcinomas, 231
Superficial pyodermas, 66, 67
Sweat-gland tumors, 232, 233
Systemic therapy, 275-304

T

Tick infestation, 51, 52
Titers, 42
Topical products, 305-318
Toxic epidermal necrolysis, 272
Transmissible venereal tumors, 233, 234
Trichoepithelioma, 234
Trombiculiasis, 58
Tuberculosis, cutaneous, 76
Tumoral calcinosis, 273
Tumors, skin, 201-235
   apocrine cysts, 203
   apocrine-gland tumors, 232, 233
   basal-cell tumor, 202
   B-cell lymphosarcoma, 213
   cutaneous histiocytosis, 208
   cysts, 202, 203
   dermoid cysts, 203
   epidermal cysts, 203
   epithelioma, intracutaneous cornifying, 210
   fibroma, 203
   fibrosarcoma, 204
   fibrous histiocytoma, 209
   follicular cysts, 203
   giant-cell tumor, 209

Index

hemangioma, 205
hemangiopericytoma, 206, 207
hemangiosarcoma, 205, 206
hepatoid-gland adenoma, 227
histiocytoma, 207, 209
intracutaneous cornifying epithelioma, 210
keratoacanthoma, 210
keratoses, 210, 211
lipoma, 211
lipomatosis, infiltrating, 212
liposarcoma, 212
lymphosarcoma, 212-215
malignant fibrous histiocytoma, 209
malignant histiocytosis, 208
mammary tumors, 215-217
mast-cell tumor, 217-219
mastocytosis, 217-219
melanoma, 219, 220
mycosis fungoides, 214
myxoma, 220, 221
myxosarcoma, 221
nasal tumors, 221, 222
nevi, 223, 224
nodular dermatofibrosis, 204, 205
oral tumors, 224-226
papilloma, 226
papillomatosis, viral, 226
perianal tumors, 227
periocular tumors, 228
pilar cysts, 203
pilomatrixoma, 228, 229
plasma-cell tumor, 229, 230
plasmacytoma, 229, 230
sebaceous-gland tumors, 230, 231
squamous-cell carcinomas, 231
sweat-gland tumors, 232, 233
T-cell-like lymphoma, 214
transmissible venereal tumors, 233, 234
trichoepithelioma, 234
warts, 226
Woringer-Kolopp disease, 215
Tyrosinemia, 256

U
Uveodermatologic syndrome, 146

V
Vasculitis, cutaneous, 243, 244
Vitamin A-responsive dermatosis, 172, 173
Vitamin E deficiency, 173
Vitiligo, 195
Vogt-Koyanagi-Harada-like syndrome, 146

W
Warts, 226
Woringer-Kolopp disease, 215

Z
Zinc-responsive dermatosis, 169-171
Zygomycosis, 89